www.harcourt-international.com

Bringing you products from all Harcourt Health Sciences companies including Baillière Tindall, Churchill Livingstone, Mosby and W.B. Saunders

○ **Browse** for latest information on new books, journals and electronic products

○ **Search** for information on over 20 000 published titles with full product information including tables of contents and sample chapters

○ **Keep up to date** with our extensive publishing programme in your field by registering with eAlert or requesting postal updates

○ **Secure online ordering** with prompt delivery, as well as full contact details to order by phone, fax or post

○ **News** of special features and promotions

If you are based in the following countries, please visit the country-specific site to receive full details of product availability and local ordering information

USA: www.harcourthealth.com

Canada: www.harcourtcanada.com

Australia: www.harcourt.com.c

D0237911

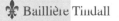

Mental Health Liaison

Dedication

We would like to dedicate this book to our children:
Hannah and Tom (SR)
James and Mary (DR)

For Baillière Tindall:

Senior Commissioning Editor: Jacqueline Curthoys
Project Development Manager: Karen Gilmour
Project Manager: Derek Robertson

Mental Health Liaison
A Handbook for Nurses and Health Professionals

Edited by

Stephen Regel MAPGDip PGCE Cert Behav Psych RMN
Senior Lecturer in Trauma Studies; Director, Centre for Traumatic Stress Research and Practice, Nottingham, UK

Dave Roberts MSc RMN RGN
Senior Lecturer in Cancer Care, Oxford Brookes University, Oxford, UK

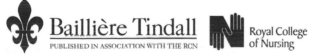

Baillière Tindall
PUBLISHED IN ASSOCIATION WITH THE RCN

Royal College of Nursing

EDINBURGH LONDON NEW YORK PHILADELPHIA ST LOUIS SYDNEY TORONTO 2002

BAILLIÈRE TINDALL
An imprint of Harcourt Publishers Limited

© Harcourt Publishers Limited 2002

✣ is a registered trademark of Harcourt Publishers Limited

The rights of Stephen Regel and Dave Roberts to be identified as
editors of this work have been asserted by them in accordance
with the Copyright, Designs and Patents Act 1988

First published 2002

ISBN 0 7020 2525 9

British Library Cataloguing in Publication Data
A catalogue record for this book is available from the British
Library

Library of Congress Cataloging in Publication Data
A catalog record for this book is available from the Library of
Congress

Note
Medical knowledge is constantly changing. As new information
becomes available, changes in treatment, procedures,
equipment and the use of drugs become necessary. The editors,
contributors and the publishers have taken care
to ensure that the information given in this text is accurate and
up-to-date. However, readers are strongly advised to confirm that
the information, especially with regard to drug usage, complies
with the latest legislation and standards of practice.

The
publisher's
policy is to use
**paper manufactured
from sustainable forests**

Printed in China

Contents

List of contributors

Phil Barker PhD RN FRCN
Professor of Psychiatric Nursing Practice, Department of Psychiatry, University of Newcastle, Royal Victoria Infirmary, Newcastle upon Tyne

Trudie Chalder SRN RMN ENB650 MSc PhD
Senior Lecturer, Department of Psychological Medicine, King's College Hospital, London

Alicia Deale PhD MSc BA(Hons) RMN Cert Behav Psych
Lecturer, Department of Psychology, Institute of Psychiatry, London

Sarah Fisher MSc PGDipHE BSc RGN
Assistant Director of Nursing, University College London Hospitals NHS Trust

David Hannigan RMN Cert Behav Psych PG Dip MSc
Cognitive Behavioural Psychotherapist, Psychological Services, West Hampshire NHS Trust, Hampshire

Angela Lavery RGN RMN BSc(Hons) Spec Pract (Mental Health)
Clinical Nurse Specialist, HIV and Mental Health, Department of Liaison Psychiatry, Leeds Hospital NHS Trust, Leeds

Rob Newell PhD BSc (Hons) RGN RMN RNT Cert Behav Psych
Professor of Nursing Research, School of Health Studies, University of Bradford

Stephen Regel MA PGDip PGCE Cert Behav Psych RMN
Senior Lecturer in Trauma Studies and Director, Centre for Traumatic Stress Research and Practice, Nottingham

Dave Roberts MSc RMN RGN
Senior Lecturer in Cancer Care, Oxford Brookes University, Oxford

Margaret Royles RMN RGN PG Dip Cert Counc
Community Psychiatric Nurse, South Oxfordshire Community Mental Health Team; *formerly* Clinical Nurse Specialist, Department of Psychological Medicine (Barnes Unit), John Radcliffe Hospital, Oxford

Robert Tunmore MA PG Dip(Ed) BSc(Hons) RMN RGN IPD Cert
Nursing Officer – Communications, Department of Health, London

Linda Whitehead BSc RMN DipN CertCogTher
Clinical Nurse Specialist, Mental Health Nursing, Department of Psychological Medicine (Barnes Unit), John Radcliffe Hospital, Oxford

Jerome Wright RGN RMN BSc (Hons)
Lecturer in Nursing, Department of Health Studies, University of York, York

Preface

Recent years have seen a rapid growth of interest in the management of psychological problems associated with physical illness and with non-mental health care settings, including the general hospital and primary care. This growth of interest has been associated with the development of new specialist mental health liaison roles, particularly in nursing. Practitioners frequently work in relative isolation from other mental health colleagues. Up to now, there has been relatively little guidance for health professionals on the practical management of mental health liaison services, and the conditions they encounter in practice. This book is an attempt to fill the gap, describing current working practices and interventions in detail. We hope this will enable practitioners to develop new services in the light of current best practice.

This book comprises contributions from leading practitioners, educators and researchers in the field of mental health nursing. Although the contributors are mental health nurses, the book is intended for use by a variety of health and social care practitioners. This will include other mental health professionals, or those working within a mental health team, including psychiatrists, social workers, occupational therapists, and physiotherapists. It will also be of interest to non-mental health nurses and doctors, working in hospitals, primary care, or specialist settings, and to counsellors and therapists.

This text is not intended to be comprehensive or exhaustive. It does, however, aim to be of practical value in the management of a range of commonly encountered clinical challenges. To this end, contributors have been encouraged to provide practice guidelines, questions for discussion, annotated reading lists and resources where these are appropriate to the subject.

The book is organised into three sections. The first, *The basis for practice,* is an overview of the major theoretical and organisational issues in contemporary mental health liaison practice. The first chapter, by Phil Barker, sets the development of liaison mental health nursing within the broad and complex philosophical context of modern health care. The following chapter outlines current thinking around working models of mental health liaison. Chapter three charts the development of contemporary liaison mental health nursing, both in the UK and in North America, and presents the findings of recent surveys of the characteristics and working practices of British nurses in this field. The fourth chapter, by Robert Tunmore, explores the potential for mental health liaison activities in primary care.

Section 2, *Generic approaches to assessment and intervention,* describes practical working approaches to three clinical areas where mental health liaison is well established: deliberate self-harm, cancer care, and HIV and AIDS. In Section 3, *Cognitive behavioural approaches,* interventions are described with a number of conditions or clinical environments commonly encountered in mental health liaison work. In all of these, cognitive behaviour therapy has a proven record of efficacy or offers a practical approach to clinical management.

We are aware that this book represents the British mental health scene. We know there are many colleagues in Europe, Australasia and the United States, who are doing innovative work in mental health liaison. As yet, our links with them have been limited. This is something we hope to remedy in the coming years, and as editors and practitioners we would welcome any observations, comments and suggestions on both this current text and any ideas for the future.

Various terms are used throughout the book to represent the people who are in receipt of our therapeutic efforts, e.g. client, patient. Each contributor has been free to use the term they feel is most familiar to them. Also, the term 'liaison' is used in a variety of different ways in the contemporary literature, and this is reflected in this book.

Acknowledgements

The idea for this book was first conceived over seven years ago. The fact that it has now come to fruition is due largely to the patience and commitment of all the contributors – we owe them our sincere thanks for all their hard work. We are also indebted to Jacqueline Curthoys and Karen Gilmour of Harcourt Health Sciences for their support and encouragement during the life of this project. Our thanks go to Professor Phil Barker for his generosity and stewardship in the early stages of the project and his support throughout.

Thanks also to the members of the Royal College of Nursing Special Interest Group in Liaison Mental Health Nursing, for all the knowledge and wisdom they have shared over the last few years, and especially to those who participated in Robert Tunmore's and Dave Roberts' and Linda Whitehead's surveys. Our thanks go to Tom Sandford for supporting the development of the group. Dave Roberts would like to thank his former colleagues at the Department of Psychological Medicine, John Radcliffe Hospital, Oxford, for all their help and support.

Figures 2.1, 2.2, and 2.3 in Chapter 2 are reproduced by kind permission of *Nursing Times*, where these figures first appeared with the article `Making the connections to aid mental health', vol. 94(15), 50–52.

Last but not least, sincere and heartfelt thanks must go to Liz Jeffrey, for typing some of the manuscripts and for `liaison' with the contributors and publishers, despite other pressing tasks!

Stephen Regel, Dave Roberts, 2002

Section 1

The basis for practice

1

Realising the promise of liaison mental health care

Phil Barker

KEY ISSUES

◆ Despite the popular affirmation of mental *health* care, especially in nursing, various political influences limit many nurses to a discrete focus on mental *illness* per se

◆ Liaison mental health care represents a genuine attempt to explore the *health* dimensions of the concept of mental health care

◆ Liaison mental health appears to embrace the concept of the 'craft of caring'

◆ The experiences gained from the person's status as a patient can play a critical role in the development of personally appropriate care in liaison mental health care

INTRODUCTION

Psychiatric services are increasingly redefined as 'mental health services' and the workers in the field conceptualise themselves as 'mental health workers'. It is interesting to note that psychiatrists are not rushing to redefine themselves as 'mental health physicians'. This is encouraging and suggests that psychiatrists might still be maintaining their professional esteem, whilst recognising that psychiatry (per se) is a part of the promotion of mental health.

Nowhere is the cosmetic manipulation of the construct of mental health more obvious than in the field of nursing where, since the publication of the Report on Mental Health Nursing (Department of Health 1994), the practice of psychiatric nursing has been officially called 'mental health nursing'.

Observation of the practice of nursing suggests, however, that the focus remains on mental *illness*.

Attention has been drawn elsewhere to the apparent 'cosmetic' nature of the change to the 'mental health' nurse's title (Barker 1999, Barker et al 1998) and the need to acknowledge the necessary balance between *psychiatric* nursing (addressing the immediate distress and disorder associated with the psychiatric crisis) and *mental health* nursing (focusing on the development of ways of living with, overcoming or otherwise recovering from mental ill health). Given the precarious balance that the liaison mental health nurse needs to strike between a specialist focus on the delivery of a mental health service and the acknowledgement that the person may be located in a non-specialist setting, the core focus of the liaison nurse appears to be more health oriented. However, given the complexity of both the constructs of health and illness and the practical realities of care delivery, this chapter includes a consideration of the social construction of health and illness and will employ the discipline of nursing as a touchstone for the actual or potential contributions of all disciplines to the field of liaison mental health care.

PSYCHIC DISTRESS: THE PROPER FOCUS OF MENTAL HEALTH NURSING?

Although discussing the practice of psychiatry, Thomas Szasz (1970) eloquently framed the dilemma of mental health nursing, when he suggested that:

> *The mental health professional who chooses to be a loyal member of his profession will thus embrace the ideology of mental health; he will teach it, apply it, refine it, distribute it as widely as possible, and, above all, defend it against those who assail it. Whereas the professional who chooses to be a critical thinker will scrutinise the ideology: he will analyse it; examine it historically, logically and sociologically; criticise it, and hence undermine it as an ideology. (p 77)*

Nursing, which for so long trailed in the wake of psychiatric medicine, has often been compromised by its loyalty to the outmoded institutional practices of psychiatry. Only recently has nursing attempted to assert itself as a unique discipline, with its own clinical focus and its own attendant philosophies and theories of practice (Barker 1999, Nolan 1993). However, such efforts to assert its independence, whilst still maintaining a relationship with medicine, require nurses to think about the potentially unique focus of their practice, a form of critical reflection that might, at least temporarily, jeopardise relations with their former medical mentors.

The redefinition of 'mental' or 'psychiatric' nursing as *mental health* nursing (Barker & Jackson 1997) implies that this branch is concerned now with mental *health*, although no consensus exists as to the meaning of the term within the practice of nursing (Altschul 1997). Contemporaneously, the strategic aim of mental health nursing has been focused officially (politically) on people with 'serious and/or enduring mental illness (*sic*)' (Department of Health 1994). Such developments raise the questions: 'What is the proper focus of nursing?' and 'What do people with mental health problems need nurses for?' (Barker 1996). Such questions may underpin the future development of mental health nursing.

In his history of British mental health nursing, Nolan (1993) concluded that nurses needed to be at the spearhead of changes in the health service, 'not lagging behind as has, sadly, been their traditional role' (p 168). In Nolan's view nurses could no longer afford to follow in the footsteps of other professional groups, 'more assertive than they [nurses] in defending their interests, since such lack of purpose could only lead to the obliteration of mental health nursing' (p 169). The expectation that nurses should refocus most, if not all, their professional energies on one ill-defined *illness* group (having redefined itself as a *health*-promoting endeavour) may signal the lack of true purpose to which Nolan referred.

THE CONSTRUCTION OF SERIOUS MENTAL ILLNESS

The need for all mental health services (including nursing) is contextual. Distress does not 'inhabit' people but exists as a complex (holistic) process involving the person's engagement with their 'world': their 'whole lived experience'. This contextual view may be employed to question the received wisdom of focusing mental *health* nursing on an 'illness', far less on a single subpopulation which, so far, has escaped satisfactory definition. The author's view is that the principal aim of mental health nursing should (obviously) be to meet the person's *nursing* needs. A viable concept of the 'severity' of such needs must involve the complex (contextual) interaction of all the factors which comprise the person's whole lived experience and cannot be defined simply as a function of some other definition – especially as a biomedical definition of illness per se.

Like all social phenomena, mental health nursing is both a social and a political construction. Language constructs the meaning of events and also constructs the person's 'identity' within, and interaction with, the situation. The power inherent in the description, classification and categorisation of phenomena, such as mental illness, cannot be underestimated, since the way in which language frames, or depicts, human experience has implications for everyone so depicted. Gergen (1990) noted how refining a language of mental states invited a process of 'enfeeblement for people labelled', with implications for patients and nurses:

> *I feel my 'clinical reality' and that of my clientele is increasingly becoming dominated by the modernist view and language of the DSM IV and I am wary of how the implications of this increased dominance will silence the development of alternative views and languages for describing the problems brought to psychotherapy. (p 54)*

Although medical classification systems offer a means of defining and distinguishing psychiatric phenomena, they were not designed as explanations. Therefore, nurses need to ask what the advantage is in knowing that a person 'suffers' from this or that disorder. How will such knowledge help determine the 'nursing needs' to be addressed?

The concept of SMI (serious and/or enduring mental illness) involves the use of quasi-psychiatric language in an effort to sharpen awareness of how people might become socially disabled or disadvantaged. Although many mental illnesses might be defined as 'serious', it is increasingly asserted that such people are most likely to have a diagnosis of schizophrenia (Repper et al 1995). This implies that all other illnesses are 'non-serious', such patients being the 'worried well' (White 1993) or the 'trivially mentally ill' (Pembroke, personal communication).

Current efforts to ensure adequate provision for SMI stem from concerns over the quality of community care. Homicides committed by people with a psychiatric diagnosis (Morall 1997) have been used by all sections of the media to argue that community care has failed and that the 'community' is now 'at risk' from the 'seriously mentally ill'. Ironically, empirical inquiry shows that people diagnosed with schizophrenia are more likely to commit suicide than homicide (Boyd 1996).

The Department of Health (DoH), mediating political concern, tried to allay public concern by making SMI a service target. In the absence of any accepted definition of SMI, which might include any age group and a range of illnesses, the DoH helped promote the view that SMI involved only people of working age with functional psychoses. Barham & Hayward (1995) argued that such a focus on the 'illness' of schizophrenia could conceal the person's 'human needs'. By narrowing the public image of SMI the media may have created a 'moral panic' (McRobbie & Thornton 1995):

> *[Moral panics are] the way in which daily events are brought to the attention of the public. They are a standard response, a familiar, sometimes weary, even ridiculous rhetoric rather than an exceptional emergency*

intervention. Used by politicians to orchestrate consent, by business to promote sales in certain niche markets, and by media to make home and social affairs newsworthy. (p 560).

The concept of SMI is enshrined in legislative and professional literature but defined in neither. When used in politically correct parlance by planners and providers of services, it may unwittingly reinforce the language of moral panic developed contemporaneously by the media. This concept may also blind us to the fact that many other people, not defined as SMI, may be experiencing significant psychic distress and attendant problems of living and may have, as a result, a significant 'need for nursing'.

LESS VISIBLE (OR MORE COMPLEX) PROBLEMS

The political, social and 'politically correct' definitions of SMI obscure the fact that many forms of mental distress might be 'serious' and that the concept of 'seriousness' is context dependent. Many groups with mental health problems, and their families, have been overshadowed by the emphasis given to schizophrenia by the term SMI. This poses an ethical dilemma for mental health nurses. If they cannot demonstrate their readiness, willingness and capability to serve all people with a need for nursing, irrespective of the origin, aetiological explanation or sociocultural construction of that need, then nurses might be criticised for neglecting people who need mental health nursing. The current concerns for people with 'serious' forms of mental illness have generated, as a side effect, a disparagement of nurses who opt to work with other client groups. One could not envisage a similar scenario in other areas of nursing. Are district nurses who deal with leg ulcers less committed than Macmillan nurses who care for people with cancer?

Although anyone might be deemed 'seriously mentally ill', depending on their context, specific groups might be classed as endangered: older people, children and adolescents and some adults with 'non-psychotic' disorders. The plight of these groups of people has been obscured, at least from a mental health nursing perspective, by the rhetoric of SMI and, more recently, the emergence of the 'epidemic' of 'personality disorders'.

Mental health nursing has, for almost a decade, affirmed its commitment to providing a public service that recognises the person's need for nursing care to be framed, positively, within a health paradigm. However, recent political influences, and their attendant policies and strategic direction, have tended to limit the practice of mental health nursing to a narrow focus on the provision of remedies for mental illness only. The need to consider mental health nursing as a broad spectrum seems long overdue.

THE SCOPE OF LIAISON MENTAL HEALTH NURSING

There are few problems of living which we otherwise define as 'illnesses', 'disabilities' or 'disorders' that did not trouble our ancestors. Of course, there are many more entries in the catalogue of human ailments and afflictions. However, at least in the case of mental health, the burgeoning list of 'illnesses and disorders' may reflect no more than a variation on one or two themes. What once was called madness or melancholia (Barker et al 1999) has been subdivided ad nauseam until almost every variant of the state of being human can be found within the pages of one diagnostic manual or another (Barker & Stevenson 2000).

Kutchins & Kirk (1997) carefully deconstructed the true misrepresentation of madness and melancholia in the contemporary business of psychiatry in their award-winning critique of the DSM IV. Ironically, this book, the latest in a long line of critiques of the value and virtue of the diagnostic process in psychiatry (Barker & Stevenson 2000, Boyle 1990, Szasz 1998), appeared at the same time as 'mental health' nurses appeared ready to embrace roles as medical diagnosticians, also aiming to add the prescribing of drugs to their clinical armamentarium. This suggests that, at least at a policy level, nursing has accepted the biomedical understanding of mental illness as a paradigm for the acquisition of mental health. Such an assumption presents some practical, as well as intellectual, challenges.

The functional core of our human problems has an enduring quality, although the linguistic content of our psychic distress may have shifted. Human distress always has seemed to involve that vague state of 'being human' and the vexed issue of 'personhood' (Forster & Stevenson 1996). Increasingly, however, we try to develop unitary explanations for serious distress, especially in terms of neuroscientific hypotheses (Dawson 1998). Whereas Freud sought to understand people by attributing their actions to various deep-seated mental concepts, 100 years later neuroscience seeks to reduce all human operations to even deeper common denominators. No less an authority than Francis Crick asserted that:

> *You, your joys and your sorrows, your memories and your ambitions, your sense of personal identity and free will, are in fact no more than the behavior of a vast assembly of nerve cells and their associated molecules. (Crick 1994, p 3)*

The layperson might be reassured to be told that distress is (merely) a function of some complex neurochemistry. They might be less enthusiastic about the idea that this theory also invalidates everything that human history has so far accepted about the state of 'being human' (Barker 1997).

Later in *The astonishing hypothesis* Crick confesses that 'The correct way to conceptualize consciousness has not yet been discovered and that we are merely groping our way toward it' (p 255). However, as Polkinghorne (1996), the particle physicist, observed, Crick's exploration might have been better conducted if he 'had not tethered himself to the ideological stake of the physically reductionist' (p 69).

Most of us, at some time, have been tempted to reduce the complex phenomena which present as distressed persons to some illness or syndrome, assuming that this name will always explain something which appears to be beyond explanation. Or we reduce the complexity of the person's experience to the function of one cognitive process or another. We talk smugly of those who, in the past, attributed human distress to the function of demons or other malicious spirits. Today, our attributions to cognitive schema (for example) are no less abstract but simply reflect the received wisdom of the present day. The name clearly is not the thing, as the map is obviously not the territory.

The phenomena associated with what are called variously life-threatening illnesses (such as AIDS), potentially dangerous forms of behaviour (such as deliberate self-harm or substance abuse) may have discrete functions but much more diffuse human meanings. These meanings involve a tangled web of fears, stigma, values, stressors, relationships, sociocultural contextual factors and the imposition of limits on ordinary, everyday living (among many others). This renders such experiences almost beyond genuine understanding. One task of the helping agent is to assist the person in exploring the specific meanings of the experience as they relate specifically to them. Although this is a significant challenge, there is reason to believe that nurses, among other disciplines, are rising to this challenge. Liaison nursing may represent one of the best examples of Peplau's now fairly aged hypothesis, that nurses do not so much address the illness or disability as the person's relationship to illness or disability (Peplau 1952).

Liaison nursing

The concept of liaison practice in psychiatry first emerged with the offer of tangible support by psychiatrists to their physician colleagues in general medicine. However, in nursing, the nature of this liaison relationship has been greatly extended and now covers a range of generic and specialist support services (Norwood 1998, Regel 1995, Roberts 1997, 1998, Tunmore 1997, Wilkinson 1998), almost spanning the life cycle (Gunstone 1999, Korczynski 1997). Liaison mental health nursing may be associated most with its discrete focus on hospital services, especially involving the support of general nursing staff in A&E (Ryan 1997, Ryrie 1997) and general medical wards (Priami 1997). However, this focus has now broadened to encompass the provision of a range of specialist supports and discrete interventions by mental health nurses to patients cared for and treated within general or specialist medical facilities (Efinger 1995, Jones 1996, Price 1995), including primary care settings (Bruce 1999, Warner 1998), across different countries (Aoun 1999, Chiu 1999, Pollard 1996) and cultures (Brown 1999).

The development of liaison mental health nursing acknowledges the complexity of people whose needs are the focus of one specific service. Although nurses have talked and written assertively about the *holistic* nature of nursing assessment and intervention, many nursing services are all too reductionist in their practice, aiming to ameliorate distress, often by the most expedient means available. The interrelationship between mind and body, which underpins the concept of holism (see Barker 1997, pp 303–308), favours an ecological perspective where everything involving the person is interconnected. This is in stark contrast to the traditional medical model which deconstructs the person, to allow the study of disease in one part of the person's functioning. Once people were viewed from the limited perspective of Newtonian physics, like a special class of billiard ball, responding passively to forces exerted upon and through the person. Now, we are beginning to acknowledge that illness and health are dynamic features of the person's total functioning and interaction with the world.

THE CRAFT OF CARING

The concept of holism suggests the influence of dualism on and in our professional as well as ordinary lives. We often talk as if 'me' was somehow separate from 'myself', in the same way that 'you' and 'me' are joined only through relationships. Yet more basically, we also talk 'as if' the world which we experience owns properties that are not inextricably part of ourselves. For example, we talk about degrees of hardness (from ashes to diamonds), yet the relative hardness we attribute to a property lies in our *relationship* with it, not in the property per se. An iron bar gripped by a child may be construed as harder than the same bar gripped by a 500-pound gorilla. The idea that life experience might teach us a 'hard' lesson implies an unnecessary dualism. This dualism is, of course, largely a function of our assumption that one event is *caused* by another (perhaps more powerful) event. In health care, the influence of the traditional medical model, with its Newtonian assumptions, has engendered a highly specific appreciation of this dualism, in our search for discrete causal relationships between phenomena that we call 'illnesses' and their discrete putative antecedents. Many people have been 'taught' important lessons about the nature of their health or illness status. Most specifically, many people learn about the extent to which they have co-constructed the experience; illness and health are rarely 'caused' by events external to the person but more often by the nature of the person's engagement with those events.

The development of a realistic 'health' orientation in nursing practice might require us to get a feel for the essential 'relativity' of experience and how people are engaged, actively, in making a reality of their own experience. As Watts (1957) noted, we do not sweat *because* it is hot – sweating (the act) *is* the heat. When we talk of the *things* with which people 'struggle', we might ask whether any such thing can exist, independent of the struggling. Inherent dualism is predominantly a peculiarity of Westernised thought. By contrast, most traditional Eastern thought finds great difficulty in separating 'knowing' and 'knowledge':

> *Life is not a situation from which anything is to be grasped or gained – as if it were something which one approaches from the outside, like a pie or a barrel of beer. To succeed is always to fail – in the sense that the more one succeeds in anything, the greater is the need to go on succeeding. To eat is to survive to be hungry. (Watts 1957, p 78)*

This very Western tradition of dualism is well established in health care, where various disciplines grapple with disorders and illnesses 'as if' they were separate from the person who is the patient and indeed, as if the patient was (systemically) separate from the health-care agent.

THE CRAFT OF THERAPY

I have written elsewhere about approaching therapy as a craft, rather than an art or science (Barker & Whitehill 1997). We talk about the 'art of nursing' but art suggests a sense of self-importance, righteousness or correctness, as if we are being 'artful', like Dickens' 'Dodger'. Artists may produce their work for a market – paintings, sculptures or operas. Arguably, they make these works primarily to satisfy themselves and to obtain funding to allow the continuation of this narcissism. At least in high art, the artist is the final arbiter of the work's quality and worth.

More recently, we have tried to emphasise the 'science of nursing'. Science also is an occupation but one that possesses a different kind of correctness, one owned, allegedly, by a universal intelligence. Unlike the artist, the scientist does not 'make' anything, but rather discovers the gods' handiwork. Again, like the artist, the scientist does not modify or adapt his work (his discovery) to suit the patron. Scientists are above this, on principle.

Craft suggests a wholly different experience, primarily because craft objects are made to satisfy discrete demands from patrons or customers. The craftsperson needs to bring together skill (art), knowledge (science) and the needs of the individual recipient to make true craft. The success or value of a crafted object is defined by the unknown gift that the person brings and bestows on the object. The meaning attached to a wedding dress, a talismanic piece of jewellery or a pot emerges from the owner (customer or patron), not from the maker. It is invisible but transformative. With the attribution of that meaning, the crafted object becomes unique, like no other, despite surface similarities.

Like other makers of craft, the liaison nurse appears to use their available skill and knowledge, most of which is common therapeutic currency, to create (metaphorically) an aesthetically pleasing thing: the nurse–patient interaction. The final meaning – the essence of the therapeutic conversation – is, however, attributed by the recipient, the patient. Like a potter, the nurse makes pots (discrete therapeutic conversations) on a regular basis for a changing clientele. Some of these relationships will be more aesthetically pleasing than others. All have the potential, however, to be effective pots, meeting the needs of the individual patient for a transformational caring experience. However, the value attached to the pots – what the patient momentarily and finally makes of the crafted object – belongs to the patient. The crafted relationship becomes a temporary and fluid receptacle to which the person may attach meaning. The patient expects that the nurse will not fuss over the therapeutic conversation or hang on to the pot after it has been finished but will surrender it to the patient to allow the will-to-meaning to be completed.

In Frankl's (1964) sense, many of these conversations between the nurse and the patient have the capacity to become 'spiritual' since they address, most of the time, the discrete meanings that the patient attaches to his life, especially when that life appears to be under threat. In that sense, much if not all illness experiences can be construed as spiritually meaningful, in either a religious or a secular sense.

THE CHAOTIC ORDER OF CARE

Although there are boundaries to the chaotic 'reflections' of our world of experience *in* our personal experience and vice versa, these boundaries exist only at the level of hypothesis. The traditional Western dualism, that split 'experience' off from that which is 'experienced', set people apart from the world and led, at least indirectly, to the notion that therapists might 'effect' change within the person's experience. Here, I have suggested that any changes that become manifest in the patient, and in the therapeutic relationship, may be likened to the 'orderly chaos' of water. These changes are understandable in terms of the fluid (tidal) exchange between patient and therapist, where the experience of one manifests itself (flows into) in the experience of the other and vice versa. This essentially Eastern construction of relationships offers a challenge to our received wisdom about the origins of 'influence' and the functional operations of the therapeutic relationship.

The concept of the craft of caring seems apposite to liaison nursing where the mental health nurse is involved in bridging two worlds: the world of the specialised knowledge of mental health and other worlds of health care, either generic services, involving children or older people, or specialised medical services (hospital or primary care) or the experience of different disorders (cancer or AIDS). The liaison mental health nurse appears to be trying to produce a form of care that is informed by certain skills, knowledge and values that belong within the mental health arena (the art and science of mental health care). At the same time they need to transform this art and science into a product that might meaningfully be used by a patient who stands outside the mental health setting. In a very special sense the liaison mental health nurse fashions (or crafts) a very special nursing product that is informed by their original field of mental health but now belongs (meaningfully) to another, non-specialised world of care.

ILLUSTRATION: THE EXPERIENCE OF CANCER

In a moving and optimistic paper Bennett (2000) described his 'journey *with* cancer', which began almost a decade ago. Bennett observed that, for many if not all, the experience of cancer was about the fear of losing: losing control over one's life and ultimately of losing life itself. Citing some lines from the Scots poet Norman MacCaig, Bennett reflected on the paradox of the cancer experience.

I give you emptiness,
I give you plenitude,
Unwrap them carefully,
One's as fragile as the other is.

This beautiful poem, like my cancer journey, conjures up the duality of emptiness and fullness at the heart of life (especially of the spirit). Nothing and fullness in union. Cancer can make you feel empty and heading for nothingness. There is no need to despair. Let your emptiness fill you up with that which is surprising, unexpected and creative. A soul calls, awaking your life to new possibilities – a transfiguration of sorts. Oh yes, my friend Cancer – there is no death to die. (Bennett 2000)

Bennett, who is nurse and therapist, was not peddling some New Age positive thinking but appeared to be acknowledging the need to capitalise on the resources of a person who is living and who never really dies. Death occurs to bodies, he seemed to be saying, not to people. Why else are we still talking about Leonardo 500 years after his demise? For Bennett, the cognitive behavioural paradigm has already proven itself (Lovejoy 2000) as a good basis to begin exploring the human resources of the person and how these can be employed in journeying with cancer. Bennett's emphasis on the potency of the experience of cancer illustrates some of the ideas about meaningful care noted earlier yet also illustrates, profoundly, how CBT can only be construed as a practical starting point, for the person's exploration of the relationship with serious illness.

Yet there remains some considerable resistance to accepting the need for meaningful care requested by Bennett. In a large part, this resistance is founded on the worldview of mental and physical health that began in earnest with Hippocrates and was cemented by Descartes. The roots of scientific psychiatry and psychology lie in the Hippocratic ethic: 'Anything not couched in physiological and physical terms (has) already touched on magic and charlatanism' (Simon 1980, p 227). Attempts to use quantum theory to capture the transactional patterns of therapy have become almost commonplace (Bass 1997, Gerstein & Bennett 1999, Kulka 1997). However, when therapists began to conjure up the metaphors of contemporary physics, in searching for possible mirrors of human complexity, Will (1986), a Scots psychiatrist and psychotherapist, wrote:

If there is one sure thing about quantum theory it is that it has no implication for the human sciences. This invocation of quantum theory is symptomatic of the phenomenon of pseudo-scientific mysticism which abounds in woolly-minded idealist discourse on the human sciences. (p 236)

There is, however, no need to employ physics (nor mysticism) to challenge the scientific orthodoxy that has bedevilled psychiatry – particularly, more recently, neuropsychiatry – which has returned, repeatedly, to a version of the Hippocratic model of insanity: searching for causes of apparent mental disturbance *in* the physical body. Bennett appears to be hoping that psychotherapy, with its fundamental interest in how people construct understandings of themselves and their lives, might be more open to the development of a holistic appreciation of the person that would include the great fuzzy concept traditionally called the spiritual process. A pragmatic approach is needed to address the human needs of people in serious states of ill health. The acute nature of their distress often demands this, as do the limits that often are imposed on available services. However, this pragmatism can be used as the launch pad for a deeper exploration (as appropriate) of the experience of illness and health, a territory of understanding known only to the person themselves.

A tension undoubtedly exists between a materialist worldview and anything approaching a spiritual perspective. The former emphasises the roles of presumed biological anomalies, coupled with psychosocial stressors, in the explanation of mental distress. The latter emphasises the search for understanding or 'will-to-meaning' (Frankl 1964) undertaken by the individual in pursuit of a personal explanation of distress. Although we are encouraged to tolerate spirituality, especially when such strivings for personal meanings are associated with religion, the materialist orthodoxy often views those with 'serious' spiritual inclinations as uneducated, suffering from a shared delusion, perhaps, or emotionally immature (Grof 1998). Psychotherapy involves an organised search for understanding. When psychotherapy tries to accommodate a spiritual pathway to understanding, it accepts that there may be many emergent 'truths' rather than one singular explanation of the 'cause' of the patient's problems. The inclusiveness of this spiritual approach to therapy involves accepting as potentially valid and therefore meaningful many of the unfamiliar experiences, especially altered states of consciousness, that traditional materialist perspectives dismiss as abnormal and potentially meaningless.

Although not all liaison nurses will construe themselves as psychotherapists, the nature of their work is arguably psychotherapeutic: helping people to acquire an understanding of their illness state that might serve to release them (albeit temporarily) from the limits illness often imposes.

CONCLUSION

Engaging the systemic reality?

The experience of being human is rarely something that can be described directly. The experience of health and illness is similar. When asked to report their feelings of illness or health, people invariably have recourse to metaphor or simile: 'The pain is *like* something gnawing at my insides' or 'Illness has sapped my confidence in myself'. Mental health is such an arch-abstraction that people in care, and those caring for them, are obliged to indulge in some of the most fanciful metaphorical allusions to express something of their engagement with the concept. The author has found the water metaphor useful in helping to explicate many of the psychotherapeutic assumptions of the chaotic order of human experience. The water metaphor raises the question: 'Have we skipped fundamental truths about action and reality, in our efforts to develop more complicated theories and constructions of *mind*?'. Human behaviour – whether action, emotion or thought – involves an exhibition of variable and irregular patterns that never repeat themselves but remain within bounded parameters (Vicenzi 1994). Water was one of the everyday enigmas that confronted Leonardo da Vinci, who sought in vain to establish its pattern. The behaviour of water continues to be one of the key challenges for contemporary chaologists.

Within the context of psychotherapy, the stable yet changing behaviour of water provides a useful metaphor for both intrapsychic and interpersonal operations. Among the countless water metaphors, these lines from Alan Watts (which illustrate the complexity of 'I' (the state of mind)) are some of the most elegant:

> *We have the impression that 'I' is something solid and still, like a tablet upon which life is writing a record. Yet the 'tablet' moves with the writing finger as the river flows along with the ripples, so that memory is like a record written on water. (Watts 1997, p 40)*

Watts recognised that this memory is not made up of graven characters but is more like waves stirred into motion by other waves, which might be called sensations and facts. Consequently, the difference between 'I' and 'me' becomes largely an illusion of memory. 'I' and 'me' possess the same nature, as part of our whole being, as the head is part of the body. When we lose our awareness of this, 'I' and 'me', the head and the body, feel at odds with one another. Watts notes:

> *'I', not understanding that it too is part of the stream of change, will try to make sense of the world and experience by attempting to fix it. (Watts 1997, p 40)*

Here, Watts raises two of the key issues for therapists: Who or what is the 'self' with which people have problems? How can we 'fix' something which, by its very metaphorical nature (water), can never be broken?

The turbulent motion of water is not only reflected in the person's experience of self but also in the exchange with the therapist. The idea of studying the process of psychotherapy as an 'event' may be misjudged. The idea of trying to judge the events within therapy as 'effective' or 'ineffective' may even be foolhardy. As Bannister (1998) noted:

> *Psychotherapy is a particular formalization of human relationships … To start from the premise that psychotherapy may not be effective is in essence to start from the premise that human relationships may not be effective and this is an absurdity. Are you really prepared to contend that your relationships, your love affairs, your enmities, your long-standing dialogue with your uncle Albert – whether the effect be good, bad or chaotic – have been, in some strange sense, 'ineffective'? (p 219)*

Therapist and patient flow, effortlessly, through each other's experience, writing the story of the session in the illusion of co-creation.

The water-borne memories that the patient brings to therapy come from the person's wider 'ocean of experience', a virtually limitless personal universe embracing surface 'currents' and 'storms' as well as 'hidden depths' and 'monsters' from the deep. These are memories since even 'now-ness' becomes history in the act of experience; the simultaneous birth and death of the moment. The fluid birth/death of the moment can be conceptualised either as what has been 'washed ashore' with the person or is part of the whole business of 'running aground', being 'all washed up' or otherwise 'on the rocks'. Therapy offers a piece of 'dry land' when the ocean of experience threatens to drown the individual. The kind of people who are the focus of the liaison nurse's attention have been storm-tossed by all manner of physical, emotional and ultimately spiritual crises. Liaison nurses' recognition that something practical must first be done, as a way of developing a means of avoiding further 'storms', is perhaps the key to the holistic emphasis of their work.

Yet the ocean is but part of a wider universe of experience, on which are written other narratives which may, in turn, become consciously incorporated into the narrative of self. Again, Watts (1957) notes the relationship between water (the subject) and the moon (the object):

> *When there is no water, there is no moon-in-the-water ... But when the moon rises, the water does not wait to receive its image, and when even the tiniest drop of water is poured out the moon does not wait to cast its reflection. (Watts 1957, p 97)*

The moon has no *intention* of casting its reflection in the water and the water does not receive this reflection *on purpose*. The reflection is caused as much by the water as by the moon. Indeed, the water *manifests* the brightness of the moon, as the moon also makes *manifest* the clarity of the water. This may serve as a paradoxical metaphor for the reflection of meaning in experience and vice versa.

David Reynolds (1984), who has employed a specific understanding of Zen in his 'Constructive Living' therapy, noted that water reflects the process of change that is fundamental to the universe:

> *...from interstellar events to the decay of atomic particles. The reality of our experience is in constant flux, too. Feelings come and go, impulses rise and disappear, thoughts flit through our minds. Our actions ... contain the possibility for influencing the course of this change ... glimmerings of our experience of playing ball on running water. (p 77)*

Although philosophical in form, these reflections are unashamedly practical in their orientation. Such metaphorical allusions help (paradoxically) to reveal some of the mystery of the illness experience. Such mysteries not only bewilder but can also strike fear into the hearts of sophisticated care staff. In her ethnographic study of the care of people who self-harm in medical admission units, Hopkins (1999) employed a Foucaldian analysis that acknowledged the complexity of the 'body' phenomenon, upon which was inscribed (literally *and* metaphorically) the self-injury. She recognised that not only was the concept of self-harm a powerful social construction but it belied arguably deeper anxieties about the body in general.

The media and press relentlessly bombard the public with images of how the 'standard' person should be, physically, mentally and emotionally. As Turner (1987) says:

> *Following Foucault, I have argued that the body has been subject to a long historical process of rationalisation and standardisation. The body has become the focus of a wide range of disciplines and forms of surveillance and control, in which the medical profession has played a critical part.*
> *(p 210)*

Bodies which do not conform to society's norms risk becoming 'other' to society. Those people who harm themselves reject the intense 'normality that society has come to demand and become a site of resistance to it. They bear witness to the fact that life is far from perfect and society is fearful of contact with them' (Hopkins 1999, p 102).

In her conclusion, Hopkins acknowledges the double-bind imposed on nurses in medical units, who are obliged (however temporarily) to care for people who self-harm. Such staff may not have the understanding of the self-harm phenomenon necessary to deliver genuine *care* or to respond to people whose life-problems appear so discordant with the care setting in which they find themselves.

> *Self harm is an act of desperation and may represent a wish to die, a wish to escape the intolerable, or an attempt to communicate intense anger. They have a deep need which requires a special kind of help. Nurses on busy medical admission units have not been asked if they want this role and, on the wards I visited, had received no special training or supervision in it.*
> *(p 109)*

Hopkins compared the plight of these nurses to the fairy-tale princess in *Rumpelstiltskin*:

> *Their greedy father (the NHS) has promised the King (society) that they can spin straw into gold. The eyes of the world are upon them – they don't know how to spin gold – but their (professional) lives are at risk if they say so. What are they to do? (Hopkins 1999, p 109)*

The liaison mental health nurse represents one discipline among several who might be able to respond to the plight of the nurses faced with what Hopkins sees as a double-bind scenario. The liaison mental health nurse might, in concert with the psychiatrist, clinical psychologist, social worker and other professionals allied to health care, offer the practical support and wise counsel that might enable those nurses to do the magic that a greedy society so urgently desires.

QUESTIONS FOR DISCUSSION

◆ Considering your own practice, to what extent is the 'health' of the patient the absence of 'illness' or the presence of something else? What do you understand by that 'something else'?

◆ How do you promote health – either directly through your own practice or indirectly through some form of support to others?

◆ Effective liaison mental health work depends greatly on interpersonal strengths. What else is essential for effective mental health liaison work?

REFERENCES

Altschul A T 1997 A personal view of psychiatric nursing. In: Tilley S (ed) The mental health nurse: views of practice and education. Blackwell Science, Oxford
Aoun S 1999 Deliberate self-harm in rural Western Australia: results of an intervention study. Aust N Z J Ment Health Nurs 8(2):65–73
Bannister D 1998 The nonsense of 'effectiveness'. Changes 16:218–220
Barham P, Hayward R 1991 Relocating madness: from the mental patient to the person. Free Association, London
Barker P 1996 The logic of experience: developing appropriate care through effective collaboration. Aust N Z J Ment Health Nurs 5:3–12
Barker P 1997 Assessment in psychiatric and mental health nursing: in search of the whole person. Stanley Thornes, Cheltenham
Barker P 1999 The philosophy and practice of psychiatric nursing. Churchill Livingstone/Harcourt Brace, London
Barker P, Jackson S 1997 Mental health nursing: making it a primary concern. Nurs Standard 11:39–42
Barker P, Stevenson C (eds) 2000 The construction of power and authority in psychiatry. Butterworth Heinemann, Oxford
Barker P, Whitehill I 1997 The craft of care: towards collaborative caring in psychiatric nursing. In: Tilley S (ed) The mental health nurse: views of practice and education. Blackwell Science, Oxford
Barker P, Walker L, Parsons S 1998 The reification of serious mental illness. Ment Health Pract 1(9):34–35
Barker P, Campbell P, Davidson B 1999 From the ashes of experience: reflections on madness, recovery and growth. Whurr, London
Bass A 1997 The status of an analogy: psychoanalysis and physics. Am Imago 54:235–256
Bennett E 2000 Cancer, you gave me the best year of my life. Paper presented to the European Association of Psychotherapy Conference, University College, Dublin, June 28.
Boyd W 1996 Report of the Confidential Inquiry into Homicides and Suicides by Mentally Ill People. Royal College of Psychiatrists, London
Boyle M 1990 Schizophrenia: a scientific delusion? Routledge, London
Brown R 1999 Indigenous mental health: the Rainbow Serpent awakening. Int J Psychiatr Nurs Res 4(3):475–481

Bruce J 1999 Dedicated psychiatric care within general practice: health outcome and service providers' views. J Adv Nurs 29(5):1060–1067.

Chiu L 1999 Psychiatric liaison nursing in Taiwan. Clin Nurse Special 13(6):311–314

Crick F 1994 The astonishing hypothesis. Simon and Schuster, New York

Dawson P J 1998 Schizophrenia and genetics: a review and critique for the psychiatric nurse. J Psychiatr Ment Health Nurs 5(4):299–308

Department of Health 1994 Working in partnership: a collaborative approach to care (report of the Mental Health Nursing Review Group). HMSO, London

Efinger J 1995 Help wanted: a quality needs assessment creates a position for a psychiatric clinical nurse specialist. J Psychosoc Nurs Ment Health Serv 33(10):24–30, 42–43

Forster S, Stevenson C 1996 Holistic thinking: personhood and the biopsychosocial model. In: Cooper N, Stevenson C, Hale G (eds) Integrating perspectives on health. Open University, Buckingham

Frankl V 1964 Man's search for meaning: an introduction to logotherapy. Hodder and Stoughton, London

Gergen K J 1990 Therapeutic professions and the diffusion of deficit. J Mind Behav 11:353–368

Gerstein L H, Bennett M 1999 Quantum physics and mental health counseling: the time is … ! J Ment Health Couns 21:255–269

Grof S 1998 The cosmic game: explorations in the frontiers of human consciousness. Newleaf, Dublin

Gunstone S 1999 Expert practice: the interventions used by a community mental health nurse with carers of dementia sufferers. J Psychiatr Ment Health Nurs 6(1):21–27

Hopkins C 1999 What does it mean to nurses on medical admission wards to have people who self harm as their patients? MSc thesis, University of Newcastle, Newcastle upon Tyne

Jones A 1996 An equal struggle (psychodynamic assessment following repeated episodes of deliberate self harm). J Psychiatr Ment Health Nurs 3(3):173–180

Korczynski J 1997 Advanced practice. Reaching out to children in need of mental health services. Nurs Spectr 9A(22):171–177

Kulka R 1997 Quantum selfhood. Psychoanal Dialogues 7:183–187

Kutchins H, Kirk S 1997 Making us crazy. Free Press, New York

Lovejoy L C 2000 Cancer-related depression: part I – neurologic alterations and cognitive-behavioural therapy. Oncol Nurs Forum 27(4):667–680

McRobbie I, Thornton J 1995 Rethinking moral panic for multi-mediated social worlds. Br J Sociol 46:559–574

Morall P 1997 Murder, madness and mental health nursing: the application of realist theory. Paper presented to the RCN Conference: Valuing Mental Health Nursing: Demonstrating Its Worth

Nolan P 1993 A history of mental health nursing. Chapman and Hall, London

Norwood S L 1998 Psychiatric consultation-liaison nursing: revisiting the role. Clin Nurse Spec 12(4):153–156

Peplau H 1952 Interpersonal relations in nursing. Putman, New York

Polkinghorne J 1996 Beyond science: the wider human context. Cambridge University Press, Cambridge

Pollard C 1996 Guest editorial. Port Arthur: from the perspective of the mental health liaison nurse. Contemp Nurse 5(4):138–140

Priami M 1997 The effectiveness of the mental health nursing interventions [sic] in a general hospital. Scand J Caring Sci 11(1):56–62

Price N 1995 The role of the consultation-liaison nurse: caring for patients with AIDS dementia complex. J Psychosoc Nurs Ment Health Serv 33(12):31–34, 40–41

Regel S 1995 The future of mental health nurses in liaison psychiatry. Br J Nurs 4(18): 052–1054, 1056

Repper J, Brooker C, Repper D 1995 Serious mental health problems: policy changes. Nurs Times 91:29–31

Reynolds D 1984 Playing ball on running water. Sheldon Press, London

Roberts D 1997 Liaison mental health nursing: origins, definition and prospects. J Adv Nurs 25(1):101–108

Roberts D 1998 Nurses' perceptions of the role of liaison mental health nurse. Nurs Times 94(43):56–57

Ryan J M 1997 Psycho-social. Role of a psychiatric liaison nurse in an A&E department. Accid Emerg Nurs 5(3):152–155

Ryrie I 1997 Liaison psychiatric nursing in an inner city accident and emergency department. J Psychiatr Ment Health Nurs 4(2):131–136

Simon B 1980 Mind and madness in ancient Greece: the classical roots of modern psychiatry. Cornell University Press, Ithaca, N Y

Szasz T S 1970 Ideology and insanity. Syracuse University Press, Syracuse, NY

Szasz T S 1998 Parity for mental illness: disparity for the mental patient. Lancet 352 (9135):1213–1215

Tunmore R 1997 Mental health liaison and consultation. Nurs Standard 11(50):46–53

Turner B S 1987 Medical power and social knowledge, 2nd edn. Sage, London

Vicenzi A E 1994 Chaos theory and some nursing considerations. Nurs Sci Quart 7:32–44

Warner L 1998 Mental health facilitators in primary care. Nurs Standard 13(6):36–40

Watts A 1957 The way of Zen. Penguin Books, Harmondsworth

Watts A 1997 The wisdom of insecurity: a message for an age of anxiety. Rider, London

White E 1993 Community psychiatric nursing 1980–90: a review of organisation, education and practice. In: Brooker C, White E (eds) Community psychiatric nursing: a research perspective, vol 2. Chapman and Hall, London

Wilkinson L 1998 Liaison service provides safety network. Nurs Times 94(37):37

Will D 1986 Science, psychotherapy and anti-psychiatry. Br J Psychother 2:230–237

2

Working models for practice

Dave Roberts

KEY ISSUES

♦ Mental health liaison is the term used to describe the activities of liaison mental health nurses and other related professionals

♦ Consultation models originated in community psychiatry and have become prominent in liaison psychiatry

♦ Consultation and liaison have been seen as alternative working models, but they are now usually seen as complementary

♦ Increasingly, working models are viewed as a collaboration between mental health liaison personnel and their non-mental health colleagues

♦ Models of liaison working are reviewed in this chapter and a collaborative approach is proposed

INTRODUCTION

Mental health liaison is a complex activity, undertaken by different health professionals in a wide range of settings. Practice cannot be standardised or prescribed but has to respond to local needs. Practitioners require a broad overview of the concepts they will be using in practice and an appreciation of the models that have been found to be effective. This chapter addresses this need and starts with a review of the theoretical background to mental health liaison.

THE THEORETICAL BACKGROUND

Liaison psychiatry: reduce, integrate or just treat?

Health-care professions follow the traditional Cartesian split of mind and body by having separate services for mental and physical illness. This distinction, also evident in theory and research, can be termed dualistic or reductionist. However, there has long been discontent at the separation of mind and body in the medical profession and at different times, an integrationist or biopsychosocial model has been advocated. During the 1920s and 1930s, an integrationist movement emerged within American psychiatry, called 'psychosomatic medicine', and this became the theoretical basis of liaison psychiatry. By the 1950s psychosomatic medicine had come to be associated with a causative relationship between mental and physical states, based in psychodynamic theory. Alexander, an American psychiatrist, proposed that a number of illnesses were 'psychosomatic' in that they represented a physical manifestation of intrapsychic conflicts. These were duodenal ulcer, bronchial asthma, ulcerative colitis, thyrotoxicosis, rheumatoid arthritis, some dermatological conditions and essential hypertension (Lipowski 1982).

As the drive for evidence-based practice has grown and the popularity of psychodynamic ideas has declined, the concept of psychosomatic illness has gone out of use. Psychosomatic medicine, however, still has currency as a term signifying the philosophical base of liaison psychiatry or the study of interrelationships between mental and physical health (Lipowski 1982). The debate about reductionism and integration has continued, without resolution. Reductionism is still a prevalent ideology in medical circles, supporting the basic Cartesian view that mental and physical substance have different properties and therefore are amenable to different forms of measurement. However, in practice, it is usually unsatisfactory (not least for the patient) to separate the different parts of the person. Some degree of integration is therefore desirable in clinical practice. Lipowski (1986) advocates the use of reductionist approaches to research and integrationist approaches to theory, practice and education.

This is all very well but does it help us to treat patients? Contemporary liaison psychiatry, certainly in the UK, takes a pragmatic approach to both research and treatment. Whereas we no longer recognise a group of illnesses called psychosomatic, there are symptoms and conditions whose presentation is primarily physical but where the aetiology is unclear and psychological factors appear to be prominent. These are called *somatoform disorders*, particularly in the USA, and are also known as *functional somatic symptoms* in the UK. Most current opinion on them suggests multifactorial, interactive causes, involving physical, psychological and social factors (Mayou et al 1995). The adoption of this biopsychosocial model is pragmatic, in that it offers a practical model for treating these complex, problematic conditions, or eclectic, in the sense that it relies on validated treatments rather than theory.

Holism

Reductionism has enjoyed little popularity in nursing and most nurses profess some loyalty to the concept of holism. This concept was introduced by Smuts in the 1920s and probably entered nursing through psychiatric nursing in the USA during the 1960s (Sarkis & Skoner 1987).

According to holism, the person is greater than the sum of their parts. This challenging concept is difficult to realise within a health-care system dominated by Cartesian dualism and the proliferation of medical and nursing specialities. Woods (1998) has pointed out that holism is evident in two forms: strong holism and weak holism. Strong holism is clearly antireductionist and supports nursing the person as a unified whole. However, it poses problems such as the point at which responsibility for nursing the person ends. How separate are their problems from the society they live in? Nursing the person as a whole puts tremendous pressure on the individual nurse to be all things to all patients. The weak version of holism is more realistic, in that it acknowledges the need to nurse the patient within a specific health-care context that changes the focus of care. The patient within a general hospital ward, for example, will be there for treatment of a specific condition. This will always be the focus of the care given, though other factors, such as the role of the family in their care, will also be important.

Holism in practice, therefore, is often an overall principle within which care is delivered, rather than a clear, unified philosophy underpinning care. It is often used as shorthand for patient-centred care or attempts to integrate (the usually separate) physical, psychological, social and spiritual aspects of care. As these are usually considered separately by the dominant health-care system, it would be more accurate to describe integrationist or integrative care than holistic care. However, these terms are rarely used in nursing, particularly in a general (i.e. non-mental health) context. Integration has a number of potential meanings: the integration of the care of mind and body, the integration of separate theoretical perspectives or, in the context of psychotherapy, the integration of differing psychotherapeutic approaches in the practice of therapy.

Mental health liaison

The theoretical divide between mind and body is mirrored in the provision of separate medical/nursing and psychiatric services. Over the course of the last century, there have been various initiatives within medicine and nursing to bridge the divide. The resulting specialisms in psychiatry and nursing are widely known as 'consultation liaison' services, describing two separate but related functions. In the United Kingdom, this is generally abbreviated to 'liaison', as in liaison psychiatry and liaison mental health nursing. To some extent this is a matter of convenience. Mental health liaison services experience problems of acceptance and legitimacy that are not helped by having a cumbersome, esoteric name. However, liaison can also be used as an umbrella term that covers the range of activities and functions undertaken by these services and consultation can be seen as a subsidiary term and function.

Mental health is a controversial term. In general, it has one of two meanings:

◆ a positive state of psychological well-being, associated with good feelings about the self, supportive relationships and a fulfilling social role
◆ an absence of mental disorder.

In recent years, the term 'mental health' has become increasingly linked with psychiatric services (i.e. 'mental health trust', 'mental health team'). This is in part because not all health-care personnel want to be defined by their association with psychiatry, but also out of a desire to shift the emphasis of care away from the traditional hospital base of psychiatry into a broader health promotion role within the wider community. In the sense of mental health services or mental health liaison, it covers the theory and practice of psychiatry, psychology, psychotherapy and mental health nursing and the contribution each of these groups makes to care and treatment.

Where services or activities are being described, particularly when they are multidisciplinary, 'mental health liaison' is preferable to 'psychiatric liaison'. There are a number of reasons for this.

◆ Liaison services have a long association with preventive psychiatry, which emphasises the promotion of health rather than solely the treatment of illness.
◆ Much of the work of liaison services deals with people who are not mentally ill, e.g. people who have taken overdoses.
◆ Nurses in the UK are generally known as mental health nurses rather than psychiatric nurses, in keeping with the *Mental Health Nursing Review* (Department of Health 1994).
◆ Many psychiatrists prefer to emphasise their links with medicine by calling themselves consultants in psychological medicine or calling their services departments of psychological medicine rather than liaison psychiatry.

Liaison psychiatry remains a discrete speciality and many psychiatrists will use this term to emphasise their psychiatric identity. Liaison psychiatrists are the dominant professional group and they play the most significant role in defining the range of psychological conditions treated within liaison teams. Lipowski (1981) defines liaison psychiatry in terms of the diagnosis, treatment, study and prevention of the following:

◆ psychiatric morbidity in the physically ill
◆ somatoform and facitious disorders
◆ psychological factors affecting physical conditions.

These are the main clinical areas for mental health liaison activity, though it is common for liaison mental health nurses (LMHNs) to focus particularly on staff-related consultation work.

MODES OF PRACTICE

The terms 'consultation', 'collaboration' and 'liaison' are commonly used in mental health liaison services. They are also widely used within a non-mental health context to describe activities carried out by clinical nurse specialists (Barbiasz et al 1982, Everson 1981). All three terms are used to denote similar activities undertaken by members of liaison teams and there is overlap between them. The following differentiates between them as modes of practice within the process of mental health liaison.

Consultation

Consultation can have a number of related and overlapping meanings within mental health liaison.

A consultation can mean a specific episode of work. This is particularly the case in the recording of liaison work for research, audit or cost-charging purposes. The nurse or psychiatrist will record a *consultation* or a *consult* as denoting a completed piece of liaison work.

Consultation can denote the working relationship between a *consultant* and a *consultee*. Consultation in this sense means responding to a request for help. This was the original model of working between mental health nurse consultants and their general nursing colleagues in the United States (Johnson 1963). Tunmore & Thomas (1992) point out that a consultant is a person who carries authority but that does not necessarily mean they are in a position of authority over the consultee. Rather, their authority is based in their specialist knowledge. The relationship can be termed 'coordinate', implying a relationship between peers or peer equivalents, with neither having power or control over the other's work (Caplan 1970). A consultant is, therefore, a specialist from outside the consultee's team, who provides expertise not available within the team. In the British context, there is the potential for confusion, as the most common health-care use of the title 'consultant' is as the senior member of a medical team.

Consultation is also a *strategy* of working to make the best use of limited mental health resources by encouraging indirect, i.e. staff-focused, work. This was the means by which consultation models originally developed in the United States, in response to a move to community-based psychiatry in the 1960s. There would not be enough psychiatric resources in the community to deal with all the potential problems, so these resources were targeted at helping those in direct contact with the patients needing help. This model has proved as useful in general hospital settings as in the community.

Consultation is most commonly seen as a *process*, with a specific focus. Caplan's (1970) model, initially developed for use in community settings, has proved transferable to hospital environments and has been influential in the development of liaison psychiatry since the 1960s.

Caplan's model of mental health consultation

This model focuses on the promotion of mental health but also involves the prevention, treatment and rehabilitation of mental disorders. It involves the work of a mental health consultant or mental health specialist and has the following features.

◆ The consultant responds to a request for help from an individual consultee or team.
◆ The help is sought for a work problem which is perceived to be outside the consultee's area of competence.
◆ The work problem involves the client or a group or category of clients of the consultee.
◆ The consultant has no authority for, nor authority over, the work of the consultee.
◆ The consultee retains responsibility for accepting or rejecting the advice given and for implementing any plan based on this advice.
◆ The consultation process is educational and should enable the consultee to manage similar situations better in future (Caplan 1970).

Caplan identifies four major types of consultation.

1. *Client-centred case consultation* focuses on the mental health needs of a client or group of clients. The consultant does an assessment and makes recommendations on how the consultee should deal with the case. These

consultations have a primary goal of recommending the best management of the client and a subsidiary goal of improving the consultee's skills in handling similar clients or situations in the future.

2. *Consultee-centred case consultation* focuses on difficulties the consultee has with the client or situation, because of a lack of skills, knowledge, confidence or professional objectivity. Helping the consultee has an indirect beneficial effect on the client.

3. *Programme-centred administrative consultation* is where the consultant is invited by the administrator (or manager) of an organisation or programme to advise on setting up or improving it. They are invited to do so on the basis of their knowledge of mental health, systems theory, administration and programme development. There is an educational component to this type of consultation.

4. *Consultee-centred administrative consultation* involves a focus on problems with running or managing a programme. This may be due to poor communication or leadership or problems of role definition or overlap (Caplan 1970).

Whatever the original intention, however, the consultant may get involved in a case and be expected to take responsibility for their own specialist contribution to the multidisciplinary team's work, thereby moving into a collaborative model of practice.

Collaboration

At the heart of all mental health liaison work is the collaboration between mental health and non-mental health professionals. It is often cited as the way in which multiprofessional groups should operate, but it is not always clear how this works in practice. Collaboration involves professionals from different specialities (or different professional groups within a speciality) working together, using different professional perspectives but with a common purpose – the improved health of the patient. In practice, collaboration may have the following components.

◆ Taking responsibility for different aspects of treatment or care but adopting a joint approach to the patient.
◆ Sharing professional skills and knowledge for the benefit of the patient.
◆ Integrating knowledge about the patient's condition, viewed from the knowledge base of each distinct professional group.
◆ Undertaking joint research into areas of common concern.

Underlying all collaboration is clarity of role and mutual professional respect. Role blurring is likely to lead to confusion about who does what. It is unlikely that colleagues will make a referral to a mental health liaison team unless they value the potential contribution they will make. Collaboration is a separate process from consultation, in which the mental health work is undertaken by someone from outside, and distinct from, the team working with the patient. However, it is harder to differentiate between collaboration and liaison.

Liaison

The original use of the term 'liaison' in the context of liaison psychiatry was to denote liaison between psychiatry (and its knowledge base) and the other branches of medicine (Lipowski 1981). Liaison psychiatry continues to have the meanings of a bridge between the branches of medicine and an integration of separate but complementary fields of medical knowledge (Lipowski 1974). Lipowski also proposes that liaison involves mediation between patients and staff and between different groups of staff. Liaison mental health nursing has similarly been described as a unifying force within nursing (Roberts 1997). In terms of theory, liaison can be viewed either as a process of integration of different, related medical and nursing knowledge or as an interpretation or translation of relevant mental health concepts and theories into a form accessible to non-mental health staff.

Like consultation, liaison can be viewed as a working relationship, a strategy for the effective use of resources or as a process.

◆ Liaison as a *relationship* involves the LMHN or psychiatrist either becoming a full member of the referring team (e.g. LHMN employed within an A&E department) or having a regular liaison attachment to a particular team, allocating a specified number of hours per week to it. The latter may, for example, involve a LMHN spending a day a week working with a bone marrow transplant service. The LMHN is then considered to be a member of the multidisciplinary haematology team.

◆ As a *strategy*, liaison allows for more effective use of mental health resources by establishing regular, timetabled contact between the referring team and the mental health worker. The referring team can plan care in the knowledge that mental health expertise will be available. Education becomes a regular part of the working relationship rather than an ad hoc arrangement. It is possible to build skills and knowledge in a more systematic way.

◆ The *process* of liaison may involve regular attendance at clinical meetings and handover meetings, and regular interdisciplinary review of cases. Education programmes cover the detection of conditions such as anxiety and depression. Staff can be offered support and supervision with difficult-to-manage cases.

Direct and indirect work

Specialist mental health care may be provided either directly (to the patient) or indirectly (to the staff) (American Nurses' Association 1990). This distinction is commonly used to describe direct and indirect consultation. In practice, the two processes work hand in hand. Direct interventions provide feedback to the referrer. The recognition and referral of mental health problems are more likely if staff have training and supervision and are familiar with the referral process. Indirect activities such as education and supervision are likely to lead to more clearly defined referrals for mental health assessment. All these activities lead to closer collaborative working relationships (Fig. 2.1). Unusually for nursing, Barbiasz et al (1982) made an additional distinction between direct, indirect and collaborative work. They describe joint interventions as part of a 'collaborative-consultative' model.

The aims of mental health liaison

The aims of mental health liaison can, therefore, be identified with direct work:

◆ the detection and treatment of mental illness and other problems that respond to psychological treatments

and with indirect work:

◆ improving and enhancing the quality of psychosocial care by working collaboratively with non-mental health colleagues.

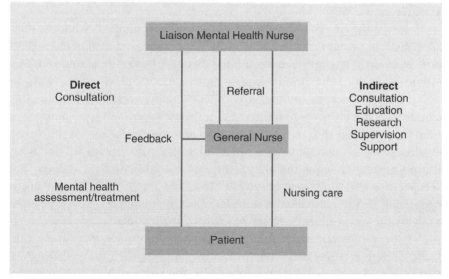

Fig. 2.1 The process of mental health liaison (Roberts 1998).

A COLLABORATIVE MODEL OF MENTAL HEALTH LIAISON

The following is a description of a working model of mental health liaison that emphasises the collaborative nature of such work (Roberts 1998). This is important in defining the operation and effects of mental health liaison services. Collaboration as a process involves mental health and non-mental health personnel, the patient within their own social context and the overall health-care environment within which this takes place. Collaboration has been recognised as an important mode of practice since the earliest report of mental health liaison by a nurse. Johnson described her role as 'a collaborator with the staff rather than an expert who tells the staff exactly what to do' (1963, p 728).

The following will describe the model within a nursing context. It could be applied within any setting where mental health professionals work collaboratively with non-mental health colleagues. Collaboration in the provision of integrative or holistic nursing care needs to acknowledge both the skills and limitations of the nursing staff within the referring team. Johnson (1963) pointed out that general staff nurses have a degree of interpersonal competence, intuitive skills and relevant concepts to use in their work. There is emerging evidence of an enhanced role for nurses in dealing with psychosocial aspects of care, particularly those working in community settings (Mead et al 1997). Specialist nurses, for example health visitors or breast care nurses, have been shown to have a significant role in the detection and management of common mental health problems such as depression (Holden et al 1989, McArdle et al 1996).

However, the specialised nature of health care sets limits on what the non-specialist can be expected to know or do. For example, education alone does not necessarily change practice for the better (Heaven & Maguire 1996). Various factors in the specific health-care environment affect the ways in which nurses conceptualise the psychosocial components of their work. This can include the attitudes of the ward sister (Wilkinson 1991), the amount of time nurses spend with individual patients and the degree of closeness they experience with them (Roberts & Snowball 1999). Also, nurses will focus on those aspects of their job that they feel they are accountable for and may not see psychosocial care as a priority if there are matters of life and death competing for their attention. It is most important, therefore, that LMHNs get to know the environments within which they work and gain an understanding of the values and working philosophies of the nurses they work with. Collaboration involves the LMHN working alongside their nurse colleagues, supporting, complementing and enhancing the work of the nursing team, whilst providing additional specialist input.

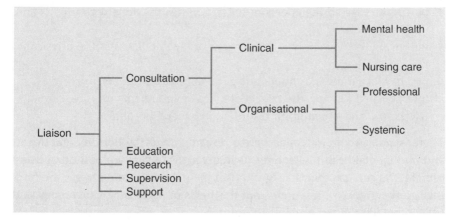

Fig. 2.2 Mental health liaison: the components of the collaborative model (Roberts 1998).

Mental health liaison activities

The core mental health liaison activities are education, research, supervision, support and consultation (Fig. 2.2).

Education

Psychosocial aspects of care are becoming more prominent in nursing education. This is particularly so in the care of chronic physical illness, such as cancer, and in acute areas of nursing, such as A&E, where difficult, violent and aggressive behaviour may occur and drug and alcohol abuse and self-harming behaviour are commonly encountered. One survey of general nurses suggests that education on anxiety and depression, alcohol dependence and suicidal behaviour would be valued (Whitehead & Mayou 1989). LMHNs are well placed to offer education to non-mental health teams, based in their own experience of managing mental health problems. This could take place either on an ad hoc basis, when a group of nurses have encountered a specific management problem, or as part of a regular staff training programme, where the staff team would be expected to attend seminars on a regular basis.

Research

In an area that is developing rapidly, on the interface between different disciplines, the LMHN is in a good position to identify areas for investigation. The role has a clear research component (American Nurses' Association 1990, Regel & Davies 1995). Areas requiring further research include:

◆ outcome studies into both the direct (i.e. therapy) and indirect (staff-related consultation, education and supervision) parts of the LMHN role

- process studies on the effects of LMHN on health-care environments and their operation
- improving the detection and treatment of mental illness in the physically ill
- psychosocial aspects of nursing (e.g. communication skills, nursing as interpersonal therapy, the effects of ward environments on care, care of psychiatric and somatoform disorders in general hospitals).

There is ample room for collaborative research involving both mental health and non-mental health personnel, as many areas of care are of mutual interest. LMHNs can use their background in mental health to interpret the findings and relevance of research from the fields of psychiatry, psychology and psychotherapy to their nursing colleagues.

Supervision and support

There is not a well-established culture of supervision in nursing and where it does exist it may be part of a process of management or appraisal (i.e. managerial supervision). Increasingly, however, supervision is seen as part of a process of professional development (Spouse 2000). Many LMHNs will be familiar with supervision models used in psychotherapy, particularly if psychotherapy is part of their role. Supervision may be the missing component that allows taught interpersonal skills to be transferred to the clinical workplace. Nurses using skills acquired in training workshops may be reluctant to try them out if they lack confidence, are uncertain of their effects or if they run into unexpected problems. A regular supervision meeting will allow them to discuss and seek resolution of these problems. Supervision should, therefore, be seen as a necessary part of educational programmes for staff.

As well as supporting the professional development of the nurses, supervision can have a supportive function. Nursing is a stressful occupation, with the sources of stress being exposure to pain, distress and suffering, high occupational demand and limited control over the health-care environment (Marshall 1980). A traditional expectation of the role of nursing is 'emotional labour', that is, the giving of the self in a very personally demanding way (Smith 1988). In extreme cases, nurses may experience 'burnout', a sense of emotional exhaustion, depersonalisation and a reduced sense of personal achievement (Duquette et al 1994). Here, support means dealing with stress, protecting against burnout and reinforcing the value of nursing work.

The mode of individual supervision may prove too time consuming for meeting the needs of all staff but could be targeted at specialist nurses whose caseloads are recognised as having a high level of interpersonal demands or of psychological morbidity. Breast care nurses and other specialist oncology roles would be particularly suitable for individual supervision. There is evidence that there are also a number of 'counselling' roles in oncology, where practitioners are working in isolated positions, with limited access to supervision (Roberts & Fallowfield 1990). Whereas it may be beyond the capacity of a LMHN to deal with the needs of all these roles, they may be in a position to give advice on other sources of support and expertise. This will help to reduce burnout among staff and ensure counsellors have at least the basic skills and support to function safely.

For many staff, group supervision will be a more suitable mode and make more effective use of limited LMHN resources. It would be particularly appropriate for ward-based groups of nurses. Many of these operate a team approach to care and this promotes a sense of group identity. This mode of supervision can draw on the existing skills and knowledge of the participants and would have the benefit of developing and enhancing a culture of mutual support within the team. Alternatively, ad hoc meetings could be arranged at times of stress and high emotional demand on staff, in the form of debriefing or defusing sessions. Staff may be more willing to accept help in this form, as they will see the immediate benefits of help when they are feeling the effects of stress. The effects of longer term support are more subtle and many staff find it hard to commit themselves to such a process. There are often problems of acceptance of support groups. Nurses may fear feeling emotionally exposed. For this reason, it is always necessary to clarify that neither supervision nor support is the same as personal therapy and to emphasise their role in professional development.

Consultation activities

Although Caplan's (1970) model has proved useful in defining the range of consultation activities, it has a number of limitations when applied within the contemporary health-care environment in the UK:

◆ Power and authority relationships are often complex and the mental health specialist may not be in a neutral position in relation to the consultee. For example, a specialist mental health nurse can be employed directly by the general hospital they work in, at a senior nursing grade. This may put them in a position of authority over the ward-based staff nurses who make referrals to them.

◆ Many services focus on mental illness and have no clear working model of mental health, so that the primary focus of consultation is psychiatric diagnosis and subsequent psychiatric or psychological treatment.

◆ It is unusual for mental health consultants to be invited into an organisation to deal with programme problems. This is now more commonly undertaken by management consultants. However, consultation within the organisation may have an organisational component.

◆ Consultation puts an emphasis on responding to an individual request for help and does not encourage the development of regular working relationships between different disciplines. Although it carries an educational component, this may not be part of a strategy of progressively developing skills and knowledge in consultees.

◆ The terminology Caplan used has limited relevance to current practice. *Case* consultation implies a rather medical model approach to consultation and *clinical* is a more widely acceptable term. The use of the term *administrative* consultation is misleading, as it has managerial connotations. Most consultations of this nature fit better within a systems theory framework and may be considered as problems of organisation rather than administration.

The following classification of consultation is proposed as an alternative working model. Consultations can be either clinical or organisational, with a further distinction depending on their focus. *Clinical* consultations can focus on the mental health of the patient or on the nursing care they are given. *Organisational* consultations may focus on professional issues or systemic factors within the health-care environment (Fig. 2.3). It is expected that in many situations, there will be overlap between these different factors or that the focus will shift at different points during the consultation process. The LMHN needs to keep an eye on the overall process of consultation and its effects on the clinical outcome for the patient, without becoming lost in the details. Lewis & Levy (1982, p 18) have pointed out that when considering the patient within the context of their illness, the process of nursing and the health-care system, the task becomes 'diagnosing the total consultation'.

Mental health consultation Mental health consultation is probably the most common form of consultation, involving a request for an assessment of the patient's mental state and current problems coping with illness. It is the main form of direct consultation, making mental health expertise directly available to the patient. The consultation involves the following components:

◆ mental health assessment
◆ psychological treatment
◆ feedback to the referrer.

The assessment itself has the potential to be therapeutic and in the case of a single contact with the patient, the first two steps are combined. The

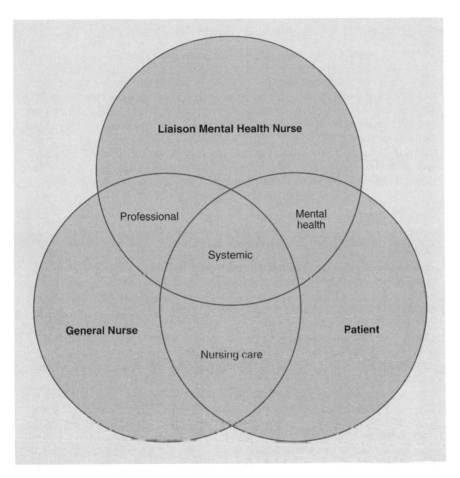

Fig. 2.3 The focus of a consultation (Roberts 1998).

consultation has an indirect form, as an educational process, in that feedback gives the referrer a framework within which to understand the nature of the patient's problems, their mental health state and the referral and consultation process. There is some evidence to suggest that this process leads over time to more patient-specific, comprehensive and psychologically (as opposed to physically) oriented referrals (Davis & Nelson 1980). The cycle of referral and feedback is a key element in the development of the collaborative working relationship. Mental health consultation is the mode of work for many nurses employed as therapists, e.g. cognitive behaviour therapists. In some cases, their contact with the referrer will be limited to a written referral and the indirect form of the work will be minimal. It is important to note that 'mental health consultation' can also refer to all consultation work undertaken by mental health teams. It is used with this meaning in Chapter 4.

> **Case Study 2.1** Mental health consultation
>
> Jackie, 27 years old, is referred routinely following an overdose. During the course of assessment, the LMHN identifies a number of recent problems coping with life, including splitting up with her boyfriend, problems with colleagues at work, running up some debts and drinking more than usual. The staff on the ward are concerned about her as she is crying a lot and they think she is depressed. They are concerned about sending her home, as they know depressed people are more at risk of suicide. The LMHN is able to tell them that she is not clinically depressed but is going through a personal crisis and will be offered follow-up as an outpatient. The staff feel reassured as they have confidence in the LMHN's abilities and they know Jackie will be monitored.

> **Case Study 2.2** Nursing care consultation
>
> Tom, 53, lives alone and has been admitted for treatment of an acute bowel obstruction. Whilst an inpatient, he becomes demanding of the nurses' time, often asking them for help with things he should be able to do himself, like dressing. At times, he makes remarks of a sexual nature. The nurses refer him to the LMHN, saying he is behaving strangely. Tom declines assessment by the LMHN and there are no specific signs of mental illness. A meeting is called with his nursing team and the staff identify feeling uncomfortable with him, wanting to respond to requests for help but feeling they are not reasonable requests. Not responding makes them feel uncomfortable, too, as they are there to help him. They say they feel Tom is lonely and that he would like them to meet his emotional needs. In discussion with the LMHN, they say they feel sad that he is lonely but they are there to deal with his acute health problem. They establish a care plan that ensures he receives the care he needs, but it is also made clear what he is expected to do as part of his own self-care and that he must treat the nurses with respect. When this is made clear to him, his behaviour becomes more reasonable.

Nursing care consultation Advice may be requested on the nursing management of a patient or group or category of patients. This can take the form of planning their nursing care or dealing with specific problems in the care of the patient. The LMHN may see the patient directly in order to contribute to the overall nursing assessment or rely on the assessments of nursing staff and contribute by sharing their mental health expertise.

Professional consultation This is advice on the management of professional matters, achieved by integrating mental health and nursing expertise and applying them to particular nursing issues. This could include advice on dealing with stress or burnout in nursing colleagues, the management of mental illness in hospital environments or strategies for dealing with interpersonal issues between staff and patients. Advice may also be given on the development of ward or hospital policy and philosophy. This may include participation in the development of in-service training programmes for staff within organisations. All these may be achieved by regular meetings at managerial level or by invitation to deal with a specified issue. Professional consultation is a wholly indirect form of consultation.

Systemic consultation Systems theory has been identified as a key theoretical element in mental health liaison work in the USA (Lewis & Levy 1982, Robinson 1987). Although systems theory has been less influential in British nursing, it is associated with organisational consultation (Campbell et al 1991). This represents the same Tavistock Clinic-based tradition that spawned the classic organisational study of British nursing, *The functioning of social systems as a defence against anxiety* (Menzies Lyth 1988). Systemic consultations include any that take account of the interaction of factors in the health-care environment that impact on the patient, their health and their

---

Case Study 2.3 Professional consultation

On the oncology ward, staff felt there were a number of problems with nurses getting close to patients. Some nurses had been meeting patients and their families socially after they were discharged. This generally happened with younger patients. The ward sister felt uneasy but found it hard to be clear about what was wrong, as she felt her staff were very keen and committed to the patients. A meeting was held with the nursing team and it became clear that not all staff felt happy with these social contacts. Some felt that it was putting pressure on all staff to become friends with patients and that this was too much to expect of them. During team discussions, the staff agreed that there was a difference between nursing and befriending patients. Nursing younger patients felt very difficult, as staff could identify with their problems and felt frustrated when they could not help. The LMHN helped them to identify the real ways in which they could help this patient group, short of befriending them.

Case Study 2.4 Systemic consultation

The LMHN is called to the A&E department to see Matthew, a man in his 30s who is drunk and being uncooperative. The sister complains that he frequently presents in A&E in this state, asking for help with his drink problem. His behaviour is often hostile or abusive. He is known to the local alcohol treatment service but the A&E staff say nothing is being done for him. The LMHN makes contact with the alcohol service and establishes that the patient has been offered a home-based detoxification programme but that he has declined it. A community mental health nurse periodically visits him at home but she too is sometimes abused verbally. The LMHN arranges an outpatient review with the alcohol team and gives the A&E staff phone numbers to contact during working hours if he presents with them. The role of the alcohol team is explained, along with the limitations of what they can do.

experience of illness. This can include dealing with problems in the interactions between different groups of staff or departments. This form of consultation can be direct, indirect or a combination of both.

CONCLUSION

Mental health liaison is the application of mental health knowledge and skills in non-mental health settings. It is a complex activity that utilises a range of mental health skills. Consultation is one of the key working practices by which liaison is carried out. A collaborative approach to liaison work ensures effective working between mental health and non-mental health colleagues.

QUESTIONS FOR DISCUSSION

◆ Is it possible to plan holistic care when there are separate teams dealing with mind and body?

◆ Who is the client served by the liaison mental health nurse: the patient or the referrer?

◆ Should liaison services be managerially separate from the teams they support?

ANNOTATED BIBLIOGRAPHY

Caplan G 1970 The theory and practice of mental health consultation. Tavistock Publications, London.

The original model of consultation developed in the USA in the 1960s and widely applied in liaison practice.

Tunmore R 1997 Mental health liaison and consultation. Ment Health Pract 1(4):29–36

Part of the Royal College of Nursing Continuing Education series. A paper that emphasises the collaborative aspects of liaison work.

Tunmore R, Thomas B 1992 Models of psychiatric consultation liaison nursing. Br J Nurs 1(9):447–451

A review of consultation models, their role within liaison mental health nursing and their potential for wider application within mental health nursing.

REFERENCES

American Nurses' Association 1990 Standards of psychiatric consultation-liaison nursing. American Nurses' Association, Kansas City, Mo

Barbiasz J, Blandford K, Byrne K et al 1982 Establishing the psychiatric liaison nurse role: collaboration with the nurse administrator. J Nurs Adm 12(1):14–18

Campbell D, Draper R, Huffington C 1991 A Systemic approach to consultation. Karnac Books, London

Caplan G 1970 The theory and practice of mental health consultation. Tavistock, London

Davis D, Nelson J 1980 Referrals to psychiatric liaison nurses. Changes in characteristics over a limited time period. Gen Hosp Psychiatry 2:41–45

Department of Health 1994 Working in partnership. The report of the Mental Health Nursing Review Team. HMSO, London

Duquette A, Kerouac S, Sandhu B K, Beaudet L 1994 Factors related to nursing burnout: a review of empirical knowledge. Issues Ment Health Nurs 15:337–358

Everson S J 1981 Integration of the role of clinical nurse specialist. J Contin Educ Nurs 12(2):16–19

Heaven C M, Maguire P 1996 Training hospice nurses to elicit patient concerns. J Adv Nurs 23:280–286

Holden J, Sagovsky R, Cox J 1989 Counselling in a general practice setting: controlled study of health visitor intervention in treatment of postnatal depression. BMJ 298:223–226

Johnson B 1963 Psychiatric nurse consultant in a general hospital. Nurs Outlook October: 728–729

Lewis A, Levy J 1982 Psychiatric liaison nursing: the theory and clinical practice. Reston Publishing, Reston, Va

Lipowski Z J 1974 Consultation-liaison psychiatry: an overview. Am J Psychiatry 131(6):623–630

Lipowski Z J 1981 Liaison psychiatry, liaison nursing, and behavioral medicine. Compr Psychiatry 22(6):554–561

Lipowski Z J 1982 Modern meaning of the terms 'psychosomatic' and 'liaison psychiatry'. In: Creed F, Pfeffer J M (eds) Medicine and psychiatry: a practical approach. Pitman Books, London, pp 3–24

Lipowski Z J 1986 To reduce or to integrate: psychiatry's dilemma. Can J Psychiatry 31:347–351

Marshall J 1980 Stress amongst nurses. In: Cooper C L, Marshall J (eds) White collar and professional stress. John Wiley, Chichester, pp 19–59

Mayou R, Bass C, Sharpe M 1995 Overview of epidemiology, classification, and aetiology. In: Mayou R, Bass C, Sharpe M (eds) Treatment of functional somatic symptoms. Oxford University Press, Oxford, pp 42–65

McArdle J, George W, McArdle C et al 1996 Psychological support for patients undergoing breast cancer surgery: a randomised study. BMJ 312.813–017

Mead N, Bower P, Gask L 1997 Emotional problems in primary care: what is the potential for increasing the role of nurses? J Adv Nurs 26:879–890

Menzies Lyth I 1988 The functioning of social systems as a defence against anxiety. A report on a study of the nursing service of a general hospital. In: Menzies Lyth I (ed) Containing anxiety in institutions. Selected essays. Vol 1. Free Association Books, London, pp 43–85

Regel S, Davies J 1995 The future of mental health nurses in liaison psychiatry. Br J Nurs 4(18):1052–1056

Roberts D 1997 Liaison mental health nursing: origins, definition and prospects. J Adv Nurs 25:101–108

Roberts D 1998 Making the connections to aid mental health. Nurs Times 94(15):50–52

Roberts D, Snowball J 1999 Psychosocial care in oncology nursing: a study of social knowledge. J Clin Nurs 8:39–47

Roberts R, Fallowfield L 1990 Who supports the cancer counsellors? Nurs Times 86:32

Robinson L 1987 Psychiatric consultation liaison nursing and psychiatric consultation doctoring: similarities and differences. Arch Psychiatr Nurs 1(2):73–80

Sarkis J M, Skoner M M 1987 An analysis of the concept of holism in nursing literature. Holist Nurs Pract 2(1):61–69

Smith P 1988 The emotional labour of nursing. Nurs Times 84(44):50–51

Spouse J 2000 Supervision of clinical practice: the nature of professional development. In: Spouse J, Redfern L (eds) Successful supervision in health care practice. Promoting professional development. Blackwell Science, Oxford, pp 126–154

Tunmore R, Thomas B 1992 Models of psychiatric consultation liaison nursing. Br J Nurs 1(9):447–451
Whitehead L, Mayou R 1989 Care of the mind. Nurs Times 85(45):49–50
Wilkinson S 1991 Factors which influence how nurses communicate with cancer patients. J Adv Nurs 16:677–688
Woods S 1998 Holism in nursing. In: Edwards S D (ed) Philosophical issues in nursing. Macmillan, London, pp 66–87

3

Liaison mental health nursing: an overview of its development and current practice

Dave Roberts   Linda Whitehead

KEY ISSUES

- Psychiatric consultation-liaison nursing and liaison mental health nursing have evolved separately in the USA and UK

- In the USA, it is recognised as a discrete subspecialist area of practice

- Most of the research has been into referral patterns

- There is evidence of theoretical and therapeutic integration in the literature

- Recent surveys of liaison mental health nurses working in the UK show wide variations in practice, but a primary focus on deliberate self-harm

INTRODUCTION

Liaison mental health nursing, and its forerunner in the USA 'psychiatric consultation-liaison nursing', have developed separately in response to different pressures and within different health-care systems.

USA:'PSYCHIATRIC CONSULTATION-LIAISON NURSING'

Psychiatric consultation-liaison nursing (formerly called 'psychiatric liaison nursing') is recognised as a subspecialist branch of psychiatric-mental health nursing in the USA (i.e. psychiatric-mental health nursing is a recognised speciality). Practitioners are prepared at Masters level and have had supervised clinical experience at graduate level (American Nurses' Association 1990). This area of subspecialist practice has evolved in response to a number of developments in health care in the USA:

◆ the development of psychiatric nursing as a speciality
◆ the establishment of university hospital-based departments of psychiatry
◆ the introduction of crisis intervention and brief therapies to psychiatry during the Second World War
◆ the community mental health movement
◆ a growing awareness within nursing of the psychosocial needs of the physically ill patient (Robinson 1982).

Johnson (1963) first described the role, working alongside general nurses as a consultant. The consultant nurse role was developed within the Duke University Medical Centre as a means of optimising the use of nursing resources and expertise. The mental health consultant was therefore one of a team of expert nurses, other examples being surgical or postoperative nurses. These roles were early examples of clinical nurse specialists. Johnson's paper identifies a number of principles from her own work that have become well established in mental health consultation-liaison practice.

◆ Much work can be done through staff, with minimal direct patient contact.
◆ General nurses often have the skills, knowledge and motivation to make therapeutic use of interpersonal relationships.
◆ The mental health consultation brings a conceptual framework within which nurses can use their skills.
◆ Consultations begin with a clarification of the role, which is primarily collaborator rather than outside expert.

Johnson's work gives us the earliest account of how the mental health nurse can work collaboratively with the general nurse to improve psychosocial aspects of care.

Theory development

Johnson's work appears to have been based on experience rather than research and no other written work is cited. A paper written the following year by Hildegard Peplau (1964) refers indirectly to literature from psychiatric nursing and psychology to identify ways in which 'psychiatric nursing skills', can benefit the general hospital patient. She identifies five 'general ideas' or 'notions', mainly originating in psychiatric nursing, that are relevant to this work.

1. All behaviour is purposeful, has meaning and can be understood.
2. Nurses must observe what is going on, interpret what is observed and decide action on the basis of those interpretations.
3. Nurses meet the needs of their patients.
4. The nurse – patient interaction (the verbal and non-verbal exchanges in a nursing situation) can influence recovery.
5. The personality of the patient is somehow involved in his illness.

These statements characterise an approach to nursing theory marking a shift from 'needs-based' models to 'interactionist' models (Kitson 1993). This shift placed a new emphasis on nurse – patient interaction as a central, therapeutic feature of nursing. Peplau's model of nursing, described in her influential book *Interpersonal Relations in Nursing* (1952), was based in psychodynamic theory, particularly through the work of Sullivan. Peplau's ideas were also influenced by 'psychosomatic medicine', which postulated a link between personality and illness. Interactionist models owe a lot to the close links between mental health and general nursing education in the USA, a situation not mirrored in the UK.

The psychiatric specialist nurse continued to develop her skills and build on experience during the 1960s. Petersen (1969) describes direct patient contact, participation in nursing assessments, helping nurses develop transferable interpersonal skills, role playing patients' experiences and translating psychiatric concepts into a form that general nurses could use.

1970s: defining the role

Nelson & Schilke (1976) pointed out that during the 1970s, psychiatric liaison nurses undertook more direct interventions with patients, rather than working through nursing staff. They offered a definition of the role as it was then being practised.

◆ Consultation to nursing staff, focused on both immediate nursing care and the longer term development of skills.
◆ Education, both formal and informal (e.g. through role modelling).
◆ Direct, specialised psychological care to patients and families.
◆ Expertise in mental illness and normal and abnormal reactions to physical illness.
◆ Understanding of the interrelationship between physical and psychological states.

- ◆ Collaboration with other mental health professionals.
- ◆ Using knowledge of systems theory and group dynamics to define problems within an organisational context.
- ◆ Working across professional boundaries, i.e. psychiatric/general nursing, nursing/psychiatry, psychiatry/medicine.

The 1970s saw other developments in psychiatric liaison nursing, as it became better established:

- ◆ subspecialisation and new practice models
- ◆ clarification of models for line management, accountability and supervision
- ◆ the development of educational programmes (Robinson 1982).

There was also an increasing reference to specific theoretical models, particularly Caplan's (1970) model of mental health consultation.

These developments included the first references to mental health nurses undertaking primary mental health assessments in the 'emergency room', i.e. A&E departments, prior to the involvement of psychiatrists or other professionals (Isaacharoff et al 1970, Severin & Becker 1974). This constituted a form of psychiatric triage later adopted, apparently independently, in the UK. Whereas this model of practice has subsequently thrived in the UK, it has declined in the USA. This may have resulted from psychiatrists' renewal of interest in emergency room work, largely motivated by the need to provide a varied experience for doctors in training (Robinson 1987).

Research into the role (USA and Canada)

There is a limited amount of research into the role and functions of the psychiatric liaison nurse in the USA. Most of it examines the referral process within the context of the general hospital. Wolff (1978) used a questionnaire to identify the reasons nurses gave for initiating a referral to the psychiatric nurse consultant. The majority of referrals were based on an observation of psychopathology, most commonly depression.

Although referred patients were more likely to evoke a negative response in staff than non-referred patients, it seemed more likely that referrals were based on assessment rather than on emotional reaction. Another study which examined referral patterns to two psychiatric liaison nurses (PLNs) over two 6-month periods showed changes in their characteristics over time. Referrals became more patient specific, more psychologically oriented and more comprehensive in their description of patients' problems (Davis & Nelson 1980). This suggested that ongoing contact with the PLNs led to an increasing sophistication and psychosocial orientation among the staff nurses who provided the bulk of their referrals.

A study by Stickney et al (1981) compared referrals to a psychiatrist and a nurse consultant in a liaison psychiatry team. A comparative analysis of 100 consecutive referrals to the psychiatrist and to the nurse showed that the nurse was more likely to see the staff alone, i.e. indirect consultations, which constituted 42% of referrals. Nurse-to-nurse referrals were more likely to be for the behavioural management of patients, rather than for specific psychological reasons. Referrals were often made informally and the referral process was helped by the nurse being perceived as available to and visible on the ward. Fincannon's (1995) analysis of a series of 102 referrals to a psychiatric consultation-liaison nurse (PCLN) showed different perceptions of patient problems (as diagnoses) between referrer and PCLN. Twenty-three percent of patients referred for depression and 52% of patients referred for anxiety met standardised diagnostic criteria for these conditions. The bulk of the remainder had a diagnosis of adjustment disorder. This discrepancy is not surprising, as adjustment disorder frequently manifests with symptoms of anxiety or depression.

A study from Canada surveyed the referring agent in a series of consecutive requests for consultation from a general hospital-based psychiatric consultation-liaison nursing service (Newton & Wilson 1990). In the great majority of cases, the referrer was satisfied or very satisfied with the service. Of particular value were ease of access and promptness of response to a request for consultation. Satisfaction with the consultation was highest when there were multiple visits by the PCLN and where this involved working with families in crisis. There was less satisfaction when the contact was brief and limited to giving advice on the management of major mental illness. This study confirms findings from other studies (Fife 1986, Roberts 1998) that ease of access and visibility in the target clinical area are highly valued by consultees. This supports the case for collaborative work and the liaison attachment style of working.

Current trends within PCLN practice in the USA include:

◆ subspecialisation, with PCLNs working in the fields of cancer, stroke, AIDS and the terminally ill
◆ working with organisational issues
◆ cost containment pressures (Norwood 1998).

Although Nelson & Schilke suggested as early as 1976 that PLNs would need to prove their worth, there is still a lack of evaluative research. Norwood (1998) notes the trend towards cost containment within the American healthcare system and suggests that the PCLNs will need to provide outcome data on their activities, including evidence of cost effectiveness. PCLNs will need to ensure that they meet the challenge of changes in the funding of health care in the USA.

UK: 'LIAISON MENTAL HEALTH NURSING'

Unlike the USA, liaison mental health nursing in the UK is not recognised as a specialist or subspecialist area of practice. Its definition is therefore more problematic (Roberts 1997). The term 'liaison mental health nursing' dates from the *Mental Health Nursing Review* (Department of Health 1994), which identified the development of mental health nursing roles within A&E departments. Prior to that, the term 'psychiatric liaison nursing' had featured in the British literature in the work of Jones (1989) and Tunmore (1989). These papers described the work of mental health nurses with medical and oncology patients and the authors made a direct link between their own work and that of their American counterparts. However, the role was already developing in response to the problem of deliberate self-harm (DSH) and rising numbers of admissions to general hospitals following overdoses during the 1960s and 1970s.

Suicide was a criminal offence in the UK until the Suicide Act of 1961. The trend before decriminalisation had been increasingly to see suicidal behaviour as a medical problem and this trend gathered pace. The Hill Report (1968) recommended setting up poisoning treatment centres in general hospitals and offering all patients a psychiatric assessment following overdose. The first British poisoning treatment centres were established in Edinburgh and Oxford. In Oxford, a working model developed, with nurses undertaking the initial mental health assessment (Catalan et al 1980a). An evaluation study showed that nurses were effective in this role (Catalan et al 1980b) and non-medical mental health assessment subsequently received government approval (Department of Health and Social Security 1984).

Two subsequent reports described community psychiatric nurses (CPNs) undertaking assessments in A&E departments following acts of self-harm (Minghella 1989) and providing a more comprehensive consultation-liaison role with A&E patients and staff (Atha et al 1989). More recent descriptions of general hospital liaison services show the predominant model is one of a small team of A&E-based mental health nurses, usually working with a liaison psychiatrist. The bulk of these nurses' work is with self-harm, but they also deal with other psychiatric problems in A&E (e.g. alcohol abuse) and provide consultation to staff (Brendon & Reet 2000, Loveridge et al 1997, Roberts & Taylor 1997, Watts 1997). Increasingly, nurses working in this field identify themselves as liaison mental health nurses (LMHNs).

Oncology and haematology

The other field which has received significant attention in the British literature is oncology. Tunmore (1989) first described this role, working at a major

British cancer centre, the Royal Marsden Hospital in London. This role was termed 'clinical nurse specialist in psychological support' but he clearly identified this with 'psychiatric liaison nursing' in the USA. Gardner (1992) later described her role working with neuro-oncology patients at the same hospital. Both Tunmore and Gardner used a combination of Rogerian counselling and cognitive behavioural techniques in their approach to clients. More recently, Edwards (1999) has described the introduction of a mental health specialist nursing role at Cookridge Hospital, another major cancer centre in Leeds. Edwards documents her work over a 1-month period, involving 131 referrals. This revealed that 53% of referrals led to direct intervention with patients involving follow-up work. A further 25% had an initial assessment but no follow-up and in 22% of the cases, the consultation was indirect, i.e. staff were given advice on management or referral elsewhere.

The one attempt at eliciting the views of consultee nurses in a British setting involved a single focus group interview with three nurses on a haematology ward (Roberts 1998). Feedback was sought on how the well-established LMHN role was viewed, initially using open questions. Participants valued the availability of the LMHN to the ward and visibility on the ward. This is consistent with the observations of PCLNs in the USA, who have also emphasised the importance of availability and visibility on wards in developing collaborative relationships and obtaining referrals (Fife 1986). Objectivity was also valued, particularly as the participants felt they got 'involved' with patients. They also felt it important that the clinical nurse specialist (CNS) had training in counselling, identifying the following counselling skills: 'to guide a conversation', 'to ask open-ended questions', 'to draw out a picture of what you're trying to establish', 'to read between the lines' and 'follow certain models'. The CNS was also felt to have expertise in supporting staff, 'setting boundaries' and the ability to 'distinguish between normal reactions and mental illness'.

THERAPEUTIC APPROACHES

Early American approaches to clinical liaison work showed a psychodynamic orientation, sometimes referring to patients' problems in terms of 'regression' or 'dependency' (Johnson 1963, Robinson 1968). Direct work focused on supportive nursing care and strengthening ego defences. Indirect work with the nursing staff involved both supporting them and providing theoretical frameworks within which they could understand the patient's behaviour. This could include attempts by the nurse consultant to identify both conscious and unconscious reasons for requesting consultation (Robinson 1968).

However, nursing theory was evolving during this period and psychodynamic theory was being modified in the light of nursing practice. Peplau

(1952) drew on Sullivan's dynamic approach to psychotherapy to develop a distinctive interpersonal model of nursing that remains influential today. Peplau's emphasis on anxiety as a focus for nursing intervention in her 1964 paper has been echoed in later papers (Dulaney & Crawford 1988, Robinson 1982).

Rather than rely on a single theoretical perspective to explain the phenomena they encounter and guide their practice, many LMHNs have combined theory in ways that they find useful. There are two main styles of doing this. Integration is an approach that incorporates new ideas if they fit within the existing philosophy of the nurse or nursing team. Eclecticism, or technical eclecticism, does not require a conceptual fit but rather some degree of proof of the effectiveness of the new idea (Roberts 1997). There is evidence for both approaches, particularly in the USA where a broad range of theory has been incorporated into the knowledge base of 'psychiatric consultation-liaison nursing'. In an interesting American paper, Dulaney & Crawford (1988) draw on their personal experience of liaison work to identify models that have proved useful in their own practice. Their eclectic model builds on dynamic theories of anxiety and Maslow's hierarchy of need. Therapeutic interventions may include 'cognitive restructuring' and more clearly nursing-based activities such as 'being with' the patient.

Other models are a clear integration of separate but complementary ideas. Lewis & Levy's (1982) 'holistic theoretical model' is an integration of nursing, stress, systems and crisis theories, with psychodynamic theories of personality development. The American Nurses' Association (1990) similarly cites nursing and mental health theory, stress, coping and adaptation theory and the integration of biological, psychological and social factors as the basis of practice.

In contrast to their American colleagues, many British writers cite specific therapy models. In deliberate self-harm work, Evans (1994) describes a psychodynamic model whereas Atha et al (1989) use a cognitive therapy-based problem-solving approach. An alternative is the integrative model described by Roberts & Mackay (1999), combining elements of crisis intervention theory, problem solving and the psychodynamic concepts of engagement and containment. LMHNs working in oncology have used an integration of Rogerian counselling and cognitive therapy (Gardner 1992, Tunmore 1989).

MANAGERIAL ARRANGEMENTS

Managerial and administrative arrangements are often described in detail in the American literature. Most of the early consultant nurse roles were employed by the nursing administration and some had educational roles.

Jackson (1969) was directly accountable to the Director of Nursing Services and Education. This link with the nursing leadership gave the role authority within the institution. Fife (1986) emphasises the importance of clarity of administrative expectations of the role but suggests that authority should be derived from professional competence and expertise. Freedom from administrative responsibilities enables the nurse to adopt a neutral consultation role in relation to nursing colleagues. However, some liaison roles have been occupied by nurses with managerial responsibilities for staff as well as their own caseload (Berarducci et al 1979). A recent survey of American clinical nurse specialists found the majority were in line management positions. Whilst this gives the authority to make changes in clinical practice, it also puts pressure on the balance of their time spent in clinical work (Scott 1999).

A group of 'psychiatric liaison nurses' from the Boston area of the USA emphasise the importance of collaboration with nurse administrators when setting up these roles (Barbiasz et al 1982). They identify the following steps.

1. *Role creation.* This involves identifying the need for the role, expectations of what the role will achieve, how the role will fit within the organisation and what support will be needed.
2. *System entry.* This requires close collaboration with the administration in arranging meetings with key personnel, becoming familiar with clinical areas and establishing working relationships.

The overall aim of the process is to establish credibility within the hospital system and this may involve investing time in the most receptive clinical units, whilst maintaining visibility in less receptive areas by regular attendance at clinical meetings.

Relationships with medical colleagues vary according to the managerial arrangements and the manner in which the role is introduced. Some problems have been reported in setting up new nursing roles that challenged the control doctors had over clinical work. Robinson's (1968) efforts to establish a nurse consultant role led to an 'armed truce' with the medical staff, who had not been adequately prepared to accommodate her work. She overcame these problems by emphasising the care rather than treatment aspect of her role and she was supported by the nursing administration. In another hospital, the introduction of nurse consultants into the emergency room caused conflict with fellow nurses, doctors and administrators (Severin & Becker 1974). Problems centred on issues of professional responsibility and the legality of clinically independent nursing practice. The nurse consultants came under a lot of pressure and nearly gave up, but were strongly supported by psychiatric colleagues. A programme of discussion about the new roles led to an improved understanding of their contribution to care and the legal framework within which this was carried out.

INTERPROFESSIONAL ISSUES

Relationships between disciplines

All LMHNs work within a multidisciplinary environment, though not all work within a mental health team. Some practitioners in the UK work alone as the sole representatives of mental health services, for example in A&E departments. The most common team composition is a mixture of psychiatrists and nurses, sometimes including psychologists and other mental health professionals. A survey of Western European consultation-liaison psychiatry services (Mayou & Huyse 1991) showed widely different patterns of service provision. Multidisciplinary consultation-liaison teams involving nurses, psychologists and social workers were the norm in Finland and The Netherlands. In many other countries, psychiatrists had access to the services of psychologists and social workers.

Lipowski (1974) identified a 'core team' of psychiatrists and nurses, with psychologists and social workers if funds allowed. He proposed the following division of labour.

Nurses
◆ Liaison attachments to areas with high psychological morbidity, e.g. oncology, critical care.
◆ Consulting with general nurses.
◆ Raising awareness of patients' psychological needs.
◆ Increasing tolerance of unusual behaviour and thereby improving the psychosocial care given to patients.
◆ This would improve the referral rate from junior medical staff, who often rely on nurses' observations to identify patients' problems.

Psychiatrists
◆ Difficult consultations requiring the integration of knowledge from different fields.
◆ Education.
◆ Research.

Psychologists
◆ Specific therapies for somatoform disorders.
◆ Research.
◆ Contributing to difficult diagnostic problems.

Given the overlap between the work of psychiatrists and psychologists, Lipowski proposed the formation of integrated divisions of psychiatry and 'behavioural medicine', i.e. psychology. There is little evidence of this having taken place, with each group keen to maintain its professional identity. This division of labour is largely redundant today, certainly within the British health-care scene where all mental health liaison staff are involved in education and research, most consultations are complex and therapists are as likely to be nurses as psychologists.

Relationships between doctors and nurses have, meanwhile, been changing, with increasing encroachment of nurses into previously medical roles. These are generally described as extended roles, in contrast to expanded roles, where nurses take on additional responsibility within a defined area of nursing practice. It could be argued, for example, that overdose assessment is an extended role, in that it was a function initially undertaken by psychiatrists. The development of this role was actively supported, if not initiated, by psychiatrists in both the USA (Isaacharoff et al 1970) and in the UK (Catalan et al 1980a). In the United States, the role has been reclaimed by psychiatry and Robinson (1987) sees this as a positive step, as she feels it might have weakened the traditional caring role of nursing. However, in the UK this role has become firmly established, with no noticeable negative effects on the profession. In many cases, it has made mental health nursing expertise directly available to A&E nurses.

Specialist and advanced nursing practice

British nursing currently suffers from a number of problems of definition of higher levels of practice. Specialist nursing practice has become associated with specific training courses and a rather artificial focus on community work (Roberts 1997). The concept of advanced practice has been debated without any clear agreement on its meaning within the British health care context. Whereas these debates may have little direct relevance for the individual practitioner, they can lead to confusion about the professional framework within which they work. This is particularly true when issues of professional accountability or legality arise. Many LMHNs work in relative isolation from fellow mental health nurses and their closest colleagues may be general nurses. Psychiatrist colleagues may assume 'medical responsibility' for some aspects of teamwork but in day-to-day practice, LMHNs will frequently have to make independent clinical decisions. In order to avoid confusion of responsibility, the following are offered as a guide.

◆ LMHNs should make a clear distinction between their own mental health assessments and the diagnostic function of psychiatrists.
◆ Advice to junior medical staff on the management of mental health problems does not carry prescriptive authority (i.e. junior doctors must accept responsibility for their own decisions based on the advice of a LMHN).

◆ In case of similar problematic situations arising in practice, local guidelines may be needed to clarify best practice.
◆ The United Kingdom Central Council for Nursing, Midwifery & Health Visiting's document *Scope of Professional Practice* (UKCC 1992) provides the framework within which nurses can undertake extended and expanded roles.
◆ Specific problems of accountability can be referred directly to the UKCC for advice (see Dowling et al 1996).

In the USA, different levels of practice are relatively well defined. There are recognised areas of specialist practice, including 'psychiatric-mental health nursing'. Psychiatric consultation-liaison nursing is a subspecialist area of practice. In addition, the title 'advanced practice nurse' is now recognised by the American Nurses' Association as describing nurse practitioners, clinical nurse specialists, nurse anaesthetists and nurse midwives (Hawkins & Thibodeau 1996). These positions are usually occupied by nurses education-ally prepared at Masters level. The legal background, however, is not so clear. The registration and licensing of nurses in the USA is dealt with by a number of different bodies, including state legislatures and state boards of nursing, and national organisations including the American Nurses' Association and the National Council of State Boards of Nursing. There is a legal definition of advanced practice in 20 states, with state boards defining the scope of profes-sional practice and no legal requirement for physicians to supervise advanced nursing practice. However, not all states recognise psychiatric-mental health nursing within these definitions (Hawkins & Thibodeau 1996).

RESULTS OF UK NATIONAL SURVEYS

Recent surveys of British LMHNs give a number of insights into current prac-tice in the UK. Tunmore (1994) undertook a postal survey of members of a national special interest group for LMHNs. Thirty-two respondents completed the questionnaire. The majority were on senior nursing grades: I grade × 4, H grade × 13, G grade × 12. A range of job titles were described, with 14 of the posts including the term 'liaison' in their title.

The majority, 19, worked within a department of liaison psychiatry or a liai-son psychiatry team and seven were based in A&E departments. In terms of areas of practice, 90% worked with deliberate self-harm and this was cited as an area of specialist practice by 40%. Other areas of specialist practice were associated with a particular physical illness (30%), e.g. cancer or acquired immune deficiency syndrome (AIDS), and 25% were specialists in specific therapeutic approaches (e.g. counselling, cognitive behaviour therapy). Most received their referrals from hospital doctors (26), general nurses (21) or psychiatrists (18). In the balance of direct and indirect work, 22 worked directly with more than 70% of their referrals and worked indirectly with less than 30% of their referrals.

The survey took a particular interest in the educational preparation of the respondents. A majority, 72%, reported some training for their role but less than half (44%) said they were satisfied with their preparation. Twenty-eight percent reported having had no specific training at all and 47% agreed with the statement that their role had developed through trial and error. Of the 32 respondents, 20 had completed postqualification English National Board (ENB) courses, 12 held or were studying for a diploma or degree, eight held or were studying for a Masters degree and 12 had no academic qualification. Of particular interest in a predominantly general hospital-based group, almost half (47%) held a registered general nurse (RGN) qualification in addition to their registration in mental nursing (RMN).

Recent developments

A more recent unpublished survey of the same specialist interest group by Roberts & Whitehead received 78 replies which reflects the growth in the numbers of British LMHNs during the period between the surveys. Again, a majority of nurses were employed on senior clinical grades. Although only one was employed at I grade, 29 were on H grade and 44 on G grade. The nurses were very experienced, with over half having more than 11 years' experience since initial qualification and 97% having 6 or more years' postqualification experience (Fig. 3.1).

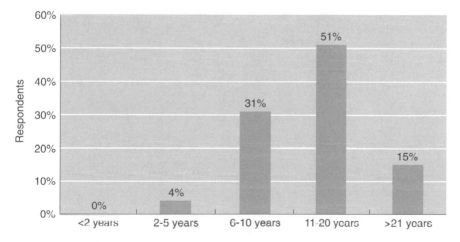

Fig. 3.1 LMHN survey: years since initial registration.

Job titles

Job titles varied considerably, though the term 'liaison' was present in the majority (56). The terms 'mental health' and 'liaison' were present in combination in 21 of the titles; for example, liaison mental health nurse and mental health liaison nurse. Psychiatric liaison nurse, liaison psychiatric nurse or a title including 'liaison psychiatry' accounted for 25 of the roles. The single term 'liaison' was present in a further 10 titles, e.g. liaison nurse, A&E liaison nurse, liaison CPN. Twenty of the titles had the word 'specialist' in them, e.g. clinical nurse specialist, nurse specialist. Community psychiatric nurse (CPN) or the word 'community' was mentioned in a further six titles and four mentioned deliberate self-harm or parasuicide. Three respondents were described as cognitive behaviour therapists.

Qualifications

Of the 78 respondents, 43% had a general nursing registration (RGN, SRN or RN) in addition to their psychiatric nursing qualification (RMN). In contrast to the earlier study, only 10 had no further qualifications. Over 40% (34) had or were working towards an ENB qualification, 16 had a Masters degree, and three a PhD. More than a third (29) had or were working towards a degree, though interestingly, only half of these were degrees in nursing (Fig. 3.2).

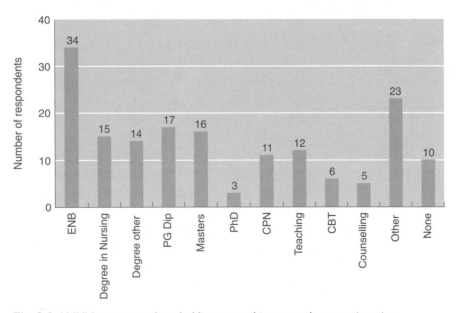

Fig. 3.2 LMHN survey: numbers holding or working towards postregistration qualifications.

Management of services

Although the majority (44%) of LMHNs were employed by mental health trusts, 22% were employed by acute, i.e. general, hospital trusts. This is very encouraging, as it indicates that liaison roles are valued by their non-mental health colleagues. A further 12% were employed by community trusts and the remainder by combined trusts. Most of the LMHNs (50) worked within multiprofessional teams, with six working only with other LMHNs and four nurses working as the only mental health professional in their setting. The majority of the respondents (61) had a nurse as line manager, 36 of these were mental health nurses, nine of them general nurses and 16 not specified. The remaining 10 who gave this information were accountable to a manager from another profession. Most of the services described were relatively newly established, with 40 of the respondents working in units operating for less than 5 years. This reflects the recent growth in liaison mental health nursing, which is probably a result of the suicide reduction targets in recent government health policies.

Clinical settings

Like the previous survey, this study records that a majority of LMHNs still work with deliberate self-harm (DSH). Fifty-nine nurses (76%) were involved in the assessment of DSH and 41 (53%) in DSH follow-up. The other major focus of clinical activity was ward consultation, reported by 47 nurses (60%), and 33 nurses (42%) worked specifically with A&E departments. Other clinical foci were: alcohol and drugs (29 nurses – 37%), obstetrics and gynaecology (15 nurses – 19%), HIV and AIDS (12 nurses – 15%) and oncology (nine nurses – 12%) (Fig. 3.3). The relatively low numbers of nurses specialising in oncology is surprising, given its prominence in the British literature, but this may be because it is limited to the small number of large cancer centres. The relatively large number of nurses working with obstetrics and gynaecology patients was also surprising, as this area of clinical focus is not widely reported in the liaison mental health nursing literature. Most respondents were generalists, working with a wide range of patients and problems, with only 10 working solely with one category of patients, examples being oncology, HIV/AIDS and psychosexual health.

Sites of clinical work included hospital wards (69 nurses – 88%), A&E departments (53 nurses – 68%) and outpatient departments (40 nurses – 51%), with 13 nurses (17%) undertaking domicillary visits. Almost all the respondents (73 nurses – 94%) worked with adults between the ages of 19 and 65 (Fig. 3.4) though a significant minority also worked with young people between 13 and 18 years. Two respondents specifically defined their role by

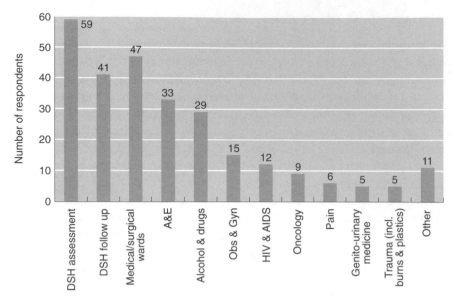

Fig. 3.3 LMHN survey: areas of clinical activity.

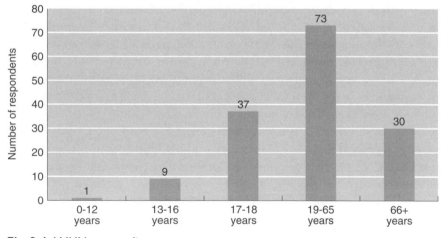

Fig. 3.4 LMHN survey: client age groups.

age group: 'liaison mental health nurse – elderly services' and 'paediatric mental health liaison nurse'. The most common source of referral was hospital doctors (61 nurses – 78%), followed by general nurses (41 nurses – 53%) and psychiatrists (38 nurses – 49%) (Fig. 3.5). The majority of respondents were involved in both direct (77 nurses) and indirect (75 nurses) work.

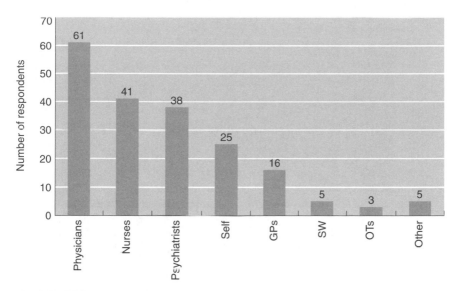

Fig. 3.5 LMHN survey: referral sources.

Therapeutic models

The most common therapeutic model in use was crisis intervention, used by 75% of the respondents. This is consistent with a high proportion of respondents working in DSH services but is surprising given the low profile the approach has in the current mental health nursing and psychiatry literature. Cognitive behaviour therapy was used by 61% and 44% used a non-specific counselling model (Fig. 3.6). The use of more than one model is consistent with the theoretical and therapeutic integration reported in the literature. The majority of respondents cited education as part of their role, with 61% actively involved in education within the general hospital.

CONCLUSION

Liaison mental health nursing has been developing over several decades in both North America and the UK. Though there have been a number of differences in their development, some common trends have emerged. LMHNs often work in small teams and in relative isolation. There are often problems introducing and establishing new roles, and relationships with other disciplines and with managers have the potential to be either supportive or problematic. The professional and legal framework within which

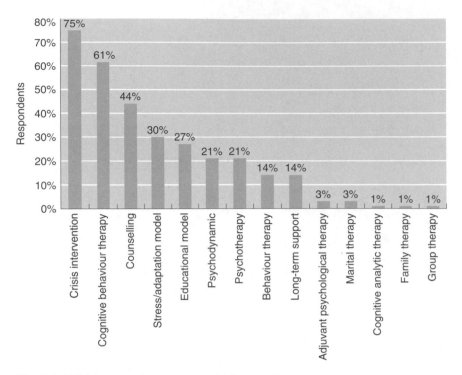

Fig. 3.6 LMHN survey: therapeutic models/approaches.

LMHNs work is generally clearer in the United States than in the UK, where higher levels of practice are still subject to debate. In the UK, the role has developed more recently and has seen a period of rapid growth in the last few years. The primary focus is on deliberate self-harm and the A&E department, but small numbers of specialists have become established with other client groups and other clinical settings. This trend is likely to continue, as clinically independent specialist nurses become more established in mental health nursing.

QUESTIONS FOR DISCUSSION

◆ Should LMHNs be mental health generalists or focus on a specific clinical problem or setting?

◆ Is LMHN a specialist area of mental health nursing practice?

◆ Should LMHNs always work with a psychiatrist?

◆ To whom is the LMHN accountable?

ANNOTATED BIBLIOGRAPHY

Catalan J, Marsack P, Hawton K, Whitwell D, Fagg J, Bancroft J 1980
Comparison of doctors and nurses in the assessment of deliberate self-
poisoning patients. Psychol Med 10:483–491

*This study of nurses doing primary overdose assessments set the scene for
clinically independent practice in LMHN.*

Department of Health 1994 Working in partnership. The Report of the
Mental Health Nursing Review Team. HMSO, London

*This major review of British mental health nursing mentioned the term 'liaison
mental health nursing' for the first time, and recommended research to
examine its potential. Puts LMHN into a broader mental health nursing
context.*

Dowling S, Martin R, Skidmore P, Doyal L, Cameron A, Lloyd S 1996 Nurses
taking on junior doctors' work: a confusion of accountability. BMJ
312(7040):1211–1214

*This paper provides a useful discussion of issues of accountability and legality
concerning nurses who work in clinically independent roles.*

Roberts D 1997 Liaison mental health nursing: origins, definition and
prospects. J Adv Nurs 25:101–108

*A paper outlining a number of issues of definition and scope of the role of
LMHN.*

UKCC 1992 The scope of professional practice. UKCC, London

*This document provides the professional framework for extended and
expanded roles in nursing in the UK.*

REFERENCES

American Nurses' Association 1990 Standards of psychiatric consultation-liaison nursing.
  American Nurses' Association, Kansas City, Mo
Atha C, Salkovskis P, Storer D 1989 Accident and emergency. Nurs Times
  85(15):28–32,(16)50–52,(17)45–47
Barbiasz J, Blandford K, Byrne K et al 1982 Establishing the psychiatric liaison nurse role:
  collaboration with the nurse administrator. J Nurs Adm 12(1):14–18
Berarducci M, Blandford K, Garant C A 1979 The psychiatric liaison nurse in the general hospital.
  Gen Hosp Psychiatry 1:66–72
Brendon S, Reet M 2000 Establishing a mental health liaison nurse service: lessons for the future.
  Nurs Standard 14(17):43–47
Caplan G 1970 The theory and practice of mental health consultation. Tavistock Publications,
  London

Catalan J, Hewett J, Kennard C, McPherson J 1980a The role of the nurse in the management of deliberate self-poisoning in the general hospital. Int J Nurs Stud 17:275–282

Catalan J, Marsack P, Hawton K, Whitwell D, Fagg J, Bancroft J 1980b Comparison of doctors and nurses in the assessment of deliberate self-poisoning patients. Psychol Med 10:483–491

Davis D S, Nelson J K N 1980 Referrals to psychiatric liaison nurses. Changes in characteristics over a limited time period. Gen Hosp Psychiatry 2:41–45

Department of Health 1994 Working in partnership. The report of the Mental Health Nursing Review Team. HMSO, London

Department of Health and Social Security 1984 The management of deliberate self harm. DHSS, London

Dowling S, Martin R, Skidmore P et al 1996 Nurses taking on junior doctors' work: a confusion of accountability. BMJ 312(7040):1211–1214

Dulaney P E, Crawford G W 1988 Ten years in liaison nursing: concepts, models, and conventional wisdom. Issues Ment Health Nurs 9:425–431

Edwards M J 1999 Providing psychological support to cancer patients. Prof Nurse 15(1):9–13

Evans M 1994 Using a psychoanalytic model to approach acts of self-harm. Nurs Times 90(42):38–40

Fife B L 1986 Establishing the mental health clinical specialist role in the medical setting. Issues Ment Health Nurs 8:15–23

Fincannon J L 1995 Analysis of psychiatric referrals and interventions in an oncology population. Oncol Nurs Forum 22(1):87–92

Gardner R 1992 Psychological care of neuro-oncology patients and their families. Br J Nurs 1(11):553–556

Hawkins J W, Thibodeau J A 1996 The advanced practice nurse. Current issues, 4th edn. Tiresias Press, New York

Hill Report 1968 Hospital treatment of acute poisoning. HMSO, London

Isaacharoff A, Godduhn J, Schneider D, Maysonnet J, Smith B 1970 Psychiatric nurses as consultants in a general hospital. Hosp Community Psychiatry 21:361–367

Jackson H A 1969 The psychiatric nurse as a mental health consultant in a general hospital. Nurs Clin North Am 4(3):527–540

Johnson B 1963 Psychiatric nurse consultant in a general hospital. Nurs Outlook October: 728–729

Jones A 1989 Liaison consultation psychiatry: the CPN as clinical nurse specialist. Community Psychiatr Nurs J April:7–14

Kitson A 1993 Formalising concepts related to nursing and caring. In: Kitson A (ed) Nursing, art and science. Chapman and Hall, London, pp. 25–47

Lewis A, Levy J 1982 Psychiatric liaison nursing: the theory and clinical practice. Reston Publishing, Reston, Va

Lipowski Z J 1974 Consultation-liaison psychiatry: an overview. Am J Psychiatry 131(6):623–630

Loveridge L, Nolan P, Carr N, White A 1997 Healing Jesus. Nurs Times 93(30):26–30

Mayou R, Huyse F 1991 Consultation-liaison psychiatry in Western Europe. Gen Hosp Psychiatry 13:188–208

Minghella E 1989 The role of the nurse in the management of parasuicide in the community. In: Wilson-Barnett J, Robinson S (eds) Directions in nursing research. Scutari Press, London, pp 85–93

Nelson J K N, Schilke D A 1976 The evolution of psychiatric liaison nursing. Perspect Psychiatr Care 14(2):60–65

Newton L, Wilson K G 1990 Consultee satisfaction with a psychiatric consultation-liaison nursing service. Arch Psychiatr Nurs 4(4):264–270

Norwood S L 1998 Psychiatric consultation-liaison nursing: revisiting the role. Clin Nurse Special 12(4):153–156

Peplau H E 1952 Interpersonal relations in nursing. Macmillan Education London

Peplau H E 1964 Psychiatric nursing skills and the general hospital patient. Nurs Forum 3(2):28–37

Petersen S 1969 The psychiatric nurse specialist in a general hospital. Nurs Outlook February: 56–58

Roberts D 1997 Liaison mental health nursing: origins, definition and prospects. J Adv Nurs 25:101–108

Roberts D 1998 Nurses' perceptions of the role of liaison mental health nurse. Nurs Times 94(43):56–57

Roberts D, Mackay G 1999 A nursing model of overdose assessment. Nurs Times 95(3):58–60

Roberts M, Taylor B 1997 Emergency action. Nurs Times 93(30):30–32

Robinson L 1968 Liaison psychiatric nursing. Perspect Psychiatr Care 4(2):87–91

Robinson 1982 Psychiatric liaison nursing 1962–1982: a review and update of the literature. Gen Hosp Psychiatry 4:139–145

Robinson L 1987 Psychiatric consultation liaison nursing and psychiatric consultation doctoring: similarities and differences. Arch Psychiatr Nurs 1(2):73–80

Scott R A 1999 A description of the roles, activities, and skills of clinical nurse specialists in the United States. Clin Nurse Special 13(4):183–190

Severin N K, Becker R F 1974 Nurses as psychiatric consultants in a general hospital emergency room. Commun Ment Health J 10(3):261–267

Stickney S K, Moir G, Gardner E R 1981 Psychiatric nurse consultation; who calls and why. J Psychosoc Nurs Ment Health Serv 19(10):22–26

Tunmore R 1989 Liaison psychiatric nursing in oncology. Nurs Times 85(33):54–56

Tunmore R 1994 Encouraging collaboration. Nurs Times 90(20):66–67

UKCC 1992 Scope of professional practice. UKCC, London

Watts D 1997 Brief encounters. Nurs Times 93(30):28–29

Wolff P I 1978 Psychiatric nursing consultation: a study of the referral process. J Psychosoc Nurs Ment Health Serv May:42–47

RESOURCES

Professional Advisory Service

United Kingdom Central Council for Nursing, Midwifery and Health Visiting

23 Portland Place

London W1N 3AF

For professional advice.

Tel: 020 7333 6541

020 7333 6550

020 7333 6553

Fax: 020 7333 6538

email: advice@ukcc.org.uk

Website:www.ukcc.org.uk

The UKCC regulates the practice of nursing in the UK and can offer advice on professional issues.

RCN special interest group in liaison mental health nursing Secretary:

Dave Roberts

School of Health Care

Clerici Building

Oxford Brookes University

Gipsy Lane

Oxford OX3 OBP

This group is a point of contact for LMHNs working across the UK. It can enable you to find other nurses working with similar client groups and settings.

4

Liaison mental health nursing in community and primary care settings

Robert Tunmore

KEY ISSUES

- Primary, secondary and tertiary prevention in primary care
- Promoting mental health in the community
- At-risk populations
- Crises and crisis intervention
- The organisation of collaborative work
- Consultation and liaison in primary care

INTRODUCTION

The National Service Framework for Mental Health (Department of Health 1999) highlights the importance of preventive strategies, suggesting that health and social services promote mental health across the population, working with individuals and communities to reduce discrimination against individuals and groups with mental health problems. This chapter addresses the use of liaison mental health nursing and mental health consultation among primary care and community services. It sets out broad common frameworks for preventive intervention and crisis management in primary care. Mental health consultation and liaison enhance collaborative clinical practice at the interface between nurses in primary care and community services and mental health nurses in primary care and mental health services.

MENTAL DISORDER IN THE COMMUNITY

Over 95% of people with mental illness are cared for in the community. The majority of mental health problems have been dealt with by primary health care services (Goldberg & Huxley 1980, 1992). Increasing emphasis on public safety, containment and risk management in psychiatric services has focused the work of the mental health nurse on the care of those with severe and enduring mental illness, notably schizophrenia, organic illness and other severe psychotic illness. The provision of care for other, more common and less severe forms of mental illness falls increasingly to the primary care team. These changing patterns in health-care provision have led to the care of the less seriously mentally ill being devolved to other areas of nursing, particularly to practice nurses who can care for those clients presenting to their GP with psychological distress (White 1993).

Anxiety, depression and alcohol use are the most common types of mental health problem in the community setting Table 4.1. Anxiety and depression account for approximately 90% of mental health problems presenting in primary care. Between 10% and 15% of women have postnatal depression after childbirth (Department of Health 1999). Somatisation disorders are more frequently encountered in primary care settings than in the general population but are still relatively rare compared to populations of patients in general hospitals (Escobar et al 1998). However, medically unexplained symptoms are common in both primary care and the general hospital (Mayou & Sharp 1995). Each GP is likely to have about 450 people registered with them who have minor mental health problems (Mann 1992). Annually about 240 people present with non-psychotic mental health problems (Mann 1992).

Table 4.1 Prevalence rates of mental illnesses in the community (Strathdee et al 1996)

Diagnosis	Per 1000 population per year	No. patients per year in a practice of 1900
Depression	30–50	60–100
Anxiety & other neuroses	335.7	70–80
Situational disturbances/ other diagnoses	26.7	50–60
Schizophrenia	2–6	4–12
Affective psychosis	3	6–7
Organic dementia	2.2	4–5
Severe personality disorder	1.1	2–3

About 33% of GP presentations have a significantly disabling mental health problem (Goldberg & Huxley 1992). Between 25% and 40% of all patients with schizophrenia are managed by the GP alone with no specialist mental health service input (Cohen 1998). Following discharge from hospital, GPs manage approximately 25% of people with schizophrenia (Melzer et al 1991). More than 90% of people with a long-term mental illness will have had contact with the primary care service over the last 12 months. They are likely to visit their GP twice as often, on average, as other members of the adult population with about eight visits per year (Kendrick et al 1994). Most visits are for routine care, for example prescriptions, sick certificates and relatively minor physical ailments. However, a number of people with mental health problems are not engaged in primary care services. About 25% of GPs do not know the numbers of people with long-term mental illness on their lists (Monkley-Poole 1995). Some mental illnesses may be underdiagnosed and go untreated. For example, depression may go unrecognised among up to half of the presentations (Wright 1993).

The National Service Framework for Mental Health (Department of Health 1999) calls for primary care groups and specialist mental health services to agree and implement assessment and management protocols across the primary care group. These protocols address the referral, assessment, treatment and management of people referred with:

◆ depression
◆ eating disorders
◆ anxiety disorders
◆ schizophrenia
◆ risk of suicide
◆ postnatal depression

Health-care policy

The recent government reforms of the National Health Service identify primary care, specialist mental health and social care as the key elements of a fully comprehensive community mental health service. The White Paper *The new NHS: modern, dependable* (Department of Health 1997a) describes a system of integrated health care introducing primary care groups (PCGs) and primary care trusts (PCTs) which bring together GPs, community nurses, local authorities and social services. The Green Paper *Developing partnerships in mental health* (Department of Health 1997b) calls for health and local authorities to work together with service users and careers so that integration of statutory, voluntary and independent bodies achieves a 'seamless mental health service'. This is a mental health service that works across geographical and organisational boundaries and which is responsive to different and changing needs. Members of the primary health-care team (PHCT) provide the majority of mental and physical health care, the specialist mental health services providing support as and when required. The PCG has greater power and influence in the development of mental health services.

The Department of Health (Department of Health 1995) emphasises how members of the PHCT should have a clear understanding of common mental health problems, their diagnosis and management and good working relationships with mental health services. Specialist mental health services involve the GP routinely in care planning meetings for clients under the care programme approach. Aftercare arrangements under Section 117 of the Mental Health Act 1983 call for mental health services and GPs to collaborate in joint planning for continuing support following discharge from secondary services (Department of Health 1990). Most general practitioners prefer the community psychiatric nurse to act as the key worker for patients with long-term mental illness rather than taking on that responsibility themselves (Kendrick et al 1991). Joint work should ensure that the GP has access to the appropriate services in case of emergency.

The main focus of mental health trusts is the provision of services for people with severe and enduring mental illness. However, they need to work very closely with the PCGs, PHCTs and PCTs to reinforce the promotion of mental health. This will involve supporting primary care staff in dealing with less severe mental health problems and equipping them to deal with the early detection of mental health problems and intervention to prevent escalation of mental health problems. 'Shared care' refers to the organisation and arrangement of primary care services, GP practices and primary and secondary mental health services. In general, the mental health service psychiatrist takes responsibility for management and treatment of the patient's mental health problems while the general practitioner is responsible for the patient's physical health problems. Consultation between community health and mental health services is an essential component of these integrated services. Mental health consultation and liaison provide models of practice which facilitate working in partnership across service boundaries.

A PREVENTIVE FRAMEWORK FOR PRIMARY CARE

In community settings the mental health nurse collaborates with non-psychiatric colleagues in the PHCT. These include health visitors, district nurses, school nurses and practice nurses as well as specialist nurses including, for example, community palliative care nurses and nurses involved in rehabilitation of patients following surgery, strokes and accidents. Practice nurses probably represent the largest group of community health workers. The Royal

College of Nursing Practice Nurses Association estimate that there are approximately 19 000 general practice nurses working in the United Kingdom (RCN 1999). With the introduction of PCGs, community and practice nurses make an important contribution to health needs assessment, strategic planning and commissioning of health services for their local population and occupy a key position in the PHCT. At the core of general practice, they are familiar with the strengths and weaknesses of primary care and a significant resource for programmes promoting mental health and preventing mental disorder in the community.

The Department of Health *Review of Mental Health Nursing* (Department of Health 1994) identifies the skills of the mental health nurse as an important resource for all members of the PHCT. The review sets out a framework for this collaborative work (Box 4.1).

Box 4.1 Working in partnership framework for collaborative working by nurses, midwives and health visitors in mental health care (Department of Health 1994)

1. Primary prevention
Work with vulnerable people or those at risk of mental illness

◆ Reducing the incidence of mental illness

◆ Approximately 250 people per thousand at risk each year

◆ Needs the work of health visitors, district nurses, school nurses, practice nurses and the specialist support of mental health nurses

2. Secondary prevention
Early detection and case finding, leading to early intervention. Work mostly carried out in the primary health care setting

◆ Early detection leading to prompt intervention

◆ Approximately 100 people per thousand at risk each year

◆ Needs the work of health visitors, district nurses, school nurses and practice nurses. Requires continuous liaison and some casework by mental health nurses

3. Tertiary prevention
Early intervention, effective treatment and rehabilitation requiring active case management

◆ Treatment and active intervention with established mental illness

◆ Approximately 24 people per thousand at risk per year

◆ Requires collaboration between mental health nurses in hospitals, residential facilities, day and community care. Needs liaison and work with health visitors, district nurses, school nurses and practice nurses

This framework for collaborative work is influenced by Caplan's conceptual model for primary prevention of mental health problems (Caplan 1964). Preventive psychiatry involves the reduction of mental disorder and the promotion of mental health in the community. It draws on theory and practice used to assess, plan and implement programmes of mental health care. Central to this approach is the assumption that mental disorders arise from dysfunctional adjustment and adaptation. Improvements in mental health are achieved by addressing relationships between the individual and his or her environment and promoting healthy adjustment through periods of crisis.

Caplan's model identifies three levels of prevention

Primary prevention

This involves reducing the incidence or rate of mental disorders in a community, i.e. lowering the number of new cases of mental disorder in the community, altering factors which lead to the disorder and reducing the risk of disorder among those who are not already mentally ill. Primary prevention aims to improve or increase helpful factors in the community and reduce factors believed to be harmful to mental health. A programme of primary prevention identifies three sets of factors:

1. harmful forces or influences
2. environmental forces which support individual resistance to harmful forces
3. environmental forces which influence the resistance of the population.

Programmes direct interventions at these factors and, by altering the dynamic relationships between them, reduce the incidence of mental disorder. Prevention involves reducing the problems and providing help.

Secondary prevention

This involves reducing the duration of established cases of mental disorders through early diagnosis and effective treatment. Early diagnosis may be achieved through several different means.

Assessment and diagnostic tools It may be possible to use assessment and diagnostic tools to identify the disorder from mild signs and symptoms. Armstrong (1998) identifies and reviews screening and assessment tools that may be used in practice settings for the care of people with psychiatric disorder in the community. Screening tools may target those populations at special risk and increased vulnerability to mental disorder (Box 4.2).

Box 4.2 Assessment tools for use in primary care (Armstrong 1998)

Assessment tool	Source
The Geriatric Depression Scale – 15-item version	Katona C et al 1995 Recognition and management of depression in late life in general practice: consensus statement. Primary Care Psychiatry 1:107–113
Goldberg General Health Questionnaire	NFER-Nelson, Darville House, 2 Oxford Road East, Windsor, Berks SL4 1BU
Hospital Anxiety and Depression Scale	NFER-Nelson, Darville House, 2 Oxford Road East, Windsor, Berks SL4 1BU
Beck Depression Inventory (full version)	France R, Robson M 1986 Behaviour therapy in primary care: a practical guide. Croom Helm, Kent
Beck Depression Inventory (short 13-item version)	Royal College of Psychiatrists, 17 Belgrave Square, London SW1X 8PG
CAGE	Ewing J A 1984 Detecting alcoholism: the CAGE questionaire. JAMA 252: 1905–1907
Edinburgh Postnatal Depression Scale	Cox J, Holden J 1994 Perinatal psychiatry. Use and misuse of the Edinburgh Scale. Gaskell, London

Health education Primary care staff need to be aware of the earlier signs and symptoms of common mental disorders and the need for further assessment and diagnostic intervention for adjustment problems that may not require specialist involvement. 'Inappropriate referrals' may indicate a need for education among the caregivers on the PHCT. They need to be equipped with the knowledge and skills to assess and identify mental health problems in order to make an appropriate referral. Knowledge of appropriate services, the referral process and point of contact should be clearly identified.

Access to services Mental health services are responsive to the needs identified by primary care staff. Early referral calls for all parties to share a clear understanding of the referral processes and systems, i.e. systems for the client's self-referral, role of family, friends, community caregivers, police, social worker and schools, etc. in the referral process.

Tertiary prevention

This involves the rehabilitation of clients into the community following mental illness.

Rehabilitation of people with mental disorder starts at the time of diagnosis and should be integrated into the programme of care from the outset. It involves identifying the range of factors that will help or hamper the client's subsequent participation in community life. This incorporates family, social, recreational and occupational relationships and the reactions of others in the client's social network.

Tertiary prevention programmes aim to reduce the negative consequences of mental disorder in a community, i.e. social deficit and impairment resulting from alienation, prejudice and stigma, and to improve integration and communication between the client and their social network.

Mental health consultation with professional and non-professional carers is an essential component of tertiary prevention programmes. Consultation takes place across a range of organisations including medical, public health, social services and welfare, education and employment services, religious, voluntary and charitable organisations. It may extend to a wider cross-section including social scientists, economists, legislators and community leaders.

POPULATIONS AT RISK

Programmes of prevention assist PHCTs to identify and plan care for populations at special risk. Those at maximum vulnerability within these populations are targeted with particular preventive interventions. In any community various populations at risk can be identified; for example, young unemployed men, those over 65 years old, children and young people. The National Service Framework for Mental Health (Department of Health 1999) identifies the following populations among those at risk of mental health problems:

◆ unemployed people – twice as likely to have depression as people in work
◆ children in the poorest households – three times more likely to have mental health problems than children in well-off households
◆ half of all women and a quarter of all men will be affected by depression at some period during their lives
◆ people who have been abused or been victims of domestic violence have higher rates of mental health problems
◆ between a quarter and a half of people using night shelters or sleeping rough may have a serious mental disorder and up to half may be alcohol dependent
◆ some black and minority ethnic groups are diagnosed as having higher rates of mental disorder than the general population; refugees are especially vulnerable
◆ there is a high rate of mental disorder in the prison population

◆ people with drug and alcohol problems have higher rates of other mental health problems
◆ people with physical illnesses have higher rates of mental health problems.

Our Healthier Nation (Department of Health 1998) highlights the effect of social and environmental factors on health status and calls for primary care services to address health promotion in three distinct populations:

1. in schools, targeting children
2. in the workplace, targeting adults
3. in the neighbourhood, targeting older people.

Our Healthier Nation (Department of Health 1998) established Health Action Zones where there are significant health problems – poor health and social deprivation – as the main focus of preventive programmes.

For example, the Health Advisory Service (1995) and the Mental Health Foundation (1999) address children and young people as a population at risk using this type of framework. They identify both harmful and helpful forces in this population. Helpful forces are those which are known to promote mental health and resilience to problems and disorder (Box 4.3). Harmful

---

Box 4.3 Mental health promoting factors

Individual	◆ Self-esteem, sociability and autonomy
	◆ Social support systems that encourage personal effort and coping
	◆ Good communication skills
	◆ A sense of humour
	◆ Religious faith
	◆ The capacity to reflect
Family (group)	◆ Family compassion, warmth and absence of parental discord
	◆ At least one good parent – child relationship
	◆ Affection
	◆ Appropriate and consistent discipline
	◆ Family support for education
Environment	◆ A wider support network within the community
	◆ Good housing
	◆ A high standard of living
	◆ A range of positive sport and leisure activities
	◆ A high morale school offering a safe and disciplined environment with strong academic and non-academic opportunities

Box 4.4 Child risk factors	
Individual risk factors	◆ Genetic influences ◆ Low IQ and learning disability ◆ Specific developmental delay ◆ Communication difficulty ◆ Difficult temperament ◆ Physical illness, especially if chronic and/or neurological ◆ Academic failure ◆ Low self-esteem
Family risk factors	◆ Overt parental conflict ◆ Family breakdown ◆ Inconsistent or unclear discipline ◆ Hostile and rejecting relationships ◆ Failure to adapt to child's changing developmental needs ◆ Abuse – physical, sexual and/or emotional ◆ Parental psychiatric illness ◆ Parental criminality, alcoholism and personality disorder ◆ Death and loss, including of friendships
Environmental risk factors	◆ Socio-economic disadvantage ◆ Homelessness ◆ Disaster ◆ Discrimination ◆ Other significant life events

forces are associated with risk factors for the population. These may predispose the population of children and young people to mental health problems and are identified in terms of the individual child or young person, their family and the wider environment (Box 4.4). The interaction of these negative and positive factors influences the outcome for the child or young person.

Identifying health-promoting and health risk factors

Prevention of mental health problems and the promotion of mental health involve the identification of factors that lead to disorder and factors that maintain and promote mental health across whole populations. The identification of factors that promote or maintain health is as important as identifying factors that increase levels of disorder. Prevention of mental health problems involves understanding the relationship between harmful and helpful factors, vulnerability and resistance and planning interventions accordingly. Preventive programmes 'depend on modifying the network of emotional influences on an individual with the hope that this will promote his active, reality based adjustment to current life difficulties rather than his being left alone to evade these by some form of irrational or regressive defence' (Caplan 1964, p 14).

Helpful and harmful factors

In order to maintain their mental health individuals need to be able to draw on a range of resources. Caplan refers to these resources as 'supplies'. Each group of supplies satisfies a particular area of need. Three broad categories are identified.

1. Physical supplies
2. Psychological supplies
3. Sociocultural supplies

The identification of supplies under these three broad headings can be used to systematically review helpful and harmful factors that affect the incidence of mental disorder among the population (Box 4.5). Helpful and harmful factors operate on these supplies at different levels: individual, group and environment. At each level some factors may be fixed and others more

---

Box 4.5 Supplies for mental health

Physical supplies	*Psychological supplies*	*Sociocultural supplies*
Meeting needs for food, water, shelter, heat, light, sensory stimulation Opportunities for exercise are necessary for bodily growth and physical development Protection from damage and physical, harm, e.g. infection and trauma	The satisfaction of interpersonal needs associated with cognitive and affective development, interaction with others, emotional involvement and continuing relationships Interpersonal needs include: 1. the need for love and affection 2. the need for boundaries, limits and controls 3. the need for participation in social activity	Influences of the culture and social structure on the individual – customs, traditions, language and values of the culture and society, expectations associated with behaviour, attitudes, position, role, progress and aspirations, rewards achievement, security

Box 4.6 Effects of inadequate supplies

Physical supplies	*Psychological supplies*	*Sociocultural supplies*
Brain trauma and infection	Disturbed parent–child relationships	Cultural uprooting and isolation, e.g. refugees and immigrant populations
Sensory isolation and depravation	Mother–child separation Adolescents, young people	Inadequate educational experience
Young children, older people	Lack of a confiding relationship	Lack of employment opportunities
	Interruption of close emotional relationships through, for example, illness, disability, death, separation or disillusionment	

flexible. For example, among individual factors age, sex, socioeconomic class and ethnic group are fixed while problem-solving ability and behaviour are more adaptable. A combination of inadequate provision of supplies, reduction of helpful and increase in harmful factors may increase the incidence of mental illness (Box 4.6).

Different types of supplies or resources are necessary for individual cognitive and affective development and personality development and functioning. The quality and quantity of supplies also affect individual development. The available resources influence the way the individual perceives and handles different situations. Normally, consistent and continuous provision of supplies establishes a routine for the way individuals deal with day-to-day experience. They develop adequate patterns of problem-solving behaviour to help with day-to-day living.

CRISIS

Caplan describes crisis in terms of a homeostatic process where, for most of the time, consistency and equilibrium are normally and routinely maintained. Certain situations may disrupt this continuity and alter the equilibrium, causing a problem for the individual. The individual uses tried and tested problem-solving approaches to deal with these problems and to cope with deviations from the routine. A crisis situation will arise when there is an imbalance between the size of the problem and the resources immediately available to deal with it, when harmful factors outweigh helpful factors. Caplan defines the term 'crisis' as '… psychological disequilibrium in a person who confronts a hazardous circumstance that for him constitutes an important problem which he can for the time being neither escape nor solve with his customary problem-solving resources'.

Caplan (1964) identifies four broad phases in the development of a crisis situation.

◆ *Phase 1.* The initial rise in tension from the impact of the stimulus calls forth the habitual problem-solving responses of homeostasis.

◆ *Phase 2.* Lack of success and continuation of stimulus is associated with a rise in tension and a sense of ineffectuality.

◆ *Phase 3.* Further rise in tension leads to mobilisation of internal and external resources. Calling on reserves of energy and emergency problem-solving mechanisms, the individual uses new methods to handle the problem. The problem may have abated in intensity. Perception of the problem may have altered. It may be defined in a different way more in line with previous experience and amenable to the individual's problem-solving repertoire. There may be resignation to aspects of the problem. New options and choices may be identified. The problem may be resolved and equilibrium re-established.

◆ *Phase 4.* The problem is not resolved. It cannot be solved by satisfaction of need nor avoided by resignation or changes in perception. Tension rises to breaking point leading to major disorganisation of the individual (pp 40–41).

Characteristics of crisis

◆ Crisis may lead to growth and development or deterioration in mental health.
◆ Crises are short-term phenomena, often resolved in a relatively short time.
◆ During a crisis individuals are more susceptible to influence.
◆ Crises are part of normal experience for most people and not necessarily related to psychopathology or mental disorder.
◆ Crises are unique to the individual experiencing them.
◆ A specific event or set of circumstances can be identified as causal factors in a crisis.

Common characteristics of a crisis have been identified (Caplan 1964, Geissler 1984). During a crisis situation individuals are more susceptible to influence by others. They are more open to help, support and advice and often elicit a helping response in others. Alternatively, and importantly for those disadvantaged by mental health problems, the individual may be susceptible to negative influences which exacerbate or maintain the crisis situation.

Box 4.7 Coping responses

Adaptive coping response	Maladaptive coping response
Development of new effective problem-solving skills	Evasion/avoidance of problem by individual/family
Reality-based approach to situation	Irrationality
Adaptive coping mechanisms	Manipulative behaviours
Open to support and guidance	Inadequate problem solving
Supportive relationships and family	Pathological defence mechanisms
The mastery of distressing experience	Regressive behaviour
Ability to master increasingly challenging problems	Socially unacceptable behaviour
	Antisocial behaviour
Inner strength, self-confidence, reliance and assurance	Social exclusion, alienation and isolation
Increased resistance to mental disorder	Increased vulnerability to mental disorder

---

The crisis is seen as a transition period in personality development. It may give opportunities for personal growth or it may be a harmful episode leading to a reduced resistance and increased vulnerability to mental disorder. The individual's response to the crisis may be either adaptive, where the situation is seen as providing opportunities for personal growth and development, or maladaptive, where the situation is a threat to the individual with increased vulnerability to mental disorder (Box 4.7).

Types of crisis

Different types of crisis can be identified (Box 4.8). They include 'developmental crises' and 'accidental crises' (Erikson 1959).

◆ Developmental crises are those associated with changing patterns of behaviour over the stages of a lifespan. They include role transitions through birth, puberty and adolescence, young adulthood, climacteric, old age, illness and death.
◆ Accidental crises are associated with life events often experienced as a sudden loss, the threat of loss and challenges to safety and stability. They include, for example, starting or finishing school or college, redundancy, starting a new job, moving house, etc.

The former are associated with a protracted time period while the latter are usually acute, relatively short-term episodes of disruption.

Box 4.8 Types of crisis (Erikson 1959, Baldwin 1978)

Accidental

Developmental

1. Dispositional crisis An acute response to an external stressor, e.g. outbursts of anger and aggression, social withdrawal and isolation

2. Crisis of anticipated life transition Normal lifespan changes that are expected and anticipated but which may be experienced as difficult to cope with or beyond the control of the individual, e.g. depression following retirement and loss of a valued role

3. Crisis resulting from trauma Caused by unexpected external events and circumstances over which the individual has little or no control and which he or she experiences as overwhelming, e.g. difficulty in being alone at home following a burglary

4. Maturational and developmental crises Unresolved psychological conflicts triggered in response to current events and circumstance, e.g. maladaptive patterns in dealing with rejection

5. Crisis reflecting psychopathology An emotional crisis triggered or perpetuated by existing mental disorder, e.g. personality disorders, severe neurosis and psychotic disorders

6. Psychiatric emergencies General functioning severely impaired to the extent that the individual is unable to assume personal responsibility. The safety of their lives and/or the lives of others is at risk, e.g. suicide attempt, overdose or alcohol intoxication, uncontrollable anger and violent behaviour

Baldwin (1978) identifies six different types of emotional crisis organised in relation to their degree of severity.

1. Dispositional crisis
2. Crisis of anticipated life transition
3. Crisis resulting from trauma
4. Maturational and developmental crises
5. Crisis reflecting psychopathology
6. Psychiatric emergencies

A framework for clinical practice

A useful framework for individual work is based on the contribution of bereavement studies to our understanding of the way individuals respond in a crisis. Goodall et al (1994) describe 'the grief wheel', a model for making sense of grief, loss and bereavement. This consists of the following four phases:

◆ shock
◆ protest
◆ disorganisation
◆ reorganisation.

Each phase is associated with a wide range of feelings and experiences that characterise the experience of coming to terms with loss of any kind: loss of health, loss due to death, divorce, loss of confidence, etc. (Box 4.9).

◆ Shock – the impact of the initial event or circumstances on the individual's experience.
◆ Protest – reaction against the loss.
◆ Disorganisation – characterised by lack of success, increased tension and upset.
◆ Reorganisation – mobilisation of internal and external resources, reserves of energy, new and different problem-solving methods, different perceptions, alignment with previous experience, new options and choices and new equilibrium.

The phases identified are not distinct, clearcut categories, but merge or over-lap with each other. The model gives a positive sense of direction, growth and development. Movement may be backwards or forwards over an unspecified time period. In general, a crisis occurs over a relatively short period of time while bereavement reactions normally have a longer duration. This model may be used to illustrate adaptive and maladaptive responses and to help clients understand their own situation, providing a sense of perspective and

Box 4.9 Common responses to crisis

Shock	Protest	Disorganisation	Reorganisation
Numbness	Sadness	Loss of interest	Return to
Lack of emotion	Anger	Hopelessness	previous levels of
Disbelief	Guilt	Helplessness	functioning
Hysteria	Fear	Loss of confidence	Changed values
Euphoria	Relief	Low self-esteem	Reinforced values
Suicidal thoughts	Preoccupation	Apathy	Different perceptions
	Physical distress	Depression	New meanings in life
	and illness	Suicidal ideas	Readjustment
		Anguish	Reequilibration
		Anxiety	
		Loneliness	
		Sadness	
		Aimlessness	
		Restlessness	
		Loss of meaning	
		Loss of faith	
		Inner tension	
		Confusion	
		Lack of	
		concentration	
		Memory loss	
		Increased physical	
		illness	
		Ineffectuality	

Box 4.10 Client's perspective of crisis

The crisis cycle involves focusing on learning from experience, in particular the issues raised by episodes of crisis in the illness experience of the individual. For example, a client's experience of reality through psychosis.

◆ How have they coped with the experience?

◆ How it has affected situations and relationships?

◆ Have they new or different understandings?

◆ What personal strengths and insights do they have?

normality (Fig. 4.1). Early interventions aim to reduce the disruption and distress of the experience.

The framework for crisis can be used as the basis for initial assessment with the client and his or her family (Box 4.10). Discussion could focus on the following factors.

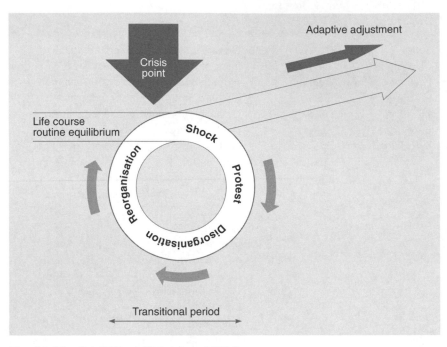

Fig. 4.1 The Grief Wheel (Goodall et al 1994)

◆ Where they see themselves on the cycle at the moment.
◆ The individual's perception of the current situation – their own story.
◆ Previous failures and successes.
◆ Identification of similarities to past problems.
◆ Identification of coping styles and practical strategies.
◆ Choices, decisions and consequences.
◆ Family involvement and other significant relationships.

Crisis interventions aim to:

◆ help the individual get their experience into perspective
◆ set a context for mental health promotion
◆ encourage expression of negative feelings
◆ influence and facilitate more adaptive, healthy coping responses
◆ maintain a reality-focused perspective
◆ empower the individual to influence preferred outcomes through their own efforts.

Family involvement is an important component of preventive programmes. The family is as likely to be part of the problem as they are to be part of the solution. Assessment and interventions should involve the family and take account of family roles, relationships, expectations, values and practices.

Clearly the crisis may extend beyond the individual and his or her immediate family to wider social networks across the community. As Caplan (1964) states, the individual 'does not usually face crisis alone, but is helped or hindered by the people around him, by his family, his friends, neighbourhood, community, and even nation'.

The crisis cycle may also be used by the PHCT to help them develop a shared understanding of primary prevention and mental health promotion as a practical means of helping clients with adaptive adjustment and healthy responses to crises. Shared understanding improves collaborative work between the primary care team and mental health services.

Crisis intervention in primary care

Various service models for crisis intervention have been identified (Cobb 1995, Joy et al 1998, Rapaport 1967). The National Service Framework for Mental Health (Department of Health 1999) identifies key factors for crisis intervention and prevention of mental health problems. These involve the mental health services working with the primary care team and other services to anticipate, prevent or respond to a mental health crisis with rapid, effective help. Key factors of preventive and crisis intervention services include:

◆ 24-hour access for emergency mental health assessment in A&E departments
◆ crisis resolution teams
◆ a crisis plan for all on the Care Programme Approach
◆ care plans to document the action to be taken in a crisis by service user, carer, GP and care coordinator
◆ crisis cards for users listing key contacts for planned crisis support
◆ crisis houses as alternatives to hospital admission
◆ rapid access to a place of safety.

THE ORGANISATION OF COLLABORATIVE WORK IN PRIMARY CARE

Close collaboration and working arrangements between mental health services and primary care, including the promotion of mental health awareness and education, are required in order that deficits in care are addressed and made good. Collaboration brings together local authorities, community and voluntary groups and local businesses, health and social services. The planning, organisation and delivery of mental health care and physical health care for individuals require integrated health and social care systems to support individuals with ongoing or continuing care needs. Members of PHCTs have become increasingly familiar with partnerships, collaboration, sharing and networking as necessary components of practice.

In the National Service Framework for Mental Health the Department of Health (1999) states that:

> *Mental health services represent a continuum from primary care to highly specialised services. For any local health and social care community mental health services will be provided by two or more organisations. No reconfiguration will unify all provision; the interfaces and boundaries must be managed effectively to provide and commission integrated services.*

The organisation and management of collaborative work at the interface of primary care and mental health services take different forms. In *Developing Partnerships*, the Department of Health (1997b) suggests that mental health nurses (and other mental health workers) may be employed directly by the primary care service to promote mental health or be employed by a community mental health team. Gask et al (1997) identify other models of practice for integrated primary care. Liaison and consultation are identified as important approaches to collaborative work in all these approaches.

Community mental health team

There has been a rapid growth in the number of community mental health teams (CMHTs) providing multidisciplinary mental health care and treatment across sectors of the community The CMHT may take clinical responsibility for the needs of the severely mentally ill and also for people with relatively minor disorders. It may focus on crisis intervention in acute episodes as well as providing continuing care services. This breadth of practice gives rise to a range of collaborative working arrangements and many opportunities for consultation and liaison work (Boardman et al 1987, Falloon & Fadden 1993, Jackson et al 1993, Onyett et al 1994, Woof et al 1986).

Generally CMHTs provide:

◆ a single point of referral
◆ multidisciplinary treatment and care
◆ rapid assessment services
◆ GP contact as a requirement of the Care Programme Approach.

Shifted outpatient clinics

This is a common arrangement among psychiatrists working in primary care. Run like the hospital outpatient clinic, it involves a visiting psychiatrist or other mental health professional providing a clinic at the health centre or in the practice setting. The mental health worker may be fairly independent of the other members of the primary care team, providing treatment to individuals with little involvement from PHCT members (Darling & Tyrer 1990). There may be little formal contact between the two parties and consultation and liaison activities may be informal, based on, for example, individual interest and personal motivation of the individuals involved (Balestrieri et al 1988, Brown et al 1988, Tyrer 1984, Tyrer et al 1994).

Attached mental health workers or 'link workers'

This model involves links between a mental health professional and primary care. The mental health professionals are often employed by secondary care services but work in the general practice setting. Often perceived as a member of the team, they may be a CPN, a counsellor, a psychologist or mental health facilitator. The link worker may be involved in both direct and indirect types of mental health consultation (Armstrong 1998, Thomas & Corney 1992). The organisation of the link is often flexible and shaped by local circumstances and policies, health strategies and resources.

The National Service Framework for Mental Health (Department of Health 1999) states that 'Specialist mental health services should establish liaison arrangements to support the general practices in the primary care group, including continuing professional development to enable all relevant staff to identify, assess and manage mental health problems'. The nature of the relationship between primary and secondary care services influences the provision of care and varies with each of these models.

The clinical effectiveness of interventions, the needs of primary care staff (Box 4.11), professional expertise among both PHCT and mental health services and the views of mental health service users (Box 4.12) are significant factors that shape the relationship between mental health services and the PHCT. The outcome of decisions about which clients are best treated in what setting and who is best placed to provide what sort of intervention will depend upon the organisation of services, including rapid assessment, acute and/or crisis intervention and continuing care services. Explicit lines of professional accountability and clinical responsibility are also required. Patterns of referral also vary with each model. Referral sources and processes need to be clear, with identifiable points of contact between mental health service and PHCT.

Liaison mental health nursing in primary care

Mental health consultation and liaison are common to each of the above arrangements of collaborative work in primary care. The main aim of

Box 4.11 Needs of primary care practitioners

Fast access to mental health opinion

Rapid assessment and Mental Health Act assessment

Home assessment

Outreach service support

Treatment guidelines and protocols with clear treatment and care objectives and regular review

Crisis intervention, e.g. assessment of suicide risk

Close contact with individual mental health link worker – a named contact

Continuity of collaborative working relationship with mental health link worker

Patient information, health education and health promotion literature

Clear identification of clinical roles and responsibilities

Box 4.12 Service user views of primary care services (Lambeth, Southwark & Lewisham HA 1998)

Strengths

Users see GPs as key gatekeepers to health and social services

Most users find their GPs helpful

GPs are less likely to pathologise behaviour

Primary care consultations are less stigmatising

Primary care services are more likely to provide better continuity of care

Primary care services may be perceived as more accessible and flexible, more friendly and personal than secondary services

Weaknesses

GP treatment focuses on the use of medication rather than referral for counselling, 'talking therapies' and other specialist support

Concern over lack of information about mental health problems and treatment

Physical problems may be overlooked if mental illness is overemphasised

The importance of understanding different cultural values may not be understood

Lack of time to talk about mental health problems

consultation and liaison work is to maintain and support the care of people with minor mental disorder by the PHCT. The goals of mental health consultation in primary care (Box 4.13) incorporate mental health promotion and

Box 4.13 The goals of mental health consultation in primary care

◆ To promote mental health care in a range of different services and settings by providing a mental health service to the community

◆ To establish the effect of mental health problems on treatment and care

◆ To prevent the escalation of mental health problems and reduce psychiatric morbidity among patients

◆ To enable non-psychiatric colleagues to promote mental health as a routine part of their work

◆ To evaluate the effect on patient well-being and hospital resources when mental health problems are recognised and followed with appropriate interventions

◆ To identify areas where mental health problems go unrecognised and untreated

◆ To develop collaborative working arrangements with colleagues in other services in a range of different settings

◆ To provide mental health interventions directly, through managing a caseload, and indirectly, through mental health consultation with non-mental health primary care practitioners

the prevention of mental disorder. The liaison mental health nurse collaborates with the PHCT in the development and planning of individually focused interventions that help promote effective coping and increased resistance to mental health problems. Often the GP practice is the setting for consultation and liaison activities. Having mental health services routinely at hand in the practice setting may help to reduce the stigma associated with mental illness and its treatment (Brown et al 1988, Strathdee 1987).

Consultation and liaison may involve the mental health nurse in direct work with the client and his or her family. They also work indirectly with the client and their family, through face-to-face personal contact with members of the PHCT who, in turn, intervene with the client and his or her family. Direct work may involve the liaison mental health nurse addressing specific problems among the most vulnerable individuals, where there are particular difficulties that are currently beyond the expertise of the PHCT and require specialist intervention.

Indirect work helps members of the PHCT with their own professional development, equipping them with the skills and knowledge so that they are better able to deal with similar problems in the future. This type of mental health consultation supports the caregiver in dealing with the clients' crises. It focuses on the development and facilitation of the caregiver's skills in problem solving and delivering effective interventions. It may also help the caregiver avoid repeated experiences of failure and the subsequent likelihood of their withdrawal from 'difficult' clients.

Katon & Gonzales (1994) review the use of randomised controlled trials of consultation-liaison psychiatry in primary care. They identify how the research in this field has a dual focus:

◆ the outcome of the process of consultation for the client, i.e. client outcomes
◆ the outcome for the consultee who provides the care directly to the client.

This dual focus on direct and indirect interventions carried out by the mental health worker is a distinctive characteristic of consultation and liaison work. The client outcome, as in other means of delivering care, is clearly important but attention to the consultee outcome is a necessary feature of this work because it addresses the *process* of consultation.

The National Service Framework for Mental Health (Department of Health 1999) emphasises how collaborative work between primary care groups and specialist mental health involves:

◆ development of resources to assess mental health needs within each practice and for work with diverse groups in the population
◆ development of the skills and competencies to manage common mental health problems
◆ agreement about arrangements for referral for assessment, advice or treatment and care
◆ development of the skills and the necessary organisational systems to provide the physical health care and other primary care support needed for people with severe mental illness.

Through consultation, the liaison mental health nurse may help the caregiver on the PHCT:

◆ to differentiate mental illness from other emotional and psychological distress
◆ by advising on possible plans for future courses of action, whether psychiatric referral and treatment is appropriate
◆ with ways of understanding crisis
◆ to increase their knowledge and understanding of coping styles and patterns
◆ to understand adaptive and maladaptive responses
◆ with assessment, identification of interventions, planning and implementation of a programme of care
◆ through support and clinical supervision.

Consultation and liaison between the primary care staff involved may lead to:

◆ assessment by a mental health worker
◆ referral to a psychiatrist or mental health services
◆ care managed by PHCT
◆ feedback and management by PHCT
◆ clinical supervision through case management.

Consultation and liaison may result in:

◆ a reduction in the number of referrals from primary care services to the mental health team
◆ an increase in the number of referrals of people with serious mental illness
◆ improved mental health assessment skills among primary care staff
◆ enhanced care management skills.

The consultation relationship can be seen as a three-way dialogue between consultant, consultee and client when addressing user or carer issues and concerns as well as consultee/consultant relationships. An effective consultation may bring together different perspectives to achieve the desired outcome. This process involves:

◆ being able to stand in the other person's shoes – seeing things from their perspective
◆ seeing where they want to get to
◆ helping to identify the steps they need to take to get there
◆ facilitating reflection on any learning that takes place.

Whether working directly with the client or indirectly, collaborating with members of the PHCT, the liaison mental health nurse facilitates mental health promotion by increasing understanding of the situation through exploration and assessment.

Mental health facilitation in primary care

Mental health facilitators, sometimes referred to as link workers or mental health advisors, may be based in CMHTs, employed by trusts to liaise with primary care services or based in GP practices. Mental health facilitation involves working with members of the PHCT who do not have professional mental health qualifications. The consultation-liaison model has been identified as one of the most helpful working frameworks for mental health facilitation and collaboration between PHCTs and mental health services (Gask et al 1997).

Focusing on face-to-face work with members of the PHCT, the role of the mental health facilitator includes four broad areas of work (Hooker 1994):

1. health promotion
2. teamwork
3. training
4. advising.

Warner & Ford (1998) report on a survey of the role of the mental health facilitator in primary care. They identify key elements of the mental health facilitator's role:

◆ education and training for primary care staff
◆ health promotion activities
◆ development of local mental health networks
◆ making links with non-statutory sector mental health services
◆ developing links between primary care and mental health services
◆ direct work with service users
◆ research involvement.

Generally, the effective use and involvement of the mental health facilitator in primary care leads to improved communication between mental health services and PHCTs, improved use of referral processes with more appropriate referrals and more effective work with clients with complex needs.

Training needs of the PHCT

Liaison and consultation include a significant educational component where the mental health nurse helps colleagues on the PHCT to identify and meet their own training needs. Written materials alone are insufficient to meet the needs of PHCTs. The mental health nurse uses the consultation process to facilitate learning among the PHCT; for example, helping them to relate their clinical experience to an individual's adaptive and maladaptive coping strategies. Training needs relating to mental health issues for PHCT members have been identified (Turton et al 1995, Warner & Ford 1998). These include:

◆ early recognition and management of common mental health problems in primary care, e.g. signs and symptoms of disorders including anxiety, depression, postnatal depression, alcohol and substance misuse, bereavement reactions, violence and aggression, psychotic episodes
◆ recognition of mental illness in populations at special risk, e.g. elderly over 65, children and young people, unemployed and refugees
◆ protocols and guidance for treatment and support including knowledge of treatment options, administration and management of neuroleptic medication

◆ directory of mental health services, local and specialist
◆ other health needs, e.g. the physical health of people with mental illness
◆ professional development – education and training including counselling skills, psychosocial interventions, care planning, teamwork and team building, clinical supervision and support.

CONCLUSION

Liaison and consultation in primary care and community settings emphasise the need for interagency work and partnerships as a means of working across professional and organisational boundaries. Mental health liaison and consultation provide a means of organising collaborative work between mental health services and primary care groups to meet both the mental and physical health needs of the population. These approaches to the organisation and delivery of care have the potential to improve the standard of care of people with mental health problems in primary care settings. They contribute to the quality of clinical work and to the organisation and delivery of health care.

This chapter has addressed some of the key issues associated with liaison and consultation in primary care and community settings. It draws on the National Service Framework for Mental Health to set a broad context for this type of work. Primary, secondary and tertiary levels of prevention are described along with approaches to crisis and crisis management for community mental health services and primary care. The needs of PHCT members are identified in relation to collaborative clinical work, education and professional development and the benefits of liaison and consultation in primary care facilitation are identified.

QUESTIONS FOR DISCUSSION

◆ Having read through this chapter, consider the main populations of clients at risk of mental illness in your local area. Identify any preventive programmes you are familiar with for these groups. Identify any gaps in preventive services. How could you and your team work more effectively with colleagues on the primary care team to meet the mental health needs of these populations?

◆ Consider the section on the organisation of collaborative work in primary care. Which approach best describes your work situation? How does the way the service is organised affect liaison and consultation in primary care? What are the strengths and weaknesses of this approach to organisation in relation to the identified needs of primary care practitioners and service users (see Boxes 4.11 and 4.12)?

◆ Consider how the crisis cycle (Fig. 4.1) might be used in clinical practice to help:

a) primary care professionals understand the nature of common mental health problems and their management

b) clients and carers to understand their situation.

◆ Having read this chapter and others in this book, you may have some ideas for your own professional development. List your own skills and knowledge of liaison and consultation that are:

a) transferable across different settings, e.g. hospital, and community settings

b) specific to a particular setting and/or client group.

◆ What are the key areas for your own professional and career development?

ANNOTATED BIBLIOGRAPHY

Jenkins R, Ustun T B (eds) 1998 Preventing mental illness: mental health promotion in primary care. John Wiley, Chichester

This textbook is based on the proceedings of a conference organised by the Department of Health in collaboration with the Royal Institute of Public Health and Hygiene with the World Health Organisation. It covers a wide range of issues including the application of prevention in primary care, guidelines for health promotion, education of the primary care team and the community, early detection and identification, screening tools and clinical issues associated with a range of common mental health problems.

Royal College of Nursing 1999 Practice nurses handbook. Royal College of Nursing, London

This annually updated book is aimed at practice nurses but provides a range of useful information and community resources. It will give liaison mental health nurses a good idea of the types of clinical problems faced by practice nurses in their day-to-day work in addition to some helpful chapters on professional issues including quality management, policy and education in primary care settings. It also contains a regional directory of services and resources across the country.

Health Education Authority 1999 Community action for mental health. Health Education Authority, London.

This is an annual publication that identifies a wide range of case studies of mental health promotion programmes in primary care across the UK. It is

published on or around World Mental Health Day on October 10th. Each year a different team provides the focus for preventive programmes although a wide range of populations at risk are covered. Mental health promotion literature and resources are also available from the Health Education Authority (see Resources).

REFERENCES

Armstrong E 1998 Screening and assessment measures for the primary care teams. Int Rev Psychiatry 10:110–113

Baldwin B 1978 A paradigm for the classification of emotional crises: implications for crisis intervention. Am J Orthopsychiatry, 48(3):538–551

Balestrieri M, Williams P, Wilkinson G 1988 Specialist mental health treatment in general practice: a meta-analysis. Psychol Med 18:711–717

Boardman A, Bouras N, Cundy J 1987 The Mental Health Advice Centre in Lewisham service usage: trends for 1978–1984. Research report No. 3. National Unit for Psychiatric Research and Development, London

Brown R, Strathdee G, Christee-Brown J, Robinson P 1988 A comparison of referrals to primary care and hospital outpatient clinics. Br J Psychiatry 155:777–782

Caplan G 1964 Principles of preventative psychiatry. Basic Books, New York

Cobb A 1995 MIND's model of a 24 hour crisis service. MIND, London

Cohen A 1998 First port of call. Open Mind 89:14–15

Darling C, Tyrer P 1990 Brief encounters in general practice: liaison in general practice psychiatry clinics. Psychiatr Bull 14:592–594

Department of Health 1990 The care programme approach for people with a mental illness referred to the specialist mental health services. Joint Health/Social Services circular HC (90) 23/LASSL (90)11. HMSO, London

Department of Health 1994 Working in partnership: a collaborative approach to care. Department of Health, London

Department of Health 1995 Building bridges: a guide to inter-agency working for care and protection of severely mentally ill people. HMSO, London

Department of Health 1997a The new NHS: modern, dependable. HMSO, London

Department of Health 1997b Developing partnerships in mental health. HMSO, London

Department of Health 1998 Our healthier nation. HMSO, London

Department of Health 1999 The National Service Framework for Mental Health. Department of Health, London

Erikson E 1959 Identity and the life cycle: psychological issues. Monograph 1, No. 1. International Universities Press, New York

Escobar J I, Gara R, Cohen Silver R, Waitzkin H, Holman A, Compton W 1998 Somatisation disorder in primary care. Br J Psychiatry 173:262–266

Falloon I, Fadden G 1993 Integrated mental health care: a comprehensive community-based approach. Cambridge University Press, Cambridge

Gask L, Sibbald B, Creed F 1997 Evaluating models of working at the interface between mental health services and primary care. Br J Psychiatry 170:6–11

Geissler E M 1984 Crisis: what it is and is not. Adv Nurs Sci 6(4):1–9

Goldberg D, Huxley P 1980 Mental illness in the community: the pathway to psychiatric care. Tavistock, London

Goldberg D, Huxley P 1992 Common mental disorders – a bio-social model. Routledge, London

Goodall A, Drange T, Bell G 1994 The grief wheel. Grief Education Institute, Denver

Health Advisory Service 1995 Child and adolescent mental health services: together we stand. HMSO, London

Hooker J C 1994 Facilitating primary health care. J Adv Nurs 19:1–3

Jackson G, Gater R, Goldberg D, Loftus L, Taylor H 1993 A new community mental health team based in primary care. Br J Psychiatry 162:375–384

Joy C B, Adams C E, Rice K 1998 Crisis intervention for severe mental illnesses. Cochrane Library. Update Software, Oxford

Katon W, Gonzales J 1994 A review of randomised trials of psychiatric consultation-liaison studies in primary care. Psychosomatics 35:268–278

Kendrick T, Sibbald B, Burns T, Freeling P 1991 Role of general practitioners in the care of long term mentally ill patients. BMJ 302 (6775):508–510

Kendrick T, Burns T, Freeling P, Sibbald B 1994 Provision of care to general practice patients with disabling long term mental illness: a survey in 16 practices. Br J Gen Pract 44:301–305

Lambeth, Southwark & Lewisham Health Authority 1998 Towards primary care led mental health services. LSLHA, London

Mann A H 1992 Problems and solutions: psychiatric disorders in British general practice. Int Rev Psychiatry 4(3/4):235–236

Mayou R, Sharp M C 1995 Psychiatric illnesses associated with physical disease. Baillière's Clin Psychiatry 1:201–223

Melzer D, Hale A, Malik S, Hogman G, Wood S 1991 Community care for patients with schizophrenia one year after hospital discharge. BMJ 303:1023–1026

Mental Health Foundation 1999 The big picture. Mental Health Foundation, London

Monkley-Poole S 1995 The attitudes of British fundholding general practitioners to community psychiatric nursing services. J Adv Nurs 21:238–247

Onyett S R, Heppleston T, Bushnell D 1994 A national survey of community mental health teams. J Ment Health 3:175–194

Rapaport L 1967 Crisis oriented short term case-work. Soc Sci Rev 41:211–217

Royal College of Nursing 1999 The practice nurses handbook. Royal College of Nursing, London

Strathdee G 1987 Primary care-psychiatry interaction: a British perspective. Gen Hosp Psychiatry 9:102–110

Strathdee G, Kendrick T, Cohen A, Thompson K 1996 A general practitioner's guide to managing long term mental health disorders. Sainsbury Centre for Mental Health, London

Thomas R, Corney R 1992 A survey of links between mental health and general practice in six district health authorities. Br J Gen Pract 42:358–361

Turton P, Tylee A, Kery S 1995 Mental health training needs in general practice. Prim Care Psychiatry 1:197–199

Tyrer P 1984 Psychiatric clinics in general practice: an extension of community care. Br J Psychiatry 145:9–14

Tyrer P, Merson O, Onyett S, Johnson T 1994 The effect of personality disorder on clinical outcome. Psychol Med 24(3):731–740

Warner L, Ford R 1998 Mental health facilitators in primary care. Nurs Standard 13(6):36–40

White E 1993 Community psychiatric nursing 1980 to 1990: a review of organisation, education and practice. In: Brooker C, White E (eds) Community psychiatric nursing: a research perspective, vol 2. Chapman and Hall, London

Woof K, Goldberg D, Fryers T 1986 Patients in receipt of community psychiatric nursing care in Salford 1976–1982. Psychol Med 16:407–414

Wright A 1993 Depression: recognition and management in general practice. RCGP, London

RESOURCES

Royal College of Nursing Practice Nurses Association, 20 Cavendish Square, London WIM OAB
Tel: 020 7409 3333

National Depression Care Training Centre, Nene University College Northampton, Park Campus, Boughton Green Road, Northampton NN2 7AL

National Primary Care Facilitation Programme, Oxford Centre for Innovation, Mill Street, Oxford OX2 0JX
Tel: 01865 812011/2
e-mail: *postmaster@facilitation.org.uk*

National Primary Care Research and Development Centre, 5th Floor, Willanson Building, University of Manchester, Oxford Road, Manchester M13 9PL
Tel: 0161 275 7601
Website: *http://www.npcrdc.man.ac.uk/*

World Mental Health Day on October 10th. Contact the Health Education Authority, Trevelyan House, 30 Great Peter Street, London SW1P 2HW
Website: *http://www.wfmh.org/wmhdkit.htm*

Section 2

Generic approaches to assessment and intervention

5

Deliberate self-harm: assessment and treatment interventions

Linda Whitehead   *Margaret Royles*

KEY ISSUES

- Deliberate self-harm is a significant risk factor for completed suicide
- Serious physical illness is associated with an increased risk of suicide
- High suicide risk is not only associated with the presence of serious mental illness
- Not all acts of self-harm are associated with the wish to die
- Clinical risk assessment following deliberate self-harm requires an understanding of the specific act of self-harm as well as the identification of suicide risk factors
- The process of psychosocial assessment in itself may be therapeutic
- Short-term treatment interventions focus on reducing suicide risk by decreasing hopelessness, improving problem solving and other coping strategies
- Not all suicides can be prevented and both relatives and mental health staff may be affected by suicide
- Training and supervision are necessary for safe practice

INTRODUCTION

Deliberate self-harm (DSH) is one of the most common reasons for medical admission to general hospitals in the UK. Mental health nurses and other non-medical staff have been shown to provide effective and accurate psychosocial assessment following DSH and in many areas mental health nurses undertake the majority of such assessments. DSH is a serious risk factor for both suicide and further self-harm. Given also the link between physical illness and suicide, the ability to assess suicide risk has relevance for other areas of liaison mental health nursing. This chapter will outline the terminology associated with suicide and DSH and will review pertinent literature on assessment and treatment interventions. It will focus on the rationale and process of the initial assessment and will identify the therapeutic possibilities of this initial contact.

A second focus will be the care and treatment of adults who may be in crisis rather than mentally ill, including those who may repeatedly self-injure. Practical therapeutic strategies such as brief problem-orientated counselling and problem solving will be outlined. The specific needs of younger and older people will be identified where these differ from the adult client. The effects of completed suicide on staff and relatives will be addressed as will the need for support and supervision.

TERMINOLOGY

The terminology in this area can be misleading. Many terms previously used, such as attempted suicide, parasuicide and pseudosuicide, presuppose death as the intended outcome though research and clinical experience indicate this is only infrequently the case. Terms such as overdosing, self-poisoning and self-wounding refer to specific subtypes of behaviour but have the advantage of not prejudging motivation. Given the range of self-harming behaviours which lead to presentation at A&E units, such as self-poisoning, swallowing razor blades, stabbing, electrocution, hanging, attempted drowning, etc., there is clearly a need for a generic term. Deliberate self-harm (DSH) will be used in this chapter to refer to those acts which are intended, or might reasonably be expected, to cause physical damage to the body *whatever the stated motivation*. In this context overdoses of recreational drugs or drugs of addiction are excluded, as are acts aimed solely at sexual gratification. The term 'patient' will be used in recognition that the majority of those who self-harm are referred and assessed within the general hospital context and that the term is gender neutral.

SUICIDE

Suicide rates vary over time and cultures (Vassilas et al 1998). Approximately 5000 deaths from suicide are recorded in England and Wales each year and these account for about 1% of deaths. After a period of rising rates during the 1970s and 1980s, the UK suicide rate is again decreasing (McClure 2000). Suicide is consistently more frequent in males than in females though this gender differential is decreasing in the UK. In general, risks are higher in the elderly though rates in young men particularly have increased in recent years. The most common methods of suicide for men are hanging, car exhaust asphyxiation and self-poisoning. Women tend to use less violent means, with the most common fatal method being self-poisoning.

Those with mental disorder are at increased risk of suicide (Harris & Barraclough 1997) with diagnoses of depression, substance abuse, schizo-phrenia and personality disorder associated with the highest risk. Unsurprisingly, psychiatric inpatients and those recently discharged from care are at particularly high risk though often the risk is not recognised (Appleby et al 1999). Suicide may occur as a familial trait though the relative roles of genetics and environmental factors are not clear. Many painful, chronic or life-threatening illnesses (Harris & Barraclough 1994) are also associated with an increased risk of suicide, especially in the period following diagnosis (Table 5.1).

A relationship with unemployment has been suggested though the exact nature of the relationship is not clear (Platt 1986). Access to potentially lethal methods, sometimes associated with high-risk occupational groups such as vets, doctors and farmers, is strongly associated with higher rates of suicide. Other groups at high risk of suicide include the socially isolated and prison-ers, especially those on remand, despite apparent lack of access to means. For a fuller account of the many factors associated with completed suicide, please consult standard psychiatric texts, such as Vassilas et al (1998). Some of the key risk factors are summarised in Box 5.1.

Table 5.1 Medical conditions associated with increased suicide risk (from Harris & Barraclough 1994)

Medical condition	Relative risk
HIV/AIDS	×6.6
Huntington's disease	×2.9
Malignant neoplasms – all sites	×1.8
Multiple sclerosis	×2.4
Peptic ulcer	×2.1
Renal disease	
Haemodialysis	×14
Transplantation	×3.8
Spinal cord injuries	×3.8
Systemic lupus erythematosus	×4.3

DELIBERATE SELF-HARM

Deliberate self-harm is now one of the main reasons for presentation to A&E departments. England and Wales have one of the highest rates in Europe and these high levels of DSH have been a cause for concern in the UK since the 1960s. House et al (1998) have estimated presentations to general hospitals following DSH in the UK to be running at approximately 150 000 per year. (These figures underestimate the prevalence of self-harm in the community, as many episodes of self-harm do not lead to general hospital presentation (Arensman et al 1995).) Approximately 85% of self-harm episodes involve self-poisoning, 11% self-injury alone and 4% both and self-poisoning is more common in women than men (Hawton et al 1997). Paracetamol is taken in almost half of all overdoses despite increasing public awareness of the dangers.

DSH occurs mainly in the young, with the majority being under 35 years. Rates are slightly higher in females though again gender differences are diminishing. The problems associated with acts of self-harm are most commonly difficulties in relationships, bereavement and other losses, housing, employment or other social difficulties. Problems with drug and alcohol abuse are common and heavy alcohol consumption precedes the act of self-harm in half of all episodes. Repetition of DSH is common and usually occurs within 3 months of the initial episode. Rates of repetition within 1 year vary between 6% and 30% (House et al 1998) with a small number of individuals often responsible for a large number of episodes. Characteristics commonly associated with individuals who harm themselves are hopelessness, impulsivity, low self-esteem and poor problem solving. Many have a history of previous psychiatric contact and 30–40% are given a psychiatric diagnosis on assessment.

ASSESSMENT FOLLOWING DELIBERATE SELF-HARM

Rationale

Research in the 1960s and 1970s established the link between suicide and mental illness (Barraclough et al 1974) though recent surveys indicate that not all who kill themselves are or have been in psychiatric care (Appleby et al 1999). It has been estimated that the lifetime risk of suicide following the diagnosis of schizophrenia or depressive disorder is between 10% and 15%. Appleby (1997) suggests that 'Mental illness itself is a powerful risk factor, capable of obliterating the effect of other variables'. For a small proportion of clients, DSH may be the first indication of psychiatric disorder.

A link between DSH and suicide has also been demonstrated. In the year after an episode of DSH 1% of clients will die by suicide (Hawton & Fagg 1988). This figure increases to almost 3% within 8 years. About one quarter of those who die by suicide have attended a general hospital following DSH in the previous 12 months. High suicidal intent suggests a high future risk, especially when accompanied by hopelessness and continuing suicidal ideas. Chronic repetition of DSH is linked with eventual suicide, particularly when associated with alcohol and drug abuse. It must be noted, however, that the link between DSH and suicide is not always that of psychiatric illness. Some people kill themselves when acutely (or chronically) distressed though this distress may not amount to serious psychiatric illness. A few individuals may commit suicide in the absence of any observable distress or disorder though the concept of 'rational' suicide remains controversial.

Lastly, even in the absence of psychiatric illness, patients referred following DSH are often severely distressed and have a variety of social, psychological and medical problems that warrant intervention. Many of these patients can be described as being 'in crisis' and thus may be amenable to interventions which aim to resolve the current problems and reduce the risk of further self-harm or suicide.

Organisation of DSH services

DHSS guidelines (1984) indicate that all patients who self-harm and present to the general hospital should receive a psychosocial assessment. Not all

---

Box 5.1 Risk factors for suicide

Factors increasing risk of suicide

Individual	**Psychiatric illness related**
Divorced, widowed, separated, single	Depression
Living alone	Schizophrenia
Professions with access to lethal methods	Personality disorder especially borderline personality
Physical illness, especially chronic and painful conditions	Substance abuse
Family history of psychiatric illness or suicide	Previous history of DSH
History of bereavement in childhood	Previous inpatient care
Prisoners, especially on remand	
Social isolation	

Box 5.1 Cont'd

High-risk situations

Recent major stresses or loss
Anniversaries of losses, birthdays
Recent DSH, especially escalating
episodes
In inpatient psychiatric care
Recent discharge from psychiatric care
Recent change of psychiatric care,
e.g. day care to outpatient care
Absence of usual supports, esp. key
worker
Malignant alienation (Watts & Morgan
1994)
Easy access to lethal means

**Factors associated with act of
self-harm**

Evidence of premeditation and
pre-planning
Lethal or violent method chosen
Acts undertaken in anticipation of
death, e.g. will written, affairs set in order
Active avoidance of discovery or
intervention
Isolation at time of act
Presence of note
No actions taken to precipitate rescue
Regret at survival

Personality/mental state

Depressed mood
Suicidal ideas
Plans for suicide
Hopelessness
Marked lability of mood
Impulsivity
Hostility
Angry/aggressive behaviour
Auditory hallucinations especially
voices instructing the patient to
kill themselves

Factors reducing risk of suicide

Positive plans for the future
Previous success in coping/problem
solving
Accepting of offered help
Good social support
Confiding relationship

Successful treatment in past
Good rapport with key worker
Positive relationship with
psychiatric and other services

those attending hospital after an episode of self-harm require medical inpatient care but admission probably increases the numbers who receive psychosocial assessment. In some hospitals less than half of self-harm presentations receive an assessment partly because many presentations occur in the evening when access to psychosocial assessment may be limited. Discharge from hospital without assessment, however, has been associated with a higher risk of repetition (Crawford & Wessley 1998).

In the past psychiatrists undertook the assessments of patients selected by casualty doctors but since the huge increase in DSH during the 1970s interest has grown in developing services involving the use of non-specialist staff. Social workers (Newson-Smith & Hirsch 1979), psychiatric nurses (Catalan et al 1980b) and specially trained junior medical staff (Gardner et al 1977) have been shown to assess self-harm safely. Many services now rely on non-medical staff, predominantly mental health nurses, to undertake the majority of DSH assessments.

Suicide risk assessment

Risk assessment aims to protect both the patient and the practitioner by identifying and reducing the risk and frequency of adverse events (and their consequences) (Snowden 1997). The process can be applied to not only the risks associated with suicide and self-harm but also the risk of violence to others, self-neglect, exploitation, etc. The assessment of risk of suicide or self-harm entails the identification and weighing of those factors associated with increased risk against those that reduce it. Generally an accumulation of risk factors increases the overall risk but the relative weight given to each factor and its significance depends on the training, skill and experience of the clinician involved (Motto 1991). The result of combining knowledge of relevant risk factors with an understanding of the specific patient and their individual circumstances forms the clinical judgement of risk.

Statements of risk may include a number of elements.

◆ Nature of the specific risk in terms of behaviour or outcome, i.e. further self-harm or suicide.
◆ Timescale involved, i.e. in the next 24 hours, week, month or year.
◆ Probability or likelihood of the behaviour occurring.
◆ Potential consequences of the behaviour, e.g. death, injury.
◆ Future events which might alter the risk.

The risk assessment evolves into a risk management plan when plans are made, strategies formulated or resources deployed to reduce risk. Lack of appropriate resources may become significant at this stage and should be documented but should not affect the assessment of risk itself. It must be noted, however, that risk can never be eliminated and this may not always be desirable; for example, when devising therapeutic treatment plans.

Suicide risk assessments and risk management plans (ideally with their rationales) should be documented, as should ancillary decisions about how and to whom the assessment and plans are to be disseminated. Though issues of confidentiality and the maintenance of both patient trust and the thera-peutic alliance may arise in this context, team decision making and open discussion with the individual and family concerned may reduce, though not eliminate potential conflict.

Motivation and self-harm

Self-harming acts have meaning and purpose and are usually associated with some form of psychological distress. Stengel (1964) coined the phrase 'a cry for help' to underline his recognition that not all DSH was directed towards suicide and death. Some describe self harm as a survival strategy and an alternative to suicide.

Bancroft & Hawton (1983) suggest that self-harming acts may be under-stood in terms of two differing functions: instrumental and expressive. Instrumental motivations focus on achieving specific goals which often involve others; for example, to force the return home of an errant spouse, to make others sorry, etc. Expressive motivations are those which result from the way the individual feels at the time; for example, guilt, self-hatred or the need to escape from intolerable pain (physical or psychological). Most patients describe several levels of motivation, e.g. to express extreme distress, elicit help and to gain time out in hospital. An understanding of the complex motivations associated with a self-harming act is important in order to assess the risk of further self-harm and to ensure appropriate therapeutic intervention.

The explanations of outside observers, such as relatives, doctors and nurses, for self-harm often differ from those of the individual concerned. Self-reported attitudes of hospital staff to self-harm vary both within and between professions (Hawton et al 1981) though patients' accounts of staff attitudes and their hospital care tend to be less than favourable (Dunleavy 1992, Pembroke 1994).

The assessment of suicidal intent

The term 'serious' in the context of self-harm is often confused and misun-derstood. It is important to distinguish between the *purpose* (intent) of the act, i.e. what the patient wanted to happen (and the extent to which the objective circumstances support this) and the *effect*, i.e. the medical consequences (or potential lethality) and there is no strong correlation between the two. The intent of a specific act can be measured using the Suicidal Intent Scale (Beck et al 1974). The scale comprises 15 items, the first eight of which focus on the objective circumstances of the attempt which can be verified, such as plan-ning for the act, precautions taken against discovery, acts to gain help and presence of a suicide note. The second seven items represent the patient's subjective view such as the purpose and likely outcome of the act, the possibility of rescue and the method's lethality. The total score for both sections (range 0–30) gives a measure of suicidal intent, with higher scores (particularly on the first eight items) suggesting higher suicidal intent. This scale is a useful adjunct to clinical judgement (confirming or challenging it) rather than replacing it.

Crisis and the crisis intervention approach

The concept of crisis can be useful when both considering the circumstances leading to self-harm and identifying intervention strategies. In Caplan's view, a crisis reflects an imbalance between the perceived threat and the coping resources available. Caplan (1964) wrote:

> ...*a crisis is provoked when a patient faces an obstacle to life goals that is, for a time, insurmountable through the utilisation of customary methods of problem solving. A period of disorganisation ensues, a period of upset, during which many different abortive attempts at solution are made.*

In this context self-harm can be viewed as either an 'abortive attempt at solution' or, in the case of those who repeatedly self-harm, as a customary method of coping or even problem solving. Frequently crisis may be accompanied by a disruption in somatic and cognitive functioning, for example by poor sleep, appetite and concentration, which may sometimes mimic a depressive disorder. Hobbs (1984), in a useful review of crisis intervention, lists the characteristics of crises that have clinical implications.

◆ Crises are self-limiting. Resolution usually occurs within 4–6 weeks of the initial trauma. If resolution is incomplete or maladaptive, the individual remains at risk of further self-harm. Treatment therefore should be swift, short term and aimed at improving coping and preventing maladaptive solutions.

◆ Early attempts at coping are accompanied by help-seeking behaviour, which may be direct or indirect, and so indirect requests for help should be recognised.

◆ An individual in crisis may represent a family or other group in difficulties which underlines the importance of contact with families or 'significant others'.

◆ Crisis, itself, is not a pathological state though the outcome might be. Learning and growth are possible.

◆ Prolonged or recurrent crisis may be associated with failure to resolve old conflicts that may have little to do with the current problems. Intervention may need to be directed to the resolution of these early difficulties when crises become recurrent.

Perhaps the most clinically important aspect of crisis is that as a period of reorganisation and adjustment, there is an opportunity for intervention and change.

Nursing model of assessment following DSH

The assessment approach described below has been developing for more than 20 years in Oxford where the majority of DSH assessments are undertaken by specialist mental health nurses. The process reflects an integrative model of nursing practice, characteristic of liaison mental health nursing, which has its roots in crisis and stress adaptation theory, dynamic, cognitive and behavioural understanding as well as biopsychosocial nursing models (Roberts 1997). The DSH interview is viewed as both risk assessment (ensuring the physical and psychological safety of the patient) and a therapeutic opportunity (Roberts & Mackay 1999).

The primary aims of the risk assessment following DSH are to:

◆ establish future suicide risk
◆ establish the presence and nature of any mental illness or disorder.

Further assessment aims include the identification of alcohol and drug abuse, psychosocial problems or a state of psychosocial crisis that might benefit from intervention (Royal College of Psychiatrists 1994).

Therapeutic aspects of the assessment interview

Several characteristics of those who are referred following DSH make therapeutic use of the assessment interview desirable. Many display continuing distress, suicidal ideas, hopelessness and poor problem solving. For many, specialist aftercare may not be acceptable or available and even when services are available, compliance is frequently poor (Moller 1989). The opportunity provided by this interview may offset some of these problems.

Therapeutic aims focus on relieving immediate emotional distress, increasing coping skills and reducing suicidality. The manner of interviewing, the form and process of the assessment can be directed towards developing therapeutic rapport and improving the patient's sense of self-efficacy (Roberts & Mackay 1999). An open-ended form of questioning allows the patient to 'tell their tale' and the opportunity to both understand their own situation and be understood. The interview may be cathartic and so reduce distress and contact with a positive, empathic assessor may promote a sense of containment and decrease hopelessness. Therapeutic strategies normally associated with follow-up, e.g. motivational interviewing, problem solving, rehearsal or role play, may be utilised, albeit in a brief form. Involving relatives may aid the assessment process and promote change. The giving of advice, where appropriate, and specific information, particularly about follow-up arrangements, may also significantly improve compliance rates.

The assessment process

The process of assessment following self-harm comprises a number of elements.

1. Information from medical and nursing staff and their notes regarding their care (e.g. significant medical history, current medical state and plans for discharge). Staff may have other valuable information about the patient; for example, current mental state, behaviour since admission and contact with relatives.

2. Comprehensive psychosocial assessment interview with the patient.

3. Information from third parties, especially GP, psychiatric or social services, significant others, etc., particularly when assessing adolescents and elderly patients.

4. Case discussion with peers, team or senior clinicians especially when a high risk of suicide or mental illness is suspected. This is good practice and protects the individual clinician. Team discussion also encourages the pooling of expertise and knowledge of resources and, by the sharing of decision making and anxiety, discourages overcautious interventions.

5. Collation of information including suicide risk factors and the complete and documented risk assessment (including other risks such as self-neglect and violence).

6. Development of an aftercare plan with the patient and arrangement of follow-up where appropriate.

7. Appropriate dissemination of plan to others.

The assessment interview (Table 5.2)

Engagement

Many patients continue to be distressed following their medical treatment and may not expect to talk to anyone about their situation. If ward or A&E staff inform patients of the assessment process beforehand cooperation with assessment is usually good. The development of rapport early on in the interview not only facilitates the assessment process but may also lead to greater compliance with aftercare, should that be required.

Assessors should introduce themselves and explain the assessment process. Obstacles to the assessment procedure such as a lack of privacy or fears about confidentiality should be addressed. Only on occasions may gentle encouragement be necessary to induce the reluctant to talk. Permission to contact significant others may be sought either at the outset or towards the end of the interview though caution should be exercised in giving assurances about any outcome of the assessment.

It is important to develop an interview style which allows the patient to talk and feel they have been understood whilst the necessary information is obtained. This information may not always be obtained in a sequential manner but this drawback may be offset by the development of a positive therapeutic rapport.

Understanding the act

The events that lead to the overdose or self-injury may be elicited in chronological order or in a thematic form. Closer questioning should focus on the 24–48 hours before the self-harm. Questions should identify not only significant events but also the thoughts, feelings and behaviours associated (including the use of alcohol or drugs). The question requiring an answer is 'Why this, why now?'. If no specific precipitating events are elicited an account of recent psychological symptoms may help; for example, the recent development of persecutory hallucinations, depressive symptoms, etc. The nature, timing and meaning of the act should become clear.

Direct questioning concerning the circumstances of the act (timing, planning, precautions against discovery, etc.) and the patient's beliefs associated with the episode will be necessary to assess the intent (see Assessment of suicidal intent above). This systematic exploration of the thoughts, feelings and behaviour leading to the act can be helpful to the patient who may otherwise find the act inexplicable. Details of previous or recent acts of self-harm will help to identify any escalation of suicidal behaviour.

If the act cannot be readily understood by this approach, it is possible that the patient is withholding information or purposely giving a false picture. Alternatively other factors such as an abnormal mental state at the time of the act or during assessment (such as a toxic confusional state) are associated with higher risk and indicate the need for further, specialist psychiatric assessment.

Clarification of current difficulties

Details concerning the nature, duration and severity of each problem should be elicited, as should their individual influence on the patient at the time of self-harm. Any recent attempts to seek help for these difficulties, contacts with others, etc. should be noted and their effectiveness assessed. The loss or absence of usual supports or care structure may also be significant.

Table 5.2 Stages in the DSH assessment interview (after Hawton & Catalan 1987)

Stage	Features
Engagement and the establishment of rapport	◆ Introduction by name, professional details where appropriate. ◆ Explanation of context and purpose of interview. ◆ Explore issue of confidentiality if appropriate.
Understanding the act	◆ Detailed account of events leading to the attempt (at least the previous 24 hours) with particular emphasis on the thoughts and feelings associated and details of any efforts made to cope with the situation. ◆ Circumstances surrounding the act, degree of planning, precautions taken, suicide notes, thoughts, feelings, motivation, actions after the act and whether alcohol was involved. ◆ Explore previous acts of self-harm especially for evidence of escalation in intent or frequency.
Clarification of current difficulties	◆ Nature of problems and their duration. Attempts to cope with these difficulties and other recent changes including contacts with helping agencies. ◆ Social circumstances, employment, relationships with partner and other family members. ◆ Consumption of alcohol and drugs.
Background/significant history	◆ Family and personal history, medical and psychiatric history. ◆ Usual personality and level of self-esteem.
Coping resources	◆ Usual coping style. ◆ Coping resources, both internal and external. ◆ Relationships with friends, carers, GP, etc.
Assessment of mental state	◆ Mood, hopelessness, suicidal ideas or plans, evidence of psychosis, cognitive functioning.
List of current problems	◆ Agree problem list. ◆ Additional problems identified by assessor but not by patient, including risk of further self-harm or suicide.
Establishing what further help is required	◆ Is the patient at serious risk of suicide? ◆ Is there evidence of psychiatric illness? ◆ Is further (specialist) assessment necessary? ◆ What help does the patient want or is willing to accept? ◆ What sources of help are available (e.g. from psychiatric or medical services, statutory and non-statutory services, voluntary bodies, family and friends)?

Table 5.2 Cont'd	
Stage	**Features**
Aftercare arrangements	◆ Agree plan following discharge; include steps to be taken before attending any follow-up. ◆ Give information on crisis services. ◆ Explain who else will be informed of plan.

Background

Information should include all those areas which potentially either have a bearing on the further risk of suicide or may influence the type of treatment to be offered. Areas to be covered include previous medical and psychiatric history (which should be addressed in some detail) and family psychiatric history, especially a history of suicide, psychotic or affective disorder or substance abuse. An individual's personal history including experiences of loss, abuse or disrupted parenting may suggest vulnerability even in the absence of current difficulties in these areas. Brief details of the current social circumstances in terms of family, marital or work situation should be outlined if problems in these areas have not already been identified. Some idea of the patient's usual personality, including self-esteem, may also be obtained though this information may be more objectively provided by a third party.

Coping resources

Coping resources, both internal and external, should be identified. Past attempts at coping may be explored, especially those that proved successful. Maladaptive patterns of coping, such as avoidance and denial, along with traits such as impulsivity and aggression may be associated with repeated self-harm. Conversely, evidence of previous problem solving in crisis and personality characteristics such as flexibility, resilience and self-belief may suggest lower risk. Supportive or confiding relationships should also be identified and an assessment made of the individual's ability to make use of them. The involvement of other services such as voluntary groups, social and probation services may also be useful when planning follow-up.

Assessment of mental state at interview

Many of the objective aspects of the mental state examination may be evaluated during the interview, i.e. behaviour, form and content of thought, rapport. Other more subjective aspects require direct questioning. Mood, especially depression, should be a focus and any changes in mood observed during the interview should be noted. Particular attention should be paid to evidence of suicidal thoughts or plans and to hopelessness which is highly correlated with subsequent suicide (Dyer & Kreitman 1984). Evidence of constructive plans for the future may indicate lower immediate and short-term risk. Evidence of severe mental illness indicates high risk and the need for further specialist psychiatric assessment.

List of current problems

In order to initiate and facilitate problem solving a comprehensive problem list should be agreed between the assessor and the patient. If the assessor identifies a difficulty that the patient denies, for example drug or alcohol abuse, the assessor may wish to develop a parallel problem list. Medical or psychiatric diagnoses may be included as 'problems' if relevant to the current state or to future risk.

Establishing what further help is required

If a high risk of suicide has been identified or if evidence of psychiatric illness has been found a more formal mental health assessment may be advisable. This further assessment may confirm the need for psychiatric treatment; for example, antidepressant medication or psychiatric admission (possibly under the provisions of the Mental Health Act).

Most patients, however, do not have significant psychiatric disorders but may express the need for help. Guidance may be needed to clarify the type of intervention that is both beneficial and available. Some patients may not have problems that are amenable to intervention or help may not be wanted and a return to the GP with advice on self-help measures may be all that is necessary. Potential sources of appropriate follow-up may already be apparent from the interview. Statutory agencies that are already involved should be contacted and appropriate information about the self-harm episode shared, preferably before discharge, especially if it is intended that the patient is returning to their sole care.

Aftercare arrangements

If additional intervention is needed, e.g. specialist outpatient psychiatric or other services, the nature and practical implications of this should be agreed with the patient and, where possible, relatives. Details of any follow-up arrangements should be given, preferably before discharge, in either verbal or, ideally, written form. Compliance may be further improved if the assessor offers follow-up though the importance of continuity of care remains controversial (Moller 1989). Crisis cards containing information about local emergency services (including the Samaritans) for use in future crises may also be given.

INTERVENTIONS FOLLOWING SELF-HARM

The aims of aftercare

The aims of intervention following deliberate self-harm are:

◆ reduction of risk of suicide and further self-harm
◆ treatment of mental illness
◆ provision of brief interventions aimed at resolving psychosocial problems, including drug and alcohol use.

Admission to psychiatric hospital, possibly on an involuntary basis, may be indicated where there is evidence of mental illness and a high risk of suicide. Even in the absence of mental illness psychiatric care, including inpatient or day care, may be appropriate if patients are seriously suicidal or in a state so disorganised that they are unable to take responsibility for themselves (Bancroft 1979).

The majority of patients, however, do not have serious continuing suicidal ideas but have either considerable psychosocial difficulties or could be seen as in crisis and thus may be amenable to less intensive outpatient interventions.

Effectiveness of interventions following DSH

There is much controversy concerning the efficacy of interventions following DSH. Two recent reviews of clinical trials of treatment (Hawton et al 1998, Van der Sande et al 1997) have been published and House et al (1998) summarised their findings. Relatively few clinical trials were identified and these were often seen as flawed. Common criticisms included low sample sizes, strict selection criteria (meaning that sample groups did not represent the heterogeneity of the clinical population) and limited standard outcome measures (usually repetition). None of the intervention strategies showed a significant reduction in repetition though some appeared promising, notably dialectical behaviour therapy (DBT), use of crisis cards and problem solving.

Dialectical behaviour therapy

This is an intensive psychological treatment used with patients, frequently diagnosed as borderline personality disorder, who have repeatedly self-harmed

(Linehan et al 1991). The treatment, comprising a year of weekly individual and group therapy with access to therapists out of hours if in crisis, was shown to reduce both repetition and inpatient psychiatric bed usage. This study indicates potential treatment directions for the small group of patients who repeatedly cut or burn themselves and for whom little else has been beneficial. Several trials of this treatment approach are currently under way in the UK.

Crisis cards

The use of crisis cards detailing sources of help in future suicidal crises has been assessed for adults referred following an overdose (Morgan et al 1993). This scheme offered easy access to psychiatric assessment and possible inpatient admission in time of crisis. Few people took advantage of this offer yet repetition was lowered, though not significantly. It is possible that the option of contact provided patients with enough support to make contact unnecessary. A more recent study in the same area has unfortunately failed to confirm these findings. Experience in Oxford, as yet unevaluated, suggests the routine use of cards offering further assessment in future crises may be justified and may not lead to increased demand.

Problem-solving treatments

Problem-solving interventions are based on the recognition that many of those who self-harm or who are in crisis exhibit poor problem-solving skills (Linehan et al 1987, McLeavey et al 1987). Specific deficits in problem solving include rigidity in thinking (e.g. leading to problems with solution generation), avoidance, passivity or lack of active problem solving (Weishaar 1990). In a small study by Salkovskis et al (1990) 20 adult patients with a history of repetition were allocated to either a domicillary-based cognitive behavioural problem-solving treatment conducted by a community psychiatric nurse or to a control group of 'treatment as usual'. Improvements in target problems, hopelessness, suicidal ideation, depression and short-term repetition were found in the treatment group.

Hawton et al (1987) describe a larger study comparing brief problem-orientated outpatient counselling with referral back to GP with advice on management. The treatment focused on resolving current problems and commonly included other strategies such as exploration of the meaning of the overdose, improving communication with significant others and general problem solving. Whilst there were no significant differences in the two groups on the basis of repetition, a positive trend was noted and subgroups of women and those with dyadic problems appeared to benefit from the brief problem-orientated counselling.

The problem-orientated approach described by Hawton et al (1987) was used as the control therapy in a study by McLeavey et al (1994) which evaluated the use of interpersonal problem-solving therapy (IPPST). IPPST was described as a skills training approach which focused on improving problem-solving skills rather than resolving the current difficulties. This structured, psychoeducational model comprised training in step-by-step problem solving and utilised specific instruction, modelling, role play and homework tasks. Both groups showed reduced numbers of problems and levels of hopelessness 1 year later and though repetition was reduced in the experimental group, this did not reach significance. The experimental group, unsurprisingly, scored much higher on measures of problem solving but the study does suggest that problem-orientated interventions may be enhanced by the addition of a skills training element.

Brief problem-orientated treatment This approach, originally based on a crisis intervention model, focuses both on the resolution of current problems and on improving coping skills (Hawton & Catalan 1987). The approach is flexible and adaptable to individual circumstances and incorporates many of the elements of problem solving but also includes other useful interventions. Possible strategies include:

◆ an exploration of the meaning and consequences of the self-harm
◆ the instillation of hope and bolstering of self-esteem
◆ facilitation and support of emotional expression
◆ encouragement of appropriate communication with others
◆ modification of inflexible thinking and challenging of maladaptive beliefs and attitudes
◆ linking of past behaviour and events to present ones to aid insight and identify emotional blocks to change
◆ giving of specific information, e.g. health education, and advice, e.g. to consult a solicitor
◆ continuing assessment and monitoring of the mental state and suicidal ideas
◆ promotion of new and adaptive coping strategies aimed at preventing further self-harm
◆ a general approach to problem solving focusing on the resolution of the current problems
◆ development of a suicide prevention plan containing a hierarchy of strategies which can be used at times of future crises
◆ other specific strategies such as relaxation training, role play, rehearsal.

This approach, though usually carried out with an individual patient, may be adapted to include significant others; for example, a partner or spouse if dyadic problems are present or other family members when the identified patient is an adolescent. One to eight outpatient sessions of 30–60 minutes may be contracted with the patient. The first appointment is usually made within one week (sometimes within days) of the initial assessment. Subsequent sessions may then take place at appropriate intervals. If longer term treatment is found necessary either referral on or a renegotiation of the initial contract may be indicated.

Problem-solving therapy This is a practical psychoeducational therapy that utilises the patient's own resources to solve problems. Its aim is not only to resolve the current difficulties but also to provide a positive model for incorporation into the individual's repertoire of coping strategies for the future (McLeavey et al 1994). Deficits in problem solving may exist as 'state or trait' phenomena. Some individuals, including many adolescents, may never have acquired these skills while others may be unable to use them due to their level of arousal or to some characteristic of the problem, i.e. its nature, magnitude, potential consequences, etc.

Problem solving uses a collaborative step-by-step approach (Hawton & Kirk 1989) to problem resolution (Box 5.2). Once problems have been identified, an

---

Box 5.2 Steps in problem solving

1. Identify problems and available resources	Identifying problems in detail may aid the process of solution generation, e.g. rather than 'marital problems', use 'husband's refusal to help with the house work at weekends'.
2. Select one problem on which to focus	This may be the problem causing most distress, the easiest one to address to give early success or the one where most change might be achieved.
3. Identify goal by which to judge success of solution	Goal should be realistic in terms of resources available and the likely behaviour of others.
4. Generate a wide range of solutions to selected problem	The client should identify as many solutions as possible, perhaps using 'brainstorming'. The therapist also may need to suggest possible solutions. Judgement should be postponed even if solutions initially appear unpromising.
5. List advantages and disadvantages of each solution	The cost in terms of time, money, effort and other resources should be noted. Also, the effect on family/friends.

Box 5.2 Cont'd

6. Select one solution	Choose solution most likely to meet goal.
7. Identify and list the tasks necessary to achieve that solution	Some solutions may be achieved in one step, others in many. Breakdown large tasks into manageable steps. Role play or rehearse any potential difficulties.
8. Beginning with the first task, work through tasks towards identified goal	This can be agreed in sessions and done as homework with both successes and failures noted.
9. Review progress at each stage	Note lessons learnt from both success and failures. Identify and explore causes of failure. If necessary return to step 7.
10. Evaluate outcome against goal	Outcome may or may not correspond to goal but may be equally satisfactory. If not, return to step 6.
11. Select another problem and start process again	Process may be continued until all problems have been solved or, more realistically, when process has been learned.

appropriate, realistic goal is chosen. Particular emphasis is placed on generating multiple solutions leading to that goal and postponing judgment until the advantages and disadvantages of each have been explored. Cognitive techniques may be necessary to reveal or clarify emotional or cognitive blocks to potential solutions. Breaking down each potential solution into small manageable tasks can be helpful to those who feel overwhelmed by their difficulties. Tasks are carried out as 'homework' between sessions and progress at each stage is reviewed in subsequent sessions. If task implementation becomes blocked, obstacles are identified and strategies such as role play or rehearsal used to overcome the problem. Once the desired goal or outcome has been achieved, the cycle can be repeated with a new problem though patients may be able to continue on their own from this point.

Special groups

Adolescents

The assessment of children and adolescents following DSH is frequently the responsibility of specialist teams based in either Child and Adolescent Psychiatry or Child and Family Social Service departments. All children under

12 require this specialist assessment given the particularly serious implications of suicidal behaviour and distinct developmental needs of this age group. The general approach to assessment is similar to that of adults though more emphasis is placed on family involvement in both assessment and after-care (Hawton 1986). Self-esteem, functioning at school and relationships with friends provide other areas for assessment.

Self-harm in adolescents is associated with relatively low levels of suicidal intent (Hawton et al 1982) though levels of distress are often high and the role of depression must not be underestimated. Self-harm may be associated with the whole range of psychiatric disorders from frank psychotic illness to conduct and behavioural disorders. In adolescents self-harm is particularly associated with lack of problem-solving skills and relationship difficulties within the family, both of which are common targets during follow-up. Treatment of any psychiatric illness is clearly a priority. Crisis intervention skills may be useful to help the family contain difficult situations and training in specific problem-solving and social skills may be necessary (Brent 1997).

The elderly

Suicidal behaviour in the elderly is closely associated with depression and other psychiatric disorders (Hepple & Quinton 1997) and suicidal behaviour such as overdosing is more closely related to suicide than in younger adults. Dementia, especially in its early stages, is not thought to protect against suicide and needs to be distinguished from depression. Physical illness, often associated with chronic pain or increasing disability, is commonly present but may mask depression and lead to misdiagnosis. Loss and bereavement are common precursors of self-harm and social factors such as isolation and poverty may be major issues. Suicidal ideation and behaviour, for example, may follow change in accommodation such as a move from home to residential care. Uncertainty about an individual's ability to cope at home may warrant domiciliary assessment and contact with relatives and other carers is always advisable.

Best practice suggests that all elderly patients receive specialist psychiatric review either before general hospital discharge or shortly afterwards.

Recurrent self-injury and self-mutilation

Whilst bizarre or mutilating self-injury (for example, self-castration, self-enucleation) is often associated with serious mental illness, most self-injury presenting to hospital requires only minor medical attention. Suicidal intent may be associated with self-injury but for many, especially those who repeatedly self-harm, it is often associated with the expression or management of strong negative emotions such as self-hatred or despair. Some describe self-injury as a survival strategy and an alternative to suicide (Babiker & Arnold 1998). Some individuals engage in multiple methods of self-harm each with its own specific motivation. The experience of patients attending hospital for medical treatment, particularly following self-laceration, is frequently negative and in turn, many patients are critical and sometimes hostile to health professionals and offers of psychiatric treatment (Pembroke 1994).

Repeated or habitual self-harm (also termed self-injury, self-mutilation or self-injurious behaviour in the USA) has been associated with eating disorders, substance abuse, low self-esteem, personality disorders and sometimes psychosis (Winchel & Stanley 1991). Engagement with services can be problematic and few treatments have been shown to be effective (Linehan et al 1991). Treatment should probably aim to resolve underlying difficulties though viewing self-harm as a coping mechanism similar to an addiction may offer other treatment options. The long-term prognosis is less poor than previously believed though the behaviour may persist for considerable periods (Tantam & Whittaker 1992).

EFFECTS OF COMPLETED SUICIDE ON THE FAMILY AND PROFESSIONALS

For most people death is a major event only experienced a few times (Stedeford 1984) though general hospital nurses may be more familiar with it than many. In mental health settings, patient death in the form of suicide fortunately confronts clinicians only infrequently. Clinicians, however, have to face personal grief in the context of clinical, professional and public scrutiny. The news of a possible suicide of a patient in care is usually a shock even when the risk of suicide is known to be high.

In most mental health trusts mechanisms exist for the formal review of the care of all patients who have committed suicide whilst (or recently) in their care. These reviews do not, however, replace the need for early, more informal meetings of the team directly involved. These meetings, which ideally should take place within a week of the death, can be an opportunity for the team to share their shock and sadness whilst supporting those individuals most involved (Midence et al 1996). Contacts with GPs and other professionals involved may be supportive for all concerned. Contact with relatives may also be helpful and careful consideration should be given to individual circumstances.

For relatives and significant others the news of the suicide of a loved one may be a total surprise or something they have feared for a while. The impact of suicide cannot be underestimated whatever the circumstances. For the survivors there is often a heavy burden of guilt, shame and fear which is complicated by questions that are difficult to answer, such as 'Why did it happen? Could I have done more?'. Normal feelings of shame, guilt and fear (Worden 1991) sometimes may be directed outwards at the professionals who 'failed' to prevent the death and complaints may ensue. Whilst many families come to terms with their loss in their own way, some may need further help from organisations such as Cruse. A small number may require very specific counselling though the source of this help should be given some thought.

TRAINING, SUPPORT AND SUPERVISION

All staff involved in the assessment and management of patients following deliberate self-harm require appropriate training in addition to their professional practice (Catalan et al 1980a, Department of Health and Social Security 1984). This training should not focus solely on assessment and risk factors for suicide and self-harm but also on developing appropriate therapeutic skills in working with needy and potentially suicidal individuals. The development of positive attitudes to both those who self-harm and to the task of suicide prevention underlines good practice.

Clinical supervision is necessary to ensure both safe, effective practice and professional development for all those working with patients. Nurses especially are expected to seek clinical supervision (UKCC 1996). Supervision should ensure high standards of professional practice as well as enabling practitioners to develop skills to cope with an often distressed and distressing client group. Support in other forms, either from peers or from the multidisciplinary team, may also be necessary to maintain healthy functioning and minimise burnout.

CONCLUSION

The assessment of deliberate self-harm and the identification of suicide risk are skills necessary for many professionals working in the general hospital especially those working in A&E settings. Managing self-harm in individuals at high risk of further self-harm or suicide with or without mental illness is a core skill for all those working in liaison mental health practice. This chapter gives an overview of the complex issues involved and outlines one model of self-harm assessment and management which could be adapted to suit local needs and resources. Cooperative working between professional disciplines and between the general hospital, psychiatric and social sectors is essential for safe practice in this area especially if the government health targets on suicide are to be met.

QUESTIONS FOR DISCUSSION

◆ How can the staff of A&E departments be helped to develop positive attitudes to patients who present following self-harm?

◆ What steps can be taken to reduce the number of patients leaving A&E departments without psychosocial assessment?

◆ In what circumstances might a patient, not suffering from mental illness but at high risk of suicide, be offered psychiatric admission?

◆ In what ways does the concept of crisis help to clarify assessment and treatment issues associated with individuals whom you have assessed following self-harm?

ANNOTATED BIBLIOGRAPHY

Hawton K, Catalan J 1987 Attempted suicide: a practical guide to its nature and management, 2nd edn. Oxford University Press, Oxford

Though written some time ago and now possibly hard to obtain, this book provides a good account of the process and practical issues associated with the assessment of attempted suicide and deliberate self-harm and it contains useful case material. Copies may be obtainable from medical libraries.

House A, Owens D, Patchett L 1998 Effective health care: deliberate self harm. NHS Centre for Reviews and Dissemination, York

Though aimed at purchasers, service providers and other decision makers this short document provides an excellent review of the evidence associated with psychosocial interventions following deliberate self-harm.

Babiker G, Arnold L 1998 The language of injury – comprehending self mutilation. BPS Books, Leicester

This well-researched book is written from both a psychological and sociological perspective by authors who have had long experience of working with repeated self-harm or injury (or self-mutilation) at the Bristol Crisis Centre. It describes from a variety of standpoints, the experience of self-harm, ways of understanding the behaviour and potential treatment approaches. This is probably one of the best accounts currently available.

Pembroke L R 1994 Self harm; perspectives from personal experience. Survivors Speak Out (Mind), London

Written by a very articulate group of service users, this book gives a very personal and challenging view of the experience of self-harm. Critical of many

services providing care for those who self-harm, the authors provide many thought-provoking insights which are both salutary and useful for all professionals involved in this area of practice.

MIND publishes two leaflets relevant to suicide and self-harm entitled 'How to help someone who is suicidal' and 'Understanding self harm'. Both offer very helpful information, advice and suggested reading for the lay public including relatives and carers.

REFERENCES

Appleby L 1997 Assessment of suicide risk. Psychiatr Bull 21:193–194

Appleby L, Shaw J, Amos T et al 1999 Suicide within 12 months of contact with mental health services: national clinical survey. BMJ 318:1235–1239

Arensman E, Kerkhof A, Hengeveld M W, Mulder J D 1995 Medically treated suicide attempts: a four-year monitoring study of the epidemiology in the Netherlands. J Epidemiol Community Health 49:285–289

Babiker G, Arnold L 1998 The language of injury – comprehending self mutilation. BPS Books, Leicester

Bancroft J 1979 Crisis intervention. In: Bloch S (ed) An introduction to the psychotherapies. Oxford Medical Press, Oxford

Bancroft J, Hawton K 1983 Why people take overdoses: a study of psychiatrists' judgements. Br J Med Psychol 56:197–204

Barraclough B, Bunch J, Nelson B, Sainsbury P 1974 A hundred cases of suicide: clinical aspects. Br J Psychiatry 125:355–373

Beck A T, Schuyler D, Herman J 1974 Development of suicidal intent scales In: Beck A T, Resnick H, Lettieri D (eds) The prediction of suicide. Bowie, Maryland

Brent D A 1997 The aftercare of adolescents with deliberate self harm. J Child Psychol Psychiatry 38(3):277–286

Caplan G 1964 Principles of preventive psychiatry. Basic Books, New York

Catalan J, Hewett J, Kennard C, McPherson J 1980a The role of the nurse in the management of deliberate self poisoning in the general hospital. Int J Nurs Stud 17:275–282

Catalan J, Marsack P, Hawton K, Whitwell D, Fagg J, Bancroft J 1980b Comparison of doctors and nurses in the assessment of deliberate self-poisoning patients. Psychol Med 10:483–491

Crawford M J, Wessley S 1998 Does initial management affect the rate of repetition of deliberate self harm? Cohort study. BMJ 317:985

Department of Health and Social Security 1984 The management of deliberate self-harm. HN(84): 25. HMSO, London

Dunleavy R 1992 An adequate response to a cry for help? Parasuicide patients' perceptions of their nursing care. Prof Nurse January:213–215

Dyer J, Kreitman N 1984 Hopelessness, depression and suicidal intent in parasuicide. Br J Psychiatry 144:127–133

Gardner R, Hanka R, O'Brien V C, Page A, Rees R 1977 Psychological and social evaluation in cases of deliberate self-poisoning admitted to a general hospital. BMJ 2:1567–1570

Harris E C, Barraclough B M 1994 Suicide as an outcome for medical disorders. Medicine 73(6):281–298

Harris E C, Barraclough B M 1997 Suicide as an outcome for mental disorders – a meta-analysis. Br J Psychiatry 170:205–228

Hawton K 1986 Suicide and attempted suicide among children and adolescents. Sage, Beverly Hills

Hawton K, Catalan J 1987 Attempted suicide: a practical guide to its nature and management, 2nd edn. Oxford University Press, Oxford

Hawton K, Fagg J 1988 Suicide, and other causes of death, following attempted suicide. Br J Psychiatry 152:359–366

Hawton K, Kirk J 1989 Problem-solving. In: Hâwton K, Salkovskis P M, Kirk J, Clark D M (eds) Cognitive behaviour therapy for psychiatric problems: a practical guide. Oxford University Press, Oxford

Hawton K, Marasck P, Fagg J 1981 The attitudes of psychiatrists to deliberate self-poisoning: comparison with physicians and nurses. Br J Med Psychol 54:341–348

Hawton K, Cole D, O'Grady J, Osborn M 1982 Motivational aspects of deliberate self harm in adolescents. Br J Psychiatry 141:286–291

Hawton K, McKeown S, Day A, Martin P, O'Connor M, Yule J 1987 Evaluation of out-patient counselling compared with general practitioner care following overdoses. Psychol Med 17:751–761

Hawton K, Fagg J, Simkin S, Bale E, Bond A 1997 Trends in deliberate self harm in Oxford, 1985–1995. Br J Psychiatry 171:556–560

Hawton K, Arensman E, Townsend E et al 1998 Deliberate self harm: systematic review of efficacy of psychosocial and pharmacological treatments in preventing repetition. BMJ 317:441–447

Hepple J, Quinton C 1997 One hundred cases of attempted suicide in the elderly. Br J Psychiatry 171:42–46

Hobbs M 1984 Crisis intervention in theory and practice: a selective review. Br J Med Psychol 57:23–34

House A, Owens D, Patchett L 1998 Effective health care: deliberate self-harm. NHS Centre for Reviews and Dissemination, York

Linehan M M, Camper P, Chiles J A, Strosahl K, Shearin E 1987 Interpersonal problem solving and parasuicide. Cogn Ther Res 11(1):1–12

Linehan M M, Armstrong H E, Suarez A, Allmon D, Heard H 1991 Cognitive behavioural treatment of chronically parasuicidal borderline patients. Arch Gen Psychiatry 48:1060–1064

McClure G M G 2000 Changes in suicide in England and Wales, 1960–1997. Br J Psychiatry 176:64–67

McLeavey B C, Daly R J, Murray C M, O'Riordan J, Taylor M 1987 Interpersonal problem solving deficits in self-poisoning patients. Suicide Life Threat Behav 17:33–49

McLeavey B C, Daly R J, Ludgate J W, Murray C M 1994 Interpersonal problem-solving skills training in the treatment of self-poisoning patients. Suicide Life Threat Behav 24:382–394

Midence K, Gregory S, Stanley R 1996 The effects of patient suicide on nursing staff. J Clin Nurs 5:115–120

Moller H J 1989 Compliance. In: Kreitman N, Platt S (eds) Current research on suicide and parasuicide. Edinburgh University Press, Edinburgh, pp 164–179

Morgan H, Jones E, Owen J 1993 Secondary prevention of non-fatal deliberate self harm: the Green Card study. Br J Psychiatry 163:111–112

Motto J A 1991 An integrated approach to estimating suicide risk. Suicide Life Threat Behav 21(1):74–89

Newson-Smith J G B, Hirsch S R 1979 A comparison of social workers and psychiatrists in evaluating parasuicide. Br J Psychiatry 134:335–342

Pembroke L R 1994 Self harm: perspectives from personal experience. Survivors Speak Out, London

Platt S 1986 Parasuicide and unemployment. Br J Psychiatry 149:401–405

Roberts D 1997 Liaison mental health nursing: origins, definitions and prospects. J Adv Nurs 55(1):101–108

Roberts D, Mackay G 1999 A nursing model of overdose assessment. Nurs Times 95(3):58–60

Royal College of Psychiatrists 1994 The general hospital management of adult deliberate self-harm. Gaskell, London

Salkovskis P M, Atha C, Storer D 1990 Cognitive-behavioural problem solving in the treatment of patients who repeatedly attempt suicide – a controlled trial. Br J Psychiatry 157:871–876

Snowden P 1997 Practical aspects of clinical risk assessment and management. Br J Psychiatry Suppl. 32: 32–34

Stedeford A 1984 Facing death: patients, families and professionals. Heinemann, Oxford

Stengel E 1964 Suicide and attempted suicide. Penguin, Harmondsworth

Tantam D, Whittaker J 1992 Personality disorder and self-wounding. Br J Psychiatry 161:451–464

UKCC 1996 Position statement on clinical supervision for nursing and health visiting. United Kingdom Central Council for Nursing, Midwifery and Health Visiting, London

Van der Sande R, Buskens E, Allart E, Van der Graaf Y, Van Engeland H 1997 Psychosocial interventions following suicide attempt – a systematic review of treatment interventions. Acta Psychiatry Scand 96:43–50

Vassilas C, Morgan G, Owen J 1998 Suicide and deliberate self harm. In: Stein G, Wilkinson G (eds) Seminars in general adult psychiatry. Gaskell, London

Watts D, Morgan G 1994 Malignant alienation. Dangers for patients who are hard to like. Br. J Psychiatry 164: 11–15

Weishaar M E 1990 Cognitive risk factors in suicide. In: Salkovskis P (ed) New frontiers in cognitive therapy. Guilford, New York

Winchel R M, Stanley M 1991 Self-injurious behaviour: a review of the behaviour and biology of self-mutilation. Am J Psychiatry 148(3):306–317

Worden J W 1991 Grief counselling and grief therapy: a handbook for the mental health practitioner, 2nd edn. Routledge, London

RESOURCES

MIND
Tel: 0208 522 2122

Samaritans
Tel: 08457 909090

Age Concern
Tel: 0208 765 7200

42nd Street, Manchester
Tel: 0161 832 0170
Help for adolescents and young people.

Trust for the Study of Adolescence
Tel: 01273 693311
Information for professionals and parents.

Bristol Crisis Service for Women
PO. Box 654
Bristol BS99 1XII
Tel: 0117 925 1119
Offers advice and information for women who repeatedly self-harm.

National Self-Harm Network
PO Box 16190
London NW1 3WW
Offers training and campaigns for the rights of those who self-harm.

6

Mental health liaison in cancer care

Dave Roberts

KEY ISSUES

◆ Cancer is a common, serious illness with a significant psychological morbidity and associated psychosocial problems

◆ Liaison mental health nursing is well established in oncology

◆ Psycho-oncology services are specialist mental health teams serving cancer patients and oncology staff

◆ Collaborative working relationships with oncology staff are important in the detection and management of psychosocial problems

◆ Mental health assessment should take a broad focus, including physical condition and social context

◆ Treatment approaches in psycho-oncology should involve the patient and his or her family and a range of other therapeutic staff

INTRODUCTION

Cancer affects one in three of the UK population before the age of 75 years. There are a quarter of a million new cases of cancer diagnosed in the UK per annum. Cancer is therefore a significant health problem.

Oncology, the services for the treatment of cancer, is a well-established area for mental health liaison. There is now a significant body of research into psychological reactions to cancer and liaison services are integrated into a number of the larger British cancer centres. Psycho-oncology, the study and treatment of psychological reactions to cancer, is a mental health speciality and its working practices provide a blueprint for the development of other services for the chronically physically ill.

CANCER CARE

The prevalence of mental disorder in cancer patients is between 20% and 50%. Given the different populations and diagnostic categories used in research studies, it is hard to be precise about rates of psychological morbidity. Barraclough (1999) estimates that half of all cancer patients have no significant psychiatric symptoms or disorder. Of the other half, 30% will have an adjustment reaction, i.e. significant distress affecting their quality of life and involving symptoms of anxiety and/or depression. This usually ceases without any professional intervention but can be helped by effective professional support from oncology staff. The remaining 20% will have a psychiatric disorder. This may be adjustment disorder, anxiety or depression or could be some preexisting psychiatric condition. According to one study of prevalence in cancer patients, adjustment disorder is the most common mental illness (Derogatis et al 1983).

Cancer carries a unique stigma among chronic illnesses. It is often interpreted by the lay public as synonymous with death. Cancer presents the sufferer with a number of physical, psychological and social problems.

◆ Although the illness is not always fatal, it raises the issue of mortality for the patient and their outlook on life may be permanently changed by this.

◆ The course of the illness can be long and arduous and lead to severe disruptions of social and occupational functioning.

◆ The specific part of the body affected by cancer, i.e. the site, can have a particular meaning for the individual (e.g. breast cancer in women or testicular cancer in men) or be associated with particular problems (such as facial disfigurement in head and neck cancers).

◆ Treatments, including surgery, radiotherapy and chemotherapy, can be drastic and are associated with serious side effects (e.g. fatigue, nausea and vomiting, hair loss, infertility), loss of function and disfigurement (e.g. following mutilating surgery such as mastectomy) (Box 6.1).

◆ Many patients feel that they have lost control over their bodies and their lives and they have to live with long-term uncertainty about treatment outcome or the possibility of relapse.

◆ There can be problems of continuity of care and communication between oncology staff and patients.

Box 6.1 Psychosocial problems associated with cancer treatments

Surgery	Surgery can lead to major changes in body image in, for example: ◆ highly visible parts of the body (facial surgery for head and neck cancers) ◆ parts defining personal and sexual identity (mastectomy for breast cancer) ◆ sexual organs (testicular cancer, gynaecological cancers) ◆ colostomy or ileostomy (bowel cancer)
Radiotherapy	Radiotherapy can have the following effects: ◆ soreness and scarring to the irradiated area ◆ restricted function in irradiated area ◆ fatigue ◆ patients may experience claustrophobia when having treatment in enclosed areas ◆ depression or cognitive impairment in cranial irradiation
Chemotherapy	Chemotherapy has a number of potentially significant psychosocial effects: ◆ hair loss ◆ fatigue ◆ nausea and vomiting ◆ sterility ◆ toxic confusion states ◆ depression ◆ cognitive impairment
Bone marrow transplantation (BMT) is a treatment for haematological malignancies	BMT involves total body irradiation, followed by infusion of the patient's own or donated marrow, with long periods of protective isolation

The patient's experience of cancer

There are now a number of research studies and personal accounts that give insights into the experience of cancer and its implications for the care we provide. One of the ways in which patients' experience has been accessed is through studies of quality of life (QOL). Survival rates have improved in a number of cancer sites and as awareness of the long-term effects of illness and treatment has grown, clinicians have used QOL as a measure of treatment outcome. Often, QOL measures focus on physical disabilities and dysfunction and where they take account of psychosocial factors, these are often framed in terms of pathology, i.e. social disability and psychopathology. An example of this type of approach is the Rotterdam Symptom Checklist, which has proved popular as an all-round measure of functioning associated with serious illness (De Haes et al 1990).

However, there are problems with this approach. The first is that QOL measures are often not mirrored in patients' own evaluation of the quality of their lives. Many consider their lives following treatment to be satisfying and fulfilling in spite of residual physical disability. They may have an enhanced sense of purpose and spirituality and stronger, more meaningful relationships. Some QOL research now acknowledges that there can be both positive and negative outcomes for individuals following cancer and that these factors may co-exist independently (Fromm et al 1996). The other problem is that most QOL measures are medically generated and do not conceptualise quality in the terms of the patients themselves. The importance of this debate is that many professionals working in oncology will use these measures as their main way of understanding the patients' experience of cancer. Patients' experience is thereby taken out of its individual and social context and framed solely in terms of response to treatment and personal pathology (Costain Schou & Hewison 1999).

Communication

Communication between patients and staff has been a recurrent theme in the oncology literature. There is evidence that doctors and other health-care staff have controlled the process of communication (McIntosh 1977). This has included withholding diagnoses of cancer or news of a worsening in the patient's condition. Even when information is given, it may be presented as unrealistically optimistic (Costain Schou & Hewison 1999). Bond's (1983) observational study of nurse–patient communication in oncology suggested that nurses did not routinely assess their patients' needs for information. Instead, they made assumptions that they should help patients maintain hope by minimising openness. They were also motivated by a desire to maintain the social order of the ward. Those patients who coped by using denial fitted in with this but other patients found informal ways of getting the information they needed.

As a result of the research into nurse–patient and doctor–patient communication, there have been a number of studies of the effects of communication skills training programmes for oncology staff (Maguire 1995). These have focused on verbal behaviours that promote the disclosure of concerns, such as open questions or questions with a psychological focus, the use of empathy and summarising. They have also identified the inhibiting effect of blocking behaviours such as focusing on physical complaints, providing reassurance, giving advice and using closed or leading questions. However, training in communication skills does not necessarily translate into effective communication when nurses return to their area of practice (Heaven & Maguire 1996).

The social environment in oncology

There is further evidence that nurses' ability to use specific communication behaviours, including both negative ones such as verbal blocking and positive facilitative verbal skills, is influenced by the ward environment they work in (Wilkinson 1991). An ethnographic study of an American oncology unit explored some of the background organisational and social pressures that inhibited the provision of good nursing care, particularly psychosocial care. The nurses were very busy and prioritised the physical aspects of the work that they were most confident in. Although they recognised the limitations of their psychosocial care, they lacked control over their own workload and had difficulty coping with the stresses of the work (Germain 1979).

A British ethnographic study (Roberts & Snowball 1999) also found a relationship between the way in which psychosocial care is carried out and the working environment of the nurses. However, in this case, the new patient-centred approach to nursing was leading to problems of closeness to patients, rather than the avoidant behaviour previously reported. The authors concluded that a balance is required between the interpersonal and professional aspects of the work, to minimise both avoidance and over involvement. The optimum level of involvement with patients was a professional closeness based on assessment of their psychosocial needs.

Cancer nursing

Cancer nursing is a specialist branch of nursing that has increasingly focused on the psychosocial aspects of care. This focus is particularly well established in the care of breast cancer. Specialist breast care nurses have been proven to have a valuable role in detecting mental illness following mastectomy (Maguire et al 1980) and may also have a role in reducing psychological morbidity in this group of patients (McArdle et al 1996). However, the trend towards providing psychological support for cancer patients has not been without its problems. A survey of 'cancer counsellors' revealed that, although many were nurses, few had a counselling or psychotherapy training and the majority did not have supervision (Roberts & Fallowfield 1990).

The focus on psychosocial care has been given further impetus by the UK government-sponsored report into the provision of cancer services, the

Calman-Hine Report (Department of Health 1995). This recommends the setting up of specialist cancer units and larger regional cancer centres for the care and treatment of cancer. Although primarily a medical report, it makes a number of recommendations about the use of specialist nursing staff. Centres for cancer treatment should include specialist nurses with expertise in counselling and psychosocial support. The report makes no specific recommendations on how this could be achieved, but it has provided support for local and national initiatives in developing specialist nursing roles with a clear psychosocial component.

PSYCHO-ONCOLOGY

Psycho-oncology (sometimes called psychosocial oncology) is the branch of psychiatry and mental health services dealing with cancer patients. Its definition usually covers two separate functions:

◆ the study and treatment of psychosocial problems and mental disorder associated with cancer
◆ the study of the relationship between psychosocial factors and cancer onset and outcome.

The latter definition is not dealt with in detail in this chapter. The term 'psycho-oncology' refers to both a specialist area of psychiatric practice and the services provided to deal with this range of problems.

The organisation of services

Given the widespread interest in psychosocial issues in oncology, there are a large number of potential collaborators within oncology teams. All professional staff in oncology units can make a contribution to the psychosocial care of patients. This can include:

◆ effective communication
◆ active listening skills
◆ initial assessment of psychological problems.

Given the prominent role played by specialist nurses (e.g. breast care nurses), services can be planned to take account of their expertise in detecting the more common mental health problems (i.e. depression and anxiety) and providing psychological support. Junior medical staff have a role in the pharmacological management of more straightforward cases of depression. All these activities can be supported by psycho-oncology staff, providing consultation, education and supervision. By making the most of the contribution of oncology staff, the mental health specialist can concentrate on the more acute, severe and complex clinical referrals. Psychosocial care is thereby delivered by the whole health care team, with different staff providing different levels of intervention depending on their skills, experience and area of professional responsibility (Table 6.1).

Table 6.1 Levels of psychosocial intervention (developed from a table originally published in *Professional Nurse* by Edwards 1999, developed from work by Tunmore, *Nursing Times* 1990)

Level of intervention	Staff involved in intervention
Level 1: Basic communication and assessment skills	Ward-based oncology nursing staff
◆ Providing information	
◆ Listening and interviewing skills	
◆ Representing psychosocial needs to others	
◆ Knowing when to refer the patient on	
◆ **Support and advice regarding communication skills and psychosocial assessment**	**Psycho-oncology staff**
Level 2: Routine preventive psychosocial care	Senior/experienced ward-based nursing staff, clinical nurse specialist in oncology
◆ Establishing rapport	
◆ Facilitating emotional expression	
◆ Ability to cope with others' distress	
◆ Knowing when to refer the patient on	
◆ **Support with psychosocial aspects of assessment**	**Psycho-oncology staff**
◆ **Supervision of psychosocial interventions**	
Level 3: Specific psychological interventions	
◆ Psychological interventions (e.g. problem-solving) based on theoretical model/skills training	Clinical nurse specialist in oncology
◆ Supervised short-term work	
◆ **Comprehensive mental health assessment**	**Psycho-oncology staff**
◆ **Support and supervision of psychological interventions**	
◆ **Specific psychological interventions**	
Level 4: Psychological treatments/therapy	
◆ **Provision of recognised form of psychological therapy, e.g. cognitive behaviour therapy**	**Psycho-oncology staff**

Coordinated psychosocial care

There is also a role for non-health staff in the provision of psychosocial care and support. Fellow patients and ex-patients often give support and information to cancer sufferers, both informally and through locally and nationally organised support groups (see Resources). There is also a broad range of complementary therapies available within some of the major British cancer centres. The best working practices can be achieved through close links between complementary therapists and psycho-oncology services. This avoids competition and promotes the coordination and integration of psychosocial care (Brennan & Sheard 1994).

A common model is to have a centre for the dissemination of information on cancer and its treatment, which is also a place of contact between patients and their families, oncology staff and voluntary agencies and a point for the coordination of psychosocial support. In Oxford, this is provided by the Cancer Information Centre, located within the main city hospital treating cancer. There are close managerial and clinical links with the local psycho-oncology service, which is located on the same site. The psycho-oncology team comprises a clinical nurse specialist who works one day a week and a psychiatrist who provides input 2 days a week. Counselling sessions are given by health care professionals trained in counselling, who are paid on a sessional basis from the psycho-oncology budget. All psycho-oncology outpatient clinics are held in the Cancer Information Centre. This helps to destigmatise and normalise psychiatric referral.

The Cancer Information Centre is open to anyone to drop in and is also used for a range of outpatient clinics. Whilst patients are there, they have access to centre staff, who are mainly from health profession backgrounds, a library of information on cancer, its treatment and self-help and there is also access to on-line information sources. The centre offers a range of complementary therapies (Box 6.2). All these services are offered free at the point of delivery, though voluntary donations to the centre are invited.

Effective psychosocial care is best seen as an integration of the following sources of input.

◆ The patient, their family and friends have a role in maintaining, developing and renegotiating support during the course of illness and treatment. This is often done informally with other patients. They can also provide a useful service by giving feedback to the professionals on their experience of care and treatment, so that improvements can be made.

◆ The primary health-care team. The GP often has a long-standing relationship with the patient and may know the home situation very well. Other primary care staff (e.g. district nurses) give care at home to cancer patients and they often give valuable informal support to patients and their families.

Box 6.2 Complementary therapies offered at the Cancer Information Centre, Oxford

◆ *Aromatherapy.* Aromatherapy is a form of massage using essential oils which are believed to have beneficial effects on the mind, body and spirit. It is offered to individuals as a means of relieving the effects of stress and anxiety and inducing a state of calm and relaxation.

◆ *Art therapy.* Art therapy is offered to groups of people as a means of expressing themselves using a variety of visual media. Many people find they can express feelings through art that they cannot do using words. Part of the benefit is in sharing feelings in a safe and confiding environment that is separate from the treatment setting.

◆ *Counselling.* This is offered to individual patients and their relatives by trained counsellors with a background in the health professions. Self-referral is the usual means of access and posters around the hospital give details of the service. Supervision is offered from the psycho-oncology team, though some counsellors have other sources of supervision. This is a more private arrangement between counsellor and patient than in the psycho-oncology team. Patients are offered up to six sessions initially. In some cases this is extended.

◆ *Healing.* This is a non-religious, holistic approach to individuals that aims to support natural healing processes and to promote enhanced well-being and awareness of the inner self. It involves physical and mental relaxation and guided imagery. Healing is not offered as a cure.

◆ *Psychoeducational groups.* These take the form of groups and workshops run by the Cancer Information Centre and psycho-oncology staff and invited outside experts. Their format varies but usually includes relaxation, visualisation and a short talk. There is an emphasis on supportive relationships, self-help techniques and a holistic approach to the individual.

◆ *Reflexology.* Reflexology is a specialised form of foot massage based on the principle that different areas of the foot are connected to the body's internal organs and their operation. It is offered to individuals to help reduce tension and aid symptoms such as pain.

◆ *Relaxation.* Progressive muscle relaxation is offered to groups of patients and their carers (and staff when they can attend). Tapes are available that are recorded on site and include relaxing music and visualisation.

◆ Self-help groups. Many patients and significant others give and receive support through self-help groups. There are both local and national groups and some of these will focus on a specific cancer site (e.g. breast cancer) or groups of diseases (e.g. haematological malignancies).

◆ Charities. There are a number of charitable groups who provide material support to patients and financial support to develop services that directly benefit patients. Again, some of these are local and there are also large national groups like the Macmillan Cancer Relief Fund, which is a major source of funding for specialist palliative care services.

◆ Complementary therapists. Though the evidence base for some of these therapies is in doubt, they are popular with patients. They frequently fill in the gaps in the oncology services by providing a positive, warm and comforting experience that is in contrast to the sometimes unpleasant treatments received in hospitals. They also use a holistic model. Care is needed to ensure that therapists do not offer, and patients do not expect, a cure.

◆ Palliative care staff, including community-based Macmillan nurses.

◆ Hospital oncology staff.

◆ Psycho-oncology and other hospital-based psychosocial care staff.

Liaison mental health nurses in oncology

There are a number of descriptions of LMHN practice in oncology from both the USA and the UK. These are mainly descriptions of working practices and practice frameworks, but there are also details of referral patterns. Fincannon (1995) gives a comprehensive account of her work as a 'psychiatric consultation-liaison nurse' (PCLN) at the Johns Hopkins Oncology Centre in Baltimore, USA. She retrospectively reviewed the first 102 referrals over a one-year period, with a focus on type of psychological problem, congruence between referrer's and PCLN's assessment of the problem, and subsequent interventions.

The main reasons for referral were depression (31%), anxiety (26%) and non-compliance (13%). Other reasons included delirium, support, family issues, past psychiatric history and relaxation. After assessment, which involved the use of DSM-IV diagnostic criteria, most of the patients referred with depression were found to have either an adjustment disorder or delirium. The majority of referrals for treatment of anxiety (52%) were diagnosed as such, but a significant proportion had an adjustment disorder (37%) or had a primary physical cause for their symptoms, such as pain or hypoxia (11%). Some of the non-compliant patients were suffering from delirium. After assessment, the referrals broke down as follows: adjustment disorder (28%), anxiety (14%), delirium (14%), non-compliance and personality disorder (10%) and depression (5%). Mental health follow-up was given to 83% of the referred patients. In terms of mode of interventions, 31% were direct, with a primary focus on patients and families, 17% were indirect, with a primary focus on staff, and 52% involved a mixture of both direct and indirect interventions. Interestingly, haematology patients and patients undergoing bone marrow transplantation were proportionately overrepresented in the referrals.

The British scene

In a British setting, Edwards (1999) describes her work at Cookridge Hospital in Leeds, where she established a new LMHN service following a research project that highlighted deficiencies in psychosocial care. She reviewed 131 referrals over a 9-month period. The majority of referrals were for adjustment disorder (38%), depression (24%), anxiety (18%) and interpersonal problems (10%). Non-compliance was not given as a category, though it is possible that 'interpersonal problems' cover this. No patients were referred with delirium. Follow-up was offered to 53% of the patients after assessment. Interventions involving staff alone (i.e. indirect referrals) made up 22% of the referrals.

The potential for comparison with Fincannon's (1995) work is limited, as they are working in very different health care environments and their reports are structured differently. For example, Edwards gives diagnoses but not reasons for referral and does not specify which diagnostic criteria were used. Also, she makes a distinction between direct and indirect interventions but, unlike Fincannon, does not specify how many referrals involved both. However, some broad similarities and difference can be seen. Both offer follow-up to the majority of referrals and both offer a mixture of direct and indirect interventions. The biggest difference is between diagnoses of adjustment disorder and depression in the two reports. This is presumably because of differences in the diagnostic categories used. Also, whilst delirium constituted a significant diagnostic category in Fincannon's report, no patients had this diagnosis in Edwards'. This may again be because of differences in diagnosis. However, in the author's experience of British oncology services, delirium is often managed by oncologists, without involving mental health services.

Other descriptions of LMHNs working in oncology do not give a breakdown of referrals but describe patterns and styles of work. Both Tunmore (1989, 1990) and Gardner (1992) give accounts of their work at the Royal Marsden Hospital in London. Tunmore (1989) put particular emphasis on working with oncology nurses to clarify problems in their work with patients, i.e. indirect consultation, but also describes direct work with patients. The work of Gardner (1992) with neuro-oncology patients puts a greater emphasis on working with the patient within a family context, to help with the adjustment of all family members to the illness and its effects. This is important in a group of conditions that carry with them the potential for severe and progressive disability.

Most of the accounts of LMHN activity describe nurses working alone as single practitioners but a report from the USA gives an account of a team of three clinical nurse specialists (CNSs) working within a major cancer centre. Van Fleet & Hughes (1996) are based at the University of Texas M D Anderson Cancer Centre. Most of their work is direct patient-related interventions, including supportive psychotherapy, education, relaxation, visualisation and imagery training and hypnosis. They also offer staff consultation. There is a liaison attachment to the bone marrow transplant unit and this work involves informal contact, regular attendance at clinical meetings and running a staff support group. The CNSs accept referrals of both inpatients and outpatients.

MENTAL HEALTH ASSESSMENT

Assessment in oncology involves the application of generic mental health skills, with an awareness of the personal context of the patient and the effects of cancer and its treatment. This is best done as a collaborative effort with oncology staff. Some form of screening has to take place to determine which patients need specialist mental health assessment.

Screening

Oncology staff have a proven role in detecting mental illness and other psychological problems in cancer populations. This includes both specialist nurses (Maguire et al 1980, McArdle et al 1996) and ward-based staff (Hardman et al 1989, Pasacreta & Massie 1990). Hardman et al (1989) used complementary diagnostic tools to determine which patients on a medical oncology ward had a mental illness. Junior medical staff and ward nurses were then asked to identify those patients they thought were suffering from anxiety or depression of a mild, moderate or severe degree. They detected 79% of the anxious patients and 49% of the depressed patients. The nurses proved better at recognising both anxiety and depression than the doctors, though they also detected more false positives.

A different approach was used in a study of psychological morbidity in a major American cancer centre (Pasacreta & Massie 1990). All the nurses at work on one day shift were asked to complete a questionnaire on each patient in their care. The questionnaire listed 25 psychiatric symptoms. The nurses were asked to say whether each patient had the symptom and whether it was of a degree that warranted a psychiatric consultation. The majority of patients in the hospital (55%) were felt to have symptoms requiring psychiatric consultation. However, only 13% of the sample were actually seeing a mental health professional. This discrepancy suggests that, although nurses may feel a patient needs mental health intervention, they frequently lack the confidence to refer them. The nurses said they often did not deal with emotional issues because they were short of staff, were unsure what to do or had to prioritise physical health concerns.

There are limitations to the conclusions that can be drawn from these studies, however. Nurses asked to focus on mental health problems for the purposes of a research study are more likely to detect problems than they are in day-to-day practice. However, both these studies support the idea that, because oncology nurses spend so much time in close contact with their patients, they are more likely than other team members to detect psychological problems. However, there are a number of reasons why nurses do not refer such patients.

◆ They may lack confidence in their ability to accurately detect mental health problems. Most oncology nurses have limited training in the detection of mental illness.

◆ Nurses dealing with life-threatening illnesses will prioritise the more critical aspects of care.

◆ Not all nurses have direct access to mental health consultation. Many have to go through junior medical staff or gain their support for a referral. Problems may occur at this stage, if the medical staff disagree or do not actively pursue the referral.

It is therefore worth developing strategies to encourage and support the appropriate referral of patients by oncology nurses (Box 6.3). This can include the use of a screening tool, the Hospital Anxiety and Depression Scale (HADS) developed for the detection of mental disorder in the physically ill (Zigmond & Snaith 1983).

Box 6.3 Strategies for encouraging oncology nurses to make referrals

◆ *Support nurse-to-nurse referral.* Given their extended contact with patients, ward-based nurses are ideally placed to detect psychological problems. In many areas, however, they are not able to make direct referral to mental health specialists. They may be obliged to go through a junior doctor who is less experienced and does not know the patients so well. This may inhibit the process of referral, though discussion of each case is desirable. Ideally, the nurses should be able to make referrals directly to a LMHN.

◆ *Accept low threshold for referral.* Nurses and other oncology staff should be encouraged to refer or discuss patients they have concerns about. This may initially lead to some inappropriate referrals but the process of discussing them will be educational for the oncology staff and help the LMHN to identify the range of psychosocial problems encountered in the clinical area.

◆ *Develop referral guidelines.* It may help to develop referral guidelines, so that staff have a clear idea of how to make the best use of the LMHN.

> **Box 6.3** Cont'd
>
> ◆ *Maintain high profile within the oncology unit.* Visibility and accessibility have been found to be valued by oncology nurses and to aid the process of referral (Roberts 1998). Ward-based nursing care often takes place in a very reactive way, responding to a variety of conflicting clinical and organisational pressures. Informal contacts are often as useful as formal meetings and LMHNs should consider dropping in to clinical areas at times when nurses are together, e.g. handover periods. All contacts have the potential to generate referrals.
>
> ◆ *Hold regular psychosocial meetings.* Regular meetings are a good way to get the whole team together to focus on psychosocial aspects of treatment and care. The traditional ward round or clinical meeting can be very medically and physically orientated and exclude any detailed discussion of psychosocial care. Some wards have additional meetings with a more limited membership, e.g. nursing staff, social worker, occupational therapist, LMHN, to discuss issues around patient and family coping, rehabilitation issues and primary care overlap. These can provide a good forum for discussing the best use of health and social care expertise and are also a useful forum for providing supervision.
>
> ◆ *Hold regular educational sessions for ward staff.* Education sessions are a good way for the ward staff to learn more about psychological reactions to cancer, common psychological problems like depression and the management of anxiety. It is best if the LMHN arranges a regular contribution to existing education programmes, so that new staff are reached and psychosocial aspects of care are integrated rather than being seen as separate.
>
> ◆ *Make use of screening tools.* Staff can be encouraged to use a screening tool like the HADS (Zigmond & Snaith 1983). This could be used to routinely screen all new admissions or, more practically, as a first level of assessment prior to involving the LMHN. Screening tools should not be used without prior education and ongoing supervision. Without these, staff may become reliant on the tool without continuing to develop their own skills.

Assessment of physical condition

The physical condition of the patient is an important part of the assessment. Most of the necessary information can be obtained from the medical notes or in discussion with medical or nursing staff. There are a number of factors to be considered that may affect the patient's mental state.

◆ Fatigue associated with the illness or the effects or treatment.

◆ Weakness and exhaustion after periods of infection or other complications.
◆ 'Patient burnout' and demoralisation after long and debilitating periods of treatment (Roberts & Davis 2000).
◆ Nutritional deficiency or metabolic imbalancess.
◆ Cognitive impairment secondary to systemic chemotherapy or cranial radiotherapy.
◆ The personal and social effects of altered body image.
◆ The level of pain or discomfort.
◆ Other side effects, e.g. nausea and vomiting.

There are also a number of drug treatments that may affect the patient's mental state.

◆ Opiates, commonly used for pain control, may cloud the patient's consciousness and in higher doses cause illusory and hallucinatory experiences. Discontinuation of opiates may precipitate a withdrawal syndrome.

◆ High-dose corticosteroids (e.g. prednisolone) used in chemotherapy can cause mood and sleep disturbance. These drugs are also used in lower doses to treat cerebral oedema or to induce a sense of well-being.

◆ Interferon is used in the treatment of some haematological conditions. It can cause a depression-like syndrome.

◆ Benzodiazepines are commonly used in oncology to sedate patients undergoing investigative procedures and are used in combination with other drugs to counteract nausea.

Assessment of mental health in the physically ill

Physical illness presents a number of problems in the diagnosis of mental illness. Many features of depression, for example, are commonly experienced. Most patients will at some time feel demoralised by their prospects, the changes in their lifestyle and loss of control over their lives. It is usual for patients to have rapid and unpredictable variations of mood at times of particular stress, e.g. diagnosis, relapse, awaiting test results. At times like this, anger and irritability, frustration, feelings of anxiety and uncertainty and indecisiveness are common. Many patients will entertain suicidal ideas, either out of a sense of demoralisation and loss of meaning or as a means of taking control of the course of their lives if the future looks bleak, undignified or painful. Some will have passive ideas of suicide; that is, they lose interest and do not want to cooperate with their treatment. In most cases, these feelings are temporary but they should be monitored. Cancer sufferers are at risk of suicide, especially those with cancers of the head and neck (Harris & Barraclough 1994). At times, there is a fine line between depression and despair, and assessment must take account of the patient's experience of illness and treatment (Roberts & Davis 2000).

Another problem is that the somatic features of depression are influenced by illness and cannot be accepted uncritically as diagnostic (see Endicott 1984). These include:

◆ sleep disturbance
◆ appetite disturbance and weight loss
◆ fatigue and reduced activity
◆ loss of sexual interest.

The assessment of depression therefore needs to focus on the following features:

◆ persistence of lowered mood and lack of reactivity to events
◆ depressed or fearful appearance
◆ . reduced enjoyment or interest or social withdrawal, in excess of the restrictions imposed by the illness
◆ depressive cognitions, i.e. feelings of guilt or worthlessness, brooding self-pity or pessimism, persistent suicidal ideas.

The assessment of anxiety needs to take into account complicating factors such as pain. Anxiety is a common feature of being a patient with cancer. Anyone who has received a diagnosis of cancer must face a life fraught with uncertainty. Having a life-threatening illness challenges all our basic assumptions about life. Many patients react by getting as much information as they can, whilst others will put all their trust in hospital staff. In addition to these long-term insecurities, specific health care situations can provoke anxiety:

◆ waiting for test results
◆ waiting to undergo investigations, operations or other treatments
◆ any outpatient appointments
◆ meeting new members of staff or being unsure who the staff will be
◆ having problems contacting key members of staff.

These factors need to be taken into account, particularly when a patient is referred for the management of anxiety.

Assessment of problems and adjustment

Assessment is best seen as an interactive process, following the chronological course of the illness and treatment but able to respond to factors identified as significant by the individual patient, even if they have no apparent direct link to the illness. Personal historical factors may have a particular significance in the patient's adjustment process. For example, the assessment may give the patient their first opportunity to disclose an unhappy or abusive childhood relationship to a professional and they may be unable to deal with the cancer until this has been addressed.

The assessment should open by asking the patient about their understanding of the reasons for referral and the role of the LMHN. They can then be asked to describe their current problems in their own terms. The following can be used as a guide to identifying key problems:

◆ current disabilities and dysfunction
◆ current treatment and expectations of outcome
◆ changes in lifestyle since the illness and treatment.

It is also necessary to understand the process of adjustment the patient has gone through so far and this should start in the period before diagnosis, so that the personal and social context at this time is known. This helps to identify the scale and nature of loss the illness has brought about. The following sequence can be used as a guide.

◆ An account of their life and lifestyle prior to diagnosis.
◆ How the illness came to light, i.e. the first symptoms.
◆ The initial medical contact, i.e. first contact with GP about the symptoms.
◆ Was there a delay in diagnosis? (This can have a profound effect on subsequent relationships with health care staff.)
◆ How was the diagnosis given and by whom?
◆ Previous experience of illness in self and others
◆ Initial reaction – patient.
◆ Initial reaction – family and friends.

This information should be put into a personal context by asking more general questions about the patient's background:

◆ family history
◆ personal history
◆ usual personality
◆ usual coping and personal resources
◆ social supports.

This not only helps the LMHN make a detailed assessment but it also has two major therapeutic functions.

◆ It is the first step in building rapport between LMHN and patient.
◆ For the patient, it puts their current circumstances into a personal historical context. Past experience of illness or other crises can be

reviewed, along with reflection on how the patient coped. Did these strategies work and can they be used again?

It is important to capture the patient's experience in his or her own terms as far as this is possible. Avoid introducing psychiatric terminology unless this helps to define problems in such a way that they can be helped. The patient's own language helps to clarify the meaning of their illness in the context of their life.

THERAPEUTIC APPROACHES

Approaches to treatment in psycho-oncology

A review by Fawzy et al (1995) proposes the following categories of intervention:

◆ *Education.* Education in the context of cancer care is a strategy for involving patients in the management of their illness, with the aim of reducing feelings of helplessness and loss of control. It usually involves educational programmes, giving information on the nature of cancers and their treatment, and can also include advice on coping, emotional reactions to cancer, and stress and anxiety management. It is sometimes referred to as psychoeducational care, particularly if it is given in conjunction with psychosocial support (Devine & Westlake 1995).

◆ *Behavioural training.* This includes a range of interventions aimed at changing the individual's response to illness or to the side effects of treatment, e.g. the nausea and vomiting associated with chemotherapy. It can include the following: relaxation training, progressive muscle relaxation, guided imagery or visualisation, hypnosis, deep breathing, biofeedback and meditation (Fawzy et al 1995). Oncology staff with further training can facilitate many of these, for example, relaxation and guided imagery.

◆ *Individual psychotherapy.* Counselling and therapy are often given to cancer patients in conjunction with other interventions, e.g. education or relaxation. The outcome of intervention can be measured in reduced psychiatric symptoms and psychological distress. Most of the interventions described follow a cognitive behavioural model (Lovejoy & Matteis 1997). Adjuvant Psychological Therapy is a form of cognitive behaviour therapy designed specifically for cancer patients. This focuses on the meaning of the cancer for the individual and mobilises their coping response to it (Greer et al 1992).

◆ *Group interventions.* Therapy is frequently given to cancer patients in a group format. This maximises the social support gained from fellow patients. There is some evidence for its effectiveness in reducing psychiatric symptoms and promoting coping (Bottomley 1996) and this may be enhanced when combined with education and stress management (Fawzy & Fawzy 1994).

Management of processes of adjustment

Assessment will help to identify the meaning of the cancer and its relationship with current and past experiences and place these within the current treatment context. This includes an awareness of the significance of the side effects of treatment, as Case study 6.1 illustrates.

Management of depression

Depression is common in cancer, but so are feelings of despondency and despair. Patients commonly experience an existential crisis, when they

---

Case Study 6.1 Management of processes of adjustment

Laura, 35, works as secretary for her husband, who runs a small business. This enables her to work at home and look after her daughter aged 4, when the child is not at nursery school. Her diagnosis of breast cancer came as a shock. She had always been very fit and active and could not understand how someone of her age could have a life-threatening illness. She and her husband had been making plans to expand the business. Laura was keen to carry on as normal, to support her husband's business and keep disruption to her daughter's life to a minimum. She returned to work as soon as possible after a partial mastectomy and was now going through chemotherapy.

She was referred when she reported feeling tearful and finding work increasingly difficult to sustain. She had also lost interest in sex and was irritable at home with the child. She felt she was neither a good wife nor mother and wondered if she should stop doing the secretarial work. On assessment, Laura did not meet the full criteria for depression. However, she reported fatigue and increasing problems concentrating and this was interfering with her work. She prided herself on her ability to work as well as being a housewife and mother. She became afraid that she could not fulfil her normal role and felt she was going to lose everything. Laura said she had always had low self-esteem and felt she had to prove herself by being successful at all she did.

In discussion with Laura, the LMHN identified that fatigue, poor concentration and irritability can be side effects of chemotherapy and that if this was the cause, these were likely to improve within a few weeks of ending chemotherapy. She was relieved to hear the change was not likely to be permanent and, together with her husband, decided to hire a temporary secretary. A schedule of activity was agreed that allowed her both additional rest time and regular exercise. Within a few weeks of ending chemotherapy, she was working as normal and had renewed interest in her sex life.

Case Study 6.2 Management of depression

Mary, 64, is married and has two adult children who live with their own families. She had a recent diagnosis of cancer of the colon which was treated with surgery but did not result in a colostomy. Her current treatment was radiotherapy. The clinical oncologist referred her because she was always tearful when she came for appointments. On assessment, she met the criteria for mild clinical depression, with anhedonia (loss of enjoyment of life) and social withdrawal, feelings of guilt and sleep disturbance. Antidepressants were discussed but she did not want to take them. Mary was reluctant to discuss the cancer but was very keen to talk about events in her family during the last 2 years. During this time, she had nursed her mother following a stroke and this had put a lot of pressure on her and the rest of the family. She had been concerned that her husband and children felt neglected. Previously, she had helped a lot with her grandchildren but she had been unable to do this during her mother's illness.

Over the course of six meetings, it became apparent that Mary felt very guilty that in the end her mother had to go into a nursing home and died there. She felt she had let her mother down and that she had also let the rest of her family down by neglecting them. She was now afraid that, should she become seriously ill, none of her family would want to look after her. She was encouraged to discuss her fears with her family and found that they had actually admired her dedication to her mother and all acknowledged that she had done as much as she could. Her eldest daughter said she would care for her in her own home if this became necessary. Communication within the family became more open and they were all more able to express their concerns about her illness. Mary's mood improved significantly and she was discharged.

may lose their sense of purpose and meaning in life. It is important to view depressive symptoms within the context of the individual's experience of illness, treatment and life. If antidepressant medication is used, it is also important to deal with any factors that are maintaining the depressive state.

Management of anxiety

Strategies to manage anxiety include:

◆ group psychoeducational methods, combining support with information
◆ written advice about anxiety and stress management made available through information centres or outpatient departments
◆ relaxation training, e.g. progressive muscle relaxation
◆ individual cognitive or behavioural interventions with phobic or panic states.

Any interventions that enhance personal control will aid anxiety management.

Case Study 6.3 Management of anxiety

Brian, a 20-year-old student, was having chemotherapy for Hodgkin's disease. He was studying at university when diagnosed and returned home to stay with his parents and have treatment. Initially, he did not seem interested in his illness and spent long periods on the phone to his student friends at the university. He was spending a lot of time in bed and his parents sometimes had to encourage him to get up to go for treatment. The chemotherapy nurse noticed he seemed to be very anxious prior to treatment and when he started hyperventilating she called for help from the LMHN.

On assessment, Brian said he missed his friends and worried about losing time at university. He disliked the hospital and being with sick people. He remembered little of what he had been told about Hodgkin's disease. He had a panic attack when he thought about people dying in hospital. Hodgkin's disease was discussed, how it was a serious illness but generally had a good prognosis. The LMHN suggested to Brian that his thoughts about dying people might reflect his own worries for the future. Brian said he thought he should find out more about the illness and the LMHN took him to the Cancer Information Centre to meet the staff and see what information was available. The LMHN also discussed anxiety management and showed Brian how to manage his breathing and deal with worrying thoughts. He borrowed a relaxation tape from the Information Centre.

The next time the LMHN saw Brian he said he had talked a lot with his parents, with all of them getting quite emotional at times. He was able to control his feelings of panic and had talked more about his illness and prognosis at his last outpatient appointment. Brian declined any more appointments.

PRACTICE GUIDELINES

The first priority of mental health liaison in oncology is to establish collaborative working relationships with oncology staff. There are a number of key relationships.

◆ *Ward-based oncology nurses.* Oncology wards can be very demanding environments to work in and staff will often request or accept supervision, usually in a group format. These nurses are a potentially rich source of referrals and ideally should have direct access to a LMHN, so that they can make nurse-to-nurse referrals.

◆ *Junior medical staff.* These are often the medical staff who are in closest contact with the patient and work very closely with ward nurses. In some areas, referrals will go through them. They will manage some straightforward cases of anxiety and depression with mental health support.

◆ *Consultant and other senior medical staff,* who will include:
 – surgeons who work with cancer patients
 – clinical oncologists (specialists in radiotherapy)
 – medical oncologists (specialists in chemotherapy)

> – haematologists (who treat haematological malignancies, e.g. leukaemia, lymphoma).

Medical consultants are key people in determining the psychosocial orientation of a clinical team. Clinical protocols and referral guidelines should be devised in cooperation with them.

◆ *Specialist nursing staff* (e.g. breast care nurses, head and neck specialists, colorectal specialists). These staff provide continuity of care for patients as they go through long-term processes of treatment, sometimes involving liaison between several different clinical teams or specialities. They often have a strong psychosocial orientation and many have acquired counselling skills. They are very well placed to detect psychological problems in their patients and they need both supervision and access to mental health consultation.

◆ *Palliative care staff.* Palliative care teams (including medical and nursing staff and sometimes other therapists, e.g. occupational therapists) may get involved at early stages of treatment, providing a range of practical and emotional support, including symptom control and family support. Palliative care teams will often manage straightforward cases of anxiety and depression without involving mental health specialists. Macmillan nurses, specialist palliative care nurses who are usually community based, are trained in counselling and family support. They will benefit from access to mental health consultation and supervision.

◆ *Occupational therapists, physiotherapists, dieticians, social workers.* These health and social care specialists are often actively involved in the process of rehabilitation and may get to know the patient and family well. They can be valuable allies in providing integrated care.

◆ *Therapy radiographers.* Although radiographers may only work for brief treatment sessions with patients, they are with them at particularly vulnerable times. Some radiographers specialise in giving information and others will have training in counselling.

Fitting in

Mental health personnel may feel they are entering an alien environment when they start work in oncology. LMHNs who have trained as general nurses will have an advantage in that they will be more familiar with the general hospital environment. Some wards, for example surgical wards, can be very hectic and primarily oriented to acute care. Mental health specialists may be expected to provide quick solutions to complex psychosocial problems.

Whereas quick solutions may not be available, it is possible to provide a clear assessment and management plan that colleagues will be able to integrate into their own management of the patient. Other wards may be more psychosocially oriented but most ward environments are very busy and nursing staff are frequently frustrated in their attempts to spend uninterrupted time with vulnerable or distressed patients. This may result in unsuitable referrals unless the LMHN establishes clear criteria for referral. Staff will then also need help to clarify what they can achieve with their own limited resources. This can be done through regular supervision sessions. There are a number of common differences of expectation about what sort of problem should be referred to a mental health team (Box 6.4).

Box 6.4 Common problems of expectation of mental health care in oncology

◆ *Patients need specialist help to come to terms with diagnosis.* The majority of patients need time, information and social support in order to deal with the issues raised by their diagnosis. In the earlier stages of adjustment, it is important to reinforce existing coping strategies and social support rather than introduce a new professional. Patients also need to get to know the staff they will be working with and who will be answering their questions about the illness and treatment over the weeks and months to come. If problems of adjustment are severe or persistent, however, intervention may be needed.

◆ *Distressed patients need to see a mental health specialist.* Ward-based nurses may find it frustrating and upsetting having to deal with distressed and tearful patients when they are busy or feel ill equipped to help. They may see the mental health specialist as a source of support for these patients. However, this is not a good use of limited specialist time, nor is it necessary to 'medicalise' what is often a healthy process of adjustment. Nurses need to be aware, however, that unresolved distress or tearfulness that is long term may be a sign of mental disorder.

◆ *Depression is understandable in cancer patients and depressed patients do not need referral for specialist help.* The cause of depression is less important than how it can be helped. Given the risks associated with untreated depression (e.g. non-compliance with treatment, suicide) oncology staff should be encouraged to have a low threshold for referring depressed patients.

◆ *All patients benefit from counselling.* There is no evidence that this is the case. Medical settings can be rather prescriptive in their approach to problems. Coping and adjustment are very individual and many patients will primarily use either their own personal resources or their family and friends. It is unlikely that all those who are at risk of coping poorly will accept help (Worden & Weisman 1980). Oncology staff need help to prioritise those patients who would benefit from counselling and this includes offering suitable patients a choice.

◆ *Patients whose home circumstances are difficult need mental health intervention.* Sometimes psychosocial problems are not adequately assessed and there is an assumption that mental health personnel can help any problem. Many psychosocial problems will be better helped by a social worker or primary care team. Effective teamwork and interdisciplinary review are therefore very important to the assessment process.

Time and space

Inpatient work in oncology can be affected by the unpredictability of ward activity. Most wards have some regular routines and it is necessary to become familiar with them. However, these are always subject to change. Ward rounds or clinical meetings can be disrupted by clinical demands and attendance by nursing staff in particular can be unpredictable. Appointments with patients on wards can be disrupted by changes in the patient's physical condition, unforeseen investigations or changes to treatment schedules. It is usually best to deal directly with the patient's named nurse for that shift, who will have an awareness of likely changes to routine. This can mean phoning the ward earlier on the day of the intended visit, to save a wasted journey.

Outpatient work is usually more predictable. However, it is necessary to plan appointments around the patient's treatment schedule and this can change at short notice. For example, a complication like an infection may lead to an emergency admission to hospital. In the rush, the patient and their family may forget to tell the LMHN about the admission. Physical health priorities usually override psychosocial ones. They may also assume health care staff are constantly in touch with each other about changes of plan but this is not the case. Also, courses of treatment can be quite complex and time consuming and it is not unusual for patients to mix different appointments up.

Finding space for an interview can be a problem. Most wards have somewhere a patient can be seen but this is not always a designated interview room. In some areas, only the ward office is available and this is frequently in use. Even if there is a designated room, it may also be used by ward staff to see patients and relatives or by medical staff for outpatient work. Access to rooms may therefore need negotiation. This is helped by making it clear to the ward team that private space is a necessary part of the assessment process. Seeing a patient at the bedside is only suitable if they are in a single room.

Issues of confidentiality need to be clarified at an early stage of any working relationship with oncology teams. Information needs to be shared so that the mental health and oncology teams can work as an integrated whole. However, mental health work is psychologically and socially invasive in ways that oncology work is not. Patients may confide details, for example about their life and relationships before their illness, that are not relevant to the treatment of cancer. Some patients who are facing death will feel the need to unburden themselves of feelings and events from long ago. It is important to let the patient know which information will be shared with the oncology team and which will be withheld.

CONCLUSION

Cancer is a common, serious illness with numerous associated psychosocial problems. Effective mental health liaison in cancer care (psycho-oncology) needs to actively involve oncology staff and other therapists. The experience of cancer is very individual and care should be taken to avoid making assumptions about how a patient will react to it. Assessment should apply generic mental health skills to the specific patient, their illness and treatment and their social context.

QUESTIONS FOR DISCUSSION

- ◆ What role is there for mental health liaison teams in improving communication in oncology?
- ◆ How can we work collaboratively to improve the quality of psychosocial care given by oncology nurses?
- ◆ How can complementary therapists be integrated into the work of psycho-oncology teams?
- ◆ How do we decide what is a normal reaction to cancer?
- ◆ What is the difference between depression and despair?

ANNOTATED BIBLOGRAPHY

The experience of cancer

Costain Schou K, Hewison J 1999 Experiencing Cancer. Quality of Life in Treatment. Open University Press, Buckingham

Results of a study of quality of life in cancer, focused on the social aspects of treatment. Many insights for professionals into the patient's experience. Includes a stimulating critique of psycho-oncology.

Diamond J 1998 C. Because cowards get cancer too ... Vermillion, London

A personal account of cancer, written by a journalist.

Psycho-oncology

Barraclough J 1999 Cancer and Emotion. A practical guide to psycho-oncology, 3rd edn. John Wiley, Chichester

A good introduction to the subject and one that patients will find very accessible.

Holland J C 1998 Psycho-oncology. Oxford University Press, Oxford
A broad-ranging and comprehensive text from the USA. The essential reference book for psycho-oncology teams.

Psycho-oncology.
A journal published six times a year by John Wiley, Chichester.

Assessment

Endicott J 1984 Measurement of depression in patients with cancer. Cancer 53(10):2243–2248

Complementary therapies

Daniel R 2000 Living with Cancer. Robinson, London

Describes the work of the Bristol Cancer Help Centre. Also discusses the integration of complementary and mainstream medical approaches. Describes elements of the Bristol approach, such as diet and the channelling of energy.

REFERENCES

Barraclough J 1999 Cancer and emotion. A practical guide to psycho-oncology, 3rd edn. John Wiley, Chichester

Bond S 1983 Nurses' communications with cancer patients. In: Wilson-Barnett J (ed) Nursing research: ten studies in patient care. John Wiley, Chichester

Bottomley A 1996 Group cognitive therapy interventions with cancer patients: a review of the literature. Eur J Cancer Care 5:143–146

Brennan J, Sheard T 1994 Psychosocial support and therapy in cancer care. Eur J Palliat Care 1:136–139

Costain Schou K, Hewison J 1999 Experiencing cancer. Open University Press, Buckingham

De Haes J C J M, Van Knippenberg F C E, Neijt J P 1990 Measuring psychological and physical distress in cancer patients: structure and application of the Rotterdam Symptom Checklist. Br J Cancer 62:1034–1038

Department of Health 1995 A policy framework for commissioning cancer services. A report by the Expert Advisory Group on Cancer to the Chief Medical Officers of England and Wales. Department of Health, London

Derogatis L R, Morrow G R, Fetting J et al 1983 The prevalence of psychiatric disorders among cancer patients. JAMA 249(6):751–757

Devine E C, Westlake S K 1995 The effects of psychoeducational care provided to adults with cancer: meta-analysis of 116 studies. Oncol Nurs Forum 22(9):1369–1381

Edwards M J 1999 Providing psychological support to cancer patients. Prof Nurse 15(1):9–13

Endicott J 1984 Measurement of depression in patients with cancer. Cancer 53(10):2243–2248

Fawzy F I, Fawzy N W 1994 A structured psychoeducational intervention for cancer patients. Gen Hosp Psychiatry 16:149–192

Fawzy F I, Fawzy N W, Arndt L A, Pasnau R O 1995 Critical review of psychosocial interventions in cancer care. Arch Gen Psychiatry 52:100–113

Fincannon J L 1995 Analysis of psychiatric referrals and interventions in an oncology population. Oncol Nurs Forum 22(1):87–92

Fromm K, Andrykowski M, Hunt J 1996 Positive and negative psychosocial sequelae of bone marrow transplantation: implications for quality of life assessment. J Behav Med 19(3):221–240

Gardner R 1992 Psychological care of neuro-oncology patients and their families. Br J Nurs 1(11):553–556

Germain C P H 1979 The cancer unit: an ethnography. Nursing Resources, Wakefield, MA

Greer S, Moorey S, Baruch J D R et al 1992 Adjuvant psychological therapy for patients with cancer: a prospective randomised trial. BMJ 304:675–680

Hardman A, Maguire P, Crowther D 1989 The recognition of psychiatric morbidity on a medical ward. J Psychosom Res 33(2):235–239

Harris E C, Barraclough B M 1994 Suicide as an outcome for medical disorders. Medicine 73(6):281–298

Heaven C M, Maguire P 1996 Training hospice nurses to elicit patient concerns. J Adv Nurs 23:280–286.

Lovejoy N C, Matteis M 1997 Cognitive-behavioral interventions to manage depression in patients with cancer: research and theoretical initiatives. Cancer Nurs 20(3):155–167

Maguire P 1995 Psychosocial interventions to reduce affective disorders in cancer patients: research priorities. Psychooncology 4:113–119

Maguire P, Tait A, Brooke M, Thomas C, Sellwood R 1980 Effect of counselling on the psychiatric morbidity associated with mastectomy. BMJ 218:1268–1271

McArdle J M C, George W D, McArdle C S et al 1996 Psychological support for patients undergoing breast cancer surgery: a randomised study. BMJ 312:813–816

McIntosh J 1977 Communication and awareness in a cancer ward. Croom Helm, London

Pasacreta J V, Massie M J 1990 Nurses' reports of psychiatric complications in patients with cancer. Oncol Nurs Forum 17(3):347–353

Roberts D 1998 Nurses' perceptions of the role of liaison mental health nurse. Nurs Times 94(43):56–57

Roberts D, Davis R 2000 A man with head and neck cancer: a case of depression, patient burnout, or despair? Prim Care Cancer 20(4):41–43

Roberts D, Snowball J 1999 Psychosocial care in oncology nursing: a study of social knowledge. J Adv Nurs 8:39–47

Roberts R, Fallowfield L 1990 Who supports the cancer counsellors? Nurs Times 86(36):32–34

Tunmore R 1989 Liaison psychiatric nursing in oncology. Nurs Times 85(33):54–56

Tunmore R 1990 Liaison psychiatry. Setting the pace. Nurs Times 86(34):29–32

Van Fleet S K, Hughes M K 1996 Psychiatric CNS consultation model in a medical setting. Clin Nurse Spec 10(4):204–211

Wilkinson S 1991 Factors which influence how nurses communicate with cancer patients. J Adv Nurs 16:677–688

Worden J W, Weisman A D 1980 Do cancer patients really want counselling? Gen Hosp Psychiatry 2:100–103

Zigmond A S, Snaith R P 1983 The Hospital Anxiety and Depression Scale. Acta Psychiat Scand 67:361–370

RESOURCES

There is a large number of professional and charitable groups nationally that promote the development of cancer services, provide support and represent the needs of cancer patients. Here are details of a few of the main ones.

Bristol Cancer Help Centre
Grove House
Cornwallis Grove
Clifton
Bristol BS8 4PG
Tel: 0117 980 9500
A centre specialising in complementary approaches to cancer and its treatment.

British Psychosocial Oncology Society
Membership secretary:
Bill Fox
Primary Health Centre
Wallsend Health Centre
The Green, Wallsend
Newcastle-upon-Tyne NE28 7PB
Tel: 0191 234 5356
Website: *www.bpos.org.uk*
A group promoting knowledge of the psychological and social aspects of
cancer among health care professionals working with cancer patients.

CancerBACUP
3 Bath Place
Rivington Street
London EC2A 3DR
Information freephone: 0808 800 1234
An information service for cancer patients and their families and friends.
Telephone information, booklets and factsheets available.

Cancerlink
11–21 Northdown Street
London N1 9BN
Tel: 0207 833 2818
Groups line: 0207 520 2603
email: *cancerlink@cancerlink.org.uk*
A national resource for linking with self-help and support groups. Also
publishes booklets on living with cancer.

Macmillan Cancer Relief
Anchor House
15–19 Britten Street
London SW3 3TZ
Tel: 0207 351 7811
email: *information_line@macmillan.org.uk*
A major national charitable organisation for supporting and developing
cancer services.

National Cancer Alliance
PO Box 579
Oxford OX4 1LB
Tel: 01865 793566
email: nationalcanceralliance@btinternet.com
The NCA is an alliance of cancer patients, their relatives and friends and health
professionals, campaigning for better cancer services throughout the UK.

7

Liaison mental health nursing and HIV and AIDS

Jerome Wright Angela Lavery

KEY ISSUES

- The psychological needs of people with HIV are significantly influenced by their social context
- The impact of HIV can result in psychological and social crises at any point from diagnosis to bereavement
- Liaison mental health nurses offer a valuable contribution to the complex care required for individuals affected by HIV
- A small but significant number of people infected by HIV experience HIV-related brain impairment which can have profound psychological consequences for individuals and their carers
- Worries about HIV infection can occur for individuals awaiting HIV testing and may persist despite a negative test result
- A few people make false claims to be HIV positive and this may be a feature of underlying psychological difficulties
- People experiencing mental health problems are more likely to engage in behaviours which may increase their risk of acquiring HIV

INTRODUCTION

This chapter aims to present an overview of the current research and issues in HIV and liaison mental health nursing care and to provide guidance on the assessment and therapeutic approaches for the many and varied mental health problems experienced by people affected by HIV and AIDS. Some thought will also be paid to future challenges. A level of familiarity with HIV infection and disease progression is assumed, although references are provided in the annotated bibliography for those readers requiring further information. It is also important to recognise, however, that knowledge and treatment of HIV infection are rapidly developing and interventions need to reflect such changes.

At the beginning of the 21st century HIV remains a highly stigmatised disease and it is this, together with the complexity of client need, which has significantly influenced the development of innovative, sensitive and skilled liaison mental health nursing approaches in responding to the needs of this particular client group. The liaison mental health nurse (LMHN) is therefore required to become familiar with a broad agenda of health issues arising from physical, psychological and social influences. These include disease progression and infectivity, psychological issues such as grief, loss, coping, changes in body image, dealing with stigma and isolation and diverse social issues such as working with alienated, marginalised and stigmatised people, legal and ethical dilemmas such as confidentiality, suicide, assisted suicide, euthanasia, living wills and access to care. In the face of such complexities, a liaison mental health nursing model has proved highly effective in addressing the profound psychological, physical and social difficulties prevalent in HIV and enabling a partnership with HIV team colleagues in general hospital settings to create an effective and holistic approach to care.

HIV EPIDEMIOLOGY AND THE EMERGING LIAISON MENTAL HEALTH NURSING RESPONSE

When tracing the first presentations of what became the HIV pandemic (Centers for Disease Control 1981, Schilts 1987), including the epidemiological accident that homosexual men and intravenous drug users and their partners were the first groups of people identified as having been exposed to HIV, it is perhaps not surprising that an accompanying epidemic of stigma also arose (Herek & Glunt 1988, Weitz 1990). Groups of predominantly young adults, already stigmatised by society and subject to all kinds of prejudicial acts and omissions, were further marginalised when faced with an infectious life-threatening disease. The way in which such groups responded is testament to their tremendous courage and organisation.

Nevertheless, unique challenges remain including, for instance, dealing with life choices such as sexual behaviour in spite of continuous infectivity, the frequent tendency for peers to provide care and support rather than biological families and issues of multiple bereavement, which affects individuals and their communities (Lennon et al 1990, Nord 1996, Paradis 1992, Weiss 1989). Although the work of such groups has been to educate society about the risks and implications of HIV for everyone, with increasing challenges to raise awareness for heterosexuals as rising numbers of women, men and children become infected with HIV (AIDS Letter 2000), it is also important to ensure that attention and resources are not diverted from vulnerable groups. Such groups include the poor, the homeless, people from overseas, drug users and their partners and homosexual men, who remain the largest UK population group infected (AIDS Letter 2000). The implication for mental health nurses therefore remains that the social context in which people with HIV find themselves has a profound influence upon both their psychological and physical health.

The requirement for effective psychiatric and mental health support services has been acknowledged since the outset of the HIV pandemic, but overall the UK's mental health nursing response has remained somewhat piecemeal and limited. The poor provision of mental health services, including drug dependency services, remains a problem throughout Europe (Catalan 1993), and is mirrored by the uneven distribution and development of liaison mental health services throughout the UK. This is also reflected in the provision of HIV services, with an emphasis upon large metropolitan areas where generally there are greater numbers of people infected with HIV. In spite of this, there are examples of innovative and established systems of mental health nursing integrated within HIV care teams (Sumpter et al 1993, Wright 1992) and evidence to support the growing recognition of HIV issues in mental health nursing throughout the UK (Firn 1992, Willis 1997).

One of the greatest challenges for mental health nurses working in HIV is the social context of the epidemic, which has profound influences upon both physical and psychological health and the way in which care is organised. In practice, the LMHN may be the only mental health professional working in an essentially physically orientated care environment and must remain aware of the social context in which care is provided. As in other areas of liaison mental health nursing practice, the process can be divided into two distinct spheres: direct and indirect care (Roberts 1997).

Direct care

Providing client-centred services, which include the assessment, planning, treatment and evaluation of mental health nursing care for clients infected and affected by HIV. This is done in collaboration with other professionals in the HIV multidisciplinary team and other mental health services.

Indirect care

Incorporates promoting, supporting and advising upon the mental health interventions of other health professionals, without direct involvement with the client, which can include case discussions and clinical supervision.

THE PSYCHOSOCIAL IMPACT OF HIV

The knowledge of a person's HIV-positive status sets in motion what some have called the 'rollercoaster' of HIV. Assumed certainties are pushed aside as almost constant challenges and crises present themselves. These crises derive not just from physical but also from psychological and social influences. Clearly, people with HIV are not immune to normal life stresses, be they related to family, relationship, job, study, housing or financial issues. However, in addition to these, a number of psychological and social crisis points have been identified which trace the process or progression of HIV disease and may result in profound psychological distress and mental health problems.

Diagnosis

Not surprisingly, the first crisis point occurs following the diagnosis of HIV, with its implications for the person, their future and relationships in the past, present and future. The response to this is, of course, also affected by the person's expectations of the HIV test result, the degree of disease progression at the point of diagnosis and their perception of the meaning of being HIV positive.

Disclosure

The second crisis often follows immediately after receiving the diagnosis but may become an issue at any point in the person's life. Disclosure of HIV status raises questions of who to tell, who not to tell and when and how to do this. The stigmatising nature of HIV disease impacts most strongly and frequently leads to secrecy or 'cover stories' being used to prevent disclosure and the damaging effects of the associated stigma and prejudice. Although it is extremely rare for people with HIV never to disclose their status to anyone, selective disclosure is the norm and may even preclude disclosure to close family and friends. The person with HIV constantly has to weigh up whether they can risk telling a person about their HIV status and whether that person will in turn either keep their confidence or disclose this to others. A constant vigilance is also required to prevent accidental disclosure at work, in social settings or at health-care facilities.

Commencement of treatment

The next crisis frequently occurs when evidence of defective immune functioning or increased viral activity becomes evident. These may be indicated by blood tests showing a reduced CD4 count or increased viral load. Even where a person may not have noticed physical changes, evidence from investigations can cause catastrophic reactions, particularly where a person has made lifestyle changes to try to maintain their health. Such changes may include healthy eating, resting, taking prescribed medication accurately and exercising. A loss of the sense of control with the accompanying fear of impending ill health occurs frequently and may result in clinic phobia, a withdrawal from contact with carers or health-related hypervigilance associated with a constant need and search for reassurance.

Whilst the advent of combination HIV antiretroviral therapy has increased life expectancy and improved physical health for many HIV-positive individuals, it has also created a significant amount of psychological difficulties. These include treatment issues concerning 'whether', 'when' or 'how' to manage the drug regime and anxieties inherent in continued health monitoring and the possibilities of treatment 'failure'. Even if effective, new concerns may emerge concerning relationships, self-image, employment, finance and dealing with 'living again' (Anderson et al 2000).

Commencement of symptoms

A similar crisis point can accompany the onset of physical symptoms of HIV disease. For most people with HIV, this represents a significant change in their perception of themselves and their health and often requires a reevaluation of their previous coping style to fit this new identity. Problems arising from a changing body image, in particular weight loss, become most marked at this point. Practical difficulties also arise, such as taking medication according to the strict regimes required and indeed doing so unobtrusively, without drawing attention that might reveal their HIV status to others. Unease within both this and the previous crisis point can lead to reactions such as an avoidance of viral load testing or rejecting or not adhering to treatment regimes.

Late-stage disease

Fatigue from repeated illnesses can take its toll upon people's coping abilities and can lead to despair, as their ability to remain physically healthy is seen as beyond their control. As the possibility of death arises, feelings relating to grieving begin to present. This may include a need to resolve issues and conflicts in personal and interpersonal life and as a result, this can become a highly charged and stressful time, with both physical and emotional needs becoming heightened.

Bereavement

Finally, issues associated with bereavement itself can produce complex and complicated grief reactions. This is exacerbated by features particular to HIV, including the death of predominantly young people, fears around infectivity and contagion and the effects of stigma and isolation for those left behind, who are frequently experiencing multiple bereavements and who may also be HIV positive themselves.

This catalogue of potential crisis points may challenge us to wonder how people cope under such pressure. The resilience, coping abilities and style of people with HIV appear to be both significant and complex. Increased purposeful activity together with a reduced avoidance of HIV issues appears to improve both clients' outlook and prognosis (Kurdek & Siesky 1990, Remien et al 1992).

Broadly, the incidence of mental disorders in HIV appears to increase as HIV disease progresses (Catalan et al 1995). Therefore, while some people with asymptomatic HIV infection do experience significant psychological or adjustment problems, the proportion increases in line with the severity of illness and disability. Affective disorders, particularly depression, commonly present as reactions to loss or the fear of loss. Suicidal thoughts are not uncommon in people with HIV and whilst studies of rates of completed suicide require careful analysis, most tend to show an increased risk (Pugh et al 1993). Anxiety frequently manifests itself through generalised fears or panic attacks. Hypochondriasis is not uncommon, with a preoccupation with physical health problems and persistent and intrusive thoughts of their own death. This can lead to a desperate search for reassurance and a preoccupation with adherence to treatment or a concern for how those around them, including children, will cope without them. Sexual problems may result from the psychological reactions of guilt, reduced self-esteem and relationship problems, as well as physical diseases (Catalan et al 1995). Likewise, drug and alcohol use, if not already a major factor, may become significant as ways of coping under such pressures (Ellis et al 1994, Weiss 1989).

An awareness that partners, carers and children, whether infected or not, have been shown to experience similar psychological reactions reinforces the LMHN's role in assessing the needs of all involved in the person's care. The phenomenon of multiple bereavement may also play an important part in the mental health of people whose friends and communities are infected with HIV, leading not only to psychological distress but also to risk-taking behaviour (Barroso 1997, Lennon et al 1990, Sherr 1995).

LIAISON MENTAL HEALTH NURSING
ASSESSMENT

Whether the LMHN is assessing the needs of the client directly or through discussion with a consultee, a number of critical factors need to be determined. For the purposes of this discussion, these can be separated into physical, psychological and social aspects of the client's life, although in practice they are inextricably linked.

The LMHN is required to ascertain the following information in the past, present and future contexts. In addition to discussion with the client, it may also be useful to obtain information from partners, family, friends, carers and other statutory and non-statutory agencies involved in the client's care. It is essential, however, that this is discussed with the client and their consent obtained prior to involvement or discussion with third parties. Diagnostic checklists and scales may be used and can be extremely valuable in assessing the nature and extent of difficulties. In addition to providing a baseline against which progress can be measured, they can also assist in evaluating the effectiveness of interventions. Knowledge of crisis points may also facilitate discussion of needs and assist in reaching a joint formulation of the problem.

Physical

◆ Date of first HIV-positive test and/or probable time of infection.
◆ Previous and current health problems – HIV related and others, including results from CD4 and viral load tests.
◆ Daily activities/functioning – sleep, appetite, elimination, breathing, mobility, pain, sensory deficits, dependence level.
◆ Current medication (including antiretroviral medication) – dose, frequency, commencement dates, response and side effects, adherence and treatment plans.
◆ Drug allergies.
◆ Substance use.

Psychological

◆ Reasons for referral/presentation.
◆ Behaviour and appearance.
◆ Thoughts/feelings:
  – mood and level of risk of self-harm
  – anxiety level and panic

- knowledge of illness and diagnosis
- insight, coping strategies and their effectiveness
- health concerns and anxieties
- satisfaction/concerns regarding care and support.
◆ Previous psychiatric history.

Social

◆ Relationships, dynamics and significant life events.
◆ Domestic circumstances.
◆ Employment and finances.
◆ Sexual health.
◆ Social networks and interests.
◆ Others aware/unaware of diagnosis.
◆ Others involved in care – professionals, formal and informal carers.

LIAISON MENTAL HEALTH NURSING INTERVENTIONS

Fundamental to the practice of liaison mental health nursing is the promotion and sustaining of the nurse–client relationship. As we have seen, this can be challenging within the climate of personal crisis, the way health care is organised and the context of HIV in society generally. While the LMHN may specialise in specific counselling techniques derived from particular models, the enactment through nursing of a biopsychosocial or integrative approach is essential to be able to respond adequately and effectively to the range of problems presenting in relation to HIV.

For the LMHN practising in the field of HIV care, it is often necessary to work as a 'maverick' (Sutton & Smith 1995) at an advanced level of nursing. In this way, just as the LMHN's work spans acute hospital, mental health and community settings, it acknowledges the contributions of medicine, psychology and sociology and yet maintains the client's needs as the central focus of care.

Using advanced interpersonal and communication skills, the LMHN has an excellent foundation to work with this client group and can utilise a broad range of therapeutic interventions. Assessment and monitoring of the client's mental state, including risk assessment and response to any prescribed medication, is required in all therapeutic relationships. However, further specific interventions should relate to both the client's needs, research evidence of effectiveness and the nurse's level of skill and experience. This may involve practical support, liaison and information-giving skills as well as psychotherapeutic techniques (Wright 1994).

Possible interventions are indicated below but these are by no means exhaustive. They may either represent approaches within the repertoire of the LMHN or be a source of information from which to make appropriate referrals.

◆ Problem-solving approaches, e.g. Green & McCreaner (1996)
◆ Psychoanalytical approaches, e.g. Winiarski (1991)
◆ Cognitive behavioural approaches, e.g. Auerbach et al (1992)
◆ Interpersonal psychotherapy approaches, e.g. Markowitz et al (1993)
◆ Systemic/family therapy approaches, e.g. Bor et al (1992)
◆ Psychoeducational approaches, e.g. Antoni (1991)

It is important for the LMHN to reflect both in and upon practice, with critical appraisal of both their role and the interventions delivered. In addition to direct clinical involvement, other roles include supervision, consultation, liaison and education (Roberts 1997). The LMHN is also frequently required to provide psychological support to partners, carers, family and friends of people who are infected with HIV and who may be experiencing psychological difficulties themselves.

Case Study 7.1 Liaison mental health nursing interventions

After a period of acute physical illness, David was diagnosed HIV positive. Following treatment of physical symptoms and commencing antiviral therapy, his health improved and he returned to work. David initially appeared to be coping well and adjusting to his diagnosis but after 2 months he started experiencing generalised anxiety symptoms and panic attacks. These were particularly bad at work and he eventually had to take time off sick. David stayed at home most days, felt uneasy in the company of friends and would avoid going out whenever possible. He would wake in the morning feeling anxious and agitated and became increasingly irritable with his partner. He began to worry about his health and would interpret anxiety symptoms as evidence of the progression of his HIV disease. David began to check his body for further evidence of any symptoms and became fanatical about diet and exercise.

His partner threatened to leave if he did not get any help and David therefore referred himself to the LMHN. Assessment revealed that David had not addressed many of the issues relating to his HIV status and had a tendency to deny and avoid these. The worries about his health were related to the suddenness of his initial illness and his overwhelming fear that his death was imminent. The LMHN offered David an opportunity to express and explore his fears and taught him anxiety management techniques. Alternative and more effective coping strategies were discussed, applied and reviewed. Finally David's fear that his partner would leave him was addressed through relationship work which involved his partner.

> **Case Study 7.2** Liaison mental health nursing interventions
>
> Sarah had been diagnosed HIV positive 11 years ago. Initially she simply got on with life but was finding this increasingly difficult. She felt low in mood most days, with this being particularly bad in the mornings. She had little energy or motivation and was unable to concentrate on work. She was unhappy in her relationship with her partner but felt unable to address this and believed that if she ended the relationship, she would spend the rest of her life alone. Sarah was lacking confidence and her self-esteem was low. This was made worse by a marked weight loss and altered body image. She believed others could simply look at her and know she was HIV positive. On many occasions Sarah contemplated ending her life but believed this was sinful and felt she did not have the courage to act upon her thoughts.
>
> The LMHN had difficulty engaging Sarah in psychological work as she believed she was a 'lost cause' and continually made reference to the fact that she was wasting the nurse's time. However, by allowing time to listen and explore Sarah's experiences a trusting, therapeutic relationship was established and eventually the nurse was able to encourage Sarah to agree to an appointment with the liaison psychiatrist. Sarah was started on antidepressant medication and within 3 weeks her mood improved significantly. This enabled the LMHN to use a cognitive behavioural approach to explore and challenge many of Sarah's negative thoughts and beliefs. Consequently, while some fears for the future remained, Sarah's level of functioning and quality of life improved and she made an active decision to become more open with her partner about her worries, with a view to improving their relationship.

HIV-RELATED BRAIN IMPAIRMENT

A recognition that HIV directly affects brain functioning was highlighted in the early years of the HIV pandemic (Price & Brew 1988), although the exact method by which the virus causes neuronal damage is unclear. Despite this, the range of HIV-related functional problems has been widely described within classification systems (American Academy of Neurology AIDS Task Force 1991, WHO 1990). These problems include memory impairment and a decline in intellectual abilities and motor function.

There are disparities in the data and information relating to the incidence of HIV-related brain impairment (Catalan et al 1995) but the number of HIV-positive individuals experiencing mild to severe HIV-related brain impairment appears to range from 8% to 16% (WHO 1990). Cofactors, such as age and diet, host factors, including previous head injury, drug or alcohol use and the levels of HIV concentration may also affect an individual's potential for developing HIV-related brain impairment.

It is important to recognise that there are many causes of cognitive impairment in a person with HIV infection, many of which are not a direct effect of HIV. Where the onset of cognitive or functional difficulties is acute, the cause is most likely to be opportunistic bacterial, viral, fungal or parasitic infections, toxic confusional states or cerebrovascular lesions. Other possible causes include cerebral tumours, the effects of medication, substance use, depression or anxiety. Fatigue from repeated illnesses may also exacerbate these difficulties. Therefore, consideration of differential diagnoses is essential, particularly as a significant number of these alternative diagnoses can be successfully treated or managed. HIV-related brain impairment must therefore be a diagnosis of exclusion.

It is clear that significant brain impairment in both adults and children is rare in the absence of significant immunological decline or other physical illnesses; therefore HIV-related brain impairment is mostly confined to late-stage HIV disease. This is supported by evidence of the absence of brain impairment in asymptomatic HIV-positive people, in contrast to the poor prognosis once HIV-related brain impairment is diagnosed.

The reasons why some HIV-positive people do not experience brain impairment are unclear, although it is possible that HIV-related brain impairment may manifest in all HIV-positive individuals given time and the absence of any AIDS-related life-threatening illnesses. This raises the question of whether more HIV-related brain impairment will be seen in the future as the advent of combination anti-HIV therapy increases life expectancy. Conversely, evidence suggests that some antiviral treatments, in particular zidovudine, reduce the likelihood of HIV-related brain impairment (Muma et al 1997). Although certain antiviral drugs (some nucleoside analogues and non-nucleoside reverse transcriptase inhibitors) have been shown to cross the blood–brain barrier, none to date has proven effective in the treatment of HIV-related brain impairment (AIDS Manual 1999). Whilst it is too early to comment on the effects of other new antivirals, it is possible that other treatments which penetrate and cross the blood–brain barrier may also reduce the likelihood of HIV-related brain impairment.

For the present, HIV-related brain impairment remains a physical reality to a significant minority of HIV-positive people, whilst for the majority it represents a psychological threat.

Assessment

Accurate diagnosis of presenting problems is achieved through liaison mental health nursing assessment of psychosocial and neuropsychiatric functioning. The LMHN is frequently able to acquire the client's or carer's description of the onset and history of problems. A psychological assessment may uncover signs of disorientation, confusion, memory lapses, forgetfulness or alterations in state of consciousness. There may also be signs of focal weakness or loss of function, visual changes, headache or seizures which may indicate neurological impairment. An assessment of a client's level of functioning using a range of measures can be extremely helpful, not only in establishing the degree of disability but also by providing a baseline from which to assess improvement or deterioration.

The involvement of a psychologist who can conduct additional specialised investigations of psychological and psychomotor skills and functioning may also be beneficial. Accompanying this detailed assessment, however, simultaneous information and education also need to be provided to the client. Not surprisingly, clients or their carers may fear a catastrophic and imminent deterioration and it is important to emphasise that individual disease progression is not easy to predict and may be less damaging than anticipated. Careful explanation of procedures coupled with listening and acknowledging fears is an essential first response to ameliorate such anxieties. Physical investigation is likely to include blood tests to identify or exclude differential diagnoses and cerebrospinal fluid via lumbar puncture, an electroencephalograph and computed tomography (CT) or magnetic resonance imaging (MRI).

Management

As well as making an essential contribution to the diagnosis of HIV-related brain impairment, the LMHN is well placed to both coordinate and manage future care. This includes supporting general nurse colleagues in mental health management on general hospital wards and organising the appropriate levels of ongoing care and support at home. Clients' needs revolve around safety, through appropriate supervision, assistance with daily living tasks or implementing reminder systems to increase orientation or achieve adherence to medication if required. On occasions the use of the Mental Health Act 1983 may be necessary, especially where confusion and wandering may place the person in some danger or where the client's behaviour may jeopardise their dignity or put them at risk because of self-neglect. A package of care needs to be developed through a creative response that maximises independence, yet minimises risk. Liaising between hospital and community carers, including the GP and primary health-care team, or engaging the assistance of the generic mental health-care teams are essential aspects of this role. The LMHN is also required to respond to the psychological needs of the client and partners or carers, which may manifest in expressions of anger, grief or anxiety.

Where the provision of care at home proves impossible or unsustainable, even with the organisation of regular respite care, appropriate long-term care needs to be provided. In the absence of a specialist centre, the LMHN may be in the best position to identify and develop links with care organisations such

> **Case Study 7.3** HIV-related brain impairment
>
> John had been HIV positive for 8 years and had suffered from various opportunistic infections. He was diagnosed as having HIV-related brain impairment 18 months ago. Recently John collapsed and was admitted to hospital for assessment and investigations which indicated that he had experienced an exacerbation of neurological symptoms, possibly related to poor treatment adherence. He appeared confused and disorientated but when questioned about this, insisted he was fine. His friends and family had expressed concern to ward staff that he had been like this for some time and that recently this seemed to be getting worse. They also reported that John's house was in a neglected state and they were worried about his health and safety.
>
> The LMHN became involved in John's care and offered a more detailed mental health assessment. With John's consent, discussion with his family and friends provided a more detailed picture of the difficulties at home. Prior to discharge from hospital, a home visit with John, the occupational therapist and LMHN was arranged. John was also referred to a social worker to assist in the provision of social care and with John's consent his GP was alerted to his current needs in preparation for the likely requirement of more intensive home support in the future. The house was tidied and cleaned and various safety devices were installed. After 4 weeks, John was able to return home with regular home care. His medication was dispensed into 'dossette' boxes and a timer was programmed to remind John to take his tablets. The LMHN visited John at home regularly to monitor his mental state, treatment adherence and social situation.

as hospices, nursing or residential homes that may be able to offer this level of support. In these situations, the LMHN can support staff in a consultation/liaison and educational role, offering both regular direct client contact and educational advice on the management of care and emotional support to carers. This often includes issues regarding infection control, confidentiality and basic information on the progression of HIV disease and its management.

HIV-RELATED ANXIETY

This term refers to people with persistent beliefs that they have acquired HIV despite negative confirmatory HIV antibody testing. A number of other labels have been used to denote different presentations of essentially the same mental health problem including AIDS phobia, pseudo-AIDS and 'worried well' (Bor et al. 1992, Catalan et al 1995, Green 1996, Miller 1986). Frequently such people have been at little or no risk of becoming infected, yet their fears can be both overwhelming and incapacitating.

Clearly, the term 'HIV-related anxiety' may be applied more widely to include people with legitimate concerns that they may have become infected and such people require responses described above under liaison mental health nursing interventions. It is also vital not to prejudge a diagnosis on the basis of the number of HIV tests the person has requested, since a person may repeatedly place themselves at risk of acquiring the infection. Such concerns represent a symptom rather than a diagnosis and indicate the need for careful liaison mental health nursing assessment as described above.

Underlying psychopathology may include misunderstanding health education messages or the modes of HIV transmission and guilt feelings about sexual or drug-taking practices. This can result in reactions ranging from mild to moderate generalised anxiety, panic and hypochondriasis to obsessional compulsive disorders, somatisation, severe depression, mania or delusional disorders (Green & McCreaner 1996). Careful assessment of the level or intensity of the belief, the duration of the presenting difficulties and the verbal and non-verbal manner in which the experience is conveyed will give an indication of the likely underlying problem.

In addition, however, it must be remembered that a person's description of their risk behaviour may not match the reality, since they may choose not to describe the behaviour that is truly giving them concern. A non-judgemental, trusting and empathic approach that establishes a genuine rapport is therefore vital at the outset in order to reduce this possibility. Close liaison with pre- and post-HIV test counsellors is also invaluable in acquiring a complete history of presentation, in deciding which treatment may be deemed appropriate and determining whether this will be carried out by the LMHN or if a referral to another mental health professional is more appropriate.

Clearly where severe depressive illness or psychosis is suspected an urgent referral to a psychiatrist is most appropriate. The more common presentations of hypochondriasis and obsessional compulsive disorder are most successfully treated using cognitive or cognitive behavioural approaches (Green & McCreaner 1996). In such instances it is invariably beneficial for the client to be seen at a different location from where the test took place since, having reached a formulation as to the likely diagnosis, the LMHN needs to encourage the client to view the problem as a mental health issue rather than a physical one. Once the client accepts this, even if only for a set duration of time, work can begin to reduce the person's anxieties.

This client group above all others requires the LMHN to develop a close working relationship with professionals at HIV testing centres in order to offer support and education on the complementary roles and mechanisms for referral.

> **Case Study 7.4** HIV-related anxiety
>
> Lucy presented at the genitourinary medicine clinic requesting an HIV antibody test. She was seen by the health advisor who ascertained that Lucy was worried she may have become infected with HIV after a brief sexual encounter with her boss. After detailed exploration of the sexual behaviour involved, it was clear there could be no risk of HIV transmission. Despite this fact, Lucy remained concerned about being infected and was therefore referred to the LMHN. Assessment revealed Lucy had had seven previous HIV tests in the past following no-risk or low-risk sexual contact. On previous occasions her anxiety was relieved by negative test results but this time, because the encounter with her boss took place the previous week, she had to wait for a period of time before having a confirmatory HIV test. Lucy felt unable to cope with the waiting and had begun to drink half a bottle of vodka each day to dull her feelings of panic.
>
> The LMHN was able to offer Lucy an opportunity to explore and express her fears. As a result, Lucy began to appreciate that her anxiety had been triggered by her guilt about having been unfaithful to her partner and the belief that she would be punished by becoming infected with HIV. It also became clear that this and other sexual contacts outside her relationship only occurred when she had been drinking heavily. Lucy was taught to manage her anxiety utilising relaxation techniques. She was also educated and supported in a return to controlled drinking. Irrational beliefs were challenged and replaced with accurate information about the modes of HIV transmission. Through education and understanding Lucy was able to manage her anxiety and no longer felt an HIV test was necessary.

FEIGNED HIV DISEASE

The deliberate mimicking of physical symptoms or false reports of illness or infection by HIV have been noted in the medical literature from the early years of the HIV pandemic. The emerging multi-system disease of HIV and AIDS coupled with the specialised and highly confidential health-care service provision no doubt made HIV a 'lucrative' arena for such deception. While Munchausen AIDS has been identified (Kavalier 1989, MacDonald & Wafer 1989) and many case reports match Asher's (1951) colourful and insightful description of people 'traveling widely and telling untruths', it would be a mistake to apply this label too broadly since the diagnosis rests heavily upon perception of the person's motivation. There is also no universal agreement over the aetiology of the symptoms of Munchausen's syndrome.

King & Ford (1988) tend to view Munchausen's syndrome as a secondary behavioural manifestation of a primary disorder, pseudologica fantastica. Others make the distinction between factitious disorders and malingering, citing internal versus external incentives for such presentations (Catalan et al

1995). Attempting to mislead health professionals by altering medical records to achieve gain (Parmar 1990) appears more fraudulent than to be primarily a result of mental disorder. However, 'gain' is hugely subjective and encompasses social or interpersonal gains such as attention, prestige and influence from and over others, as much as financial gain or access to drugs (Murphy & Mulcahy 1991).

The LMHN, in particular those working closely with HIV, genitourinary medicine or sexual health clinics and A&E departments, is often the first to make a mental health assessment of clients exhibiting such behaviour. However, feigned HIV infection, like all attempts at deception, is virtually impossible to detect when a person first presents. Nevertheless, repeated refusal to donate a sample of blood for confirmatory HIV antibody testing or to check CD4 or viral load measures is the major indication that should raise suspicion. Other clues may derive from differences in collaborating history, mismatches or errors over dates and names of doctors or other medical information. The fact that such persons frequently present in crisis with a history that is both 'acute and harrowing' (Asher 1951) can make attempts at a comprehensive physical and mental health assessment difficult in practice, although such examples do reinforce the need for a careful and systematic approach to all clients.

Once factitious AIDS or Munchausen AIDS is suspected or even confirmed, the delicate task of confronting the person often falls to the LMHN. This seems highly appropriate since effective management demands the need to convey an acknowledgment of the person's physical concerns and a willingness to engage and provide support for psychological difficulties. Safeguarding the client from physical investigations or procedures is vital as is the discouragement of self-discharge before psychiatric or psychological follow-up can be offered and arranged. Maintaining the safety of the client may also be a motive for informing other genitourinary medicine and sexual health clinics or A&E departments if it appears the person is likely to travel to use other services. Such action protects the client from unwarranted and unnecessary investigations which may result in iatrogenic problems. However, caution needs to be exercised since persons in crisis are more likely to engage in risk behaviour (Simpson et al 1993, Thornton & Catalan 1993) and it is not unknown for people with a history of feigning HIV disease to become infected.

A careful balance therefore needs to be maintained in the LMHN's liaison approach with medical and nursing colleagues in educating staff about the existence of the phenomenon without reducing the professional and caring readiness of staff. Indeed, it may be said that the 'success' of a number of people feigning HIV infection and accessing care is a natural cost of creating flexible and responsive HIV services.

Case Study 7.5 Feigned HIV disease

Michael attended the local A&E department after having taken an overdose of 15 paracetamol tablets. When asked why he had done this, he stated that he was HIV positive and was unable to cope and therefore wished to end his life. He was declared medically fit and was admitted informally to a psychiatric ward. Whilst there, the staff involved in his care began to notice certain inconsistencies within the information Michael gave them. This resulted in staff becoming suspicious of his diagnosis and Michael was asked for evidence to confirm his HIV status. Despite maintaining the truth of his claims, he could not provide this and refused to have an HIV antibody test. On the same day he took his own discharge from the ward.

Staff suspected Michael was feigning his HIV status but clearly recognised the need for further assessment and possible intervention and therefore referred him to the LMHN who visited him at home. The LMHN undertook the delicate task of engaging Michael in further assessment, during which time he confirmed that he was not HIV positive. Over the next 10 weeks, a non-judgemental approach began to uncover some of the reasons that may have led to his claims to be HIV positive, including an extremely deprived early life, and this provided the foundation for further intervention. Michael was later referred for longer term psychotherapy.

HIV IN MENTAL HEALTH-CARE SETTINGS

The provision of health care is often segregated in terms of physical or psychological needs but, as has been clearly illustrated, the needs of people with HIV often span these groups. Therefore, whilst this chapter has so far focused on the psychological needs of this client group within an essentially physically orientated care environment, it is necessary to consider the needs of people with HIV in mental health-care settings.

HIV and pre-existing mental illness are not mutually exclusive and therefore mental health nurses are likely to encounter clients with HIV infection. In fact, there is evidence to suggest that clients with mental health problems are at greater risk of acquiring HIV infection because they are more likely to participate in risky behaviours (Otto-Salaj et al 1998). This is supported by evidence of higher rates of HIV infection in people with chronic mental illness (Stefan & Catalan 1995). Mental health problems resulting in emotional lability, impulsiveness, sexual disinhibition or cognitive impairment may affect an individual's ability to assess risk and make judgements. In addition, confirmation of HIV infection for clients with preexisting mental health problems is likely to exacerbate such difficulties (Firn 1992). Mental health professionals are also likely to work with clients with substance-related problems and 'dual diagnosis' where again, higher rates of HIV infection are likely (Gournay et al 1997). Finally, as has been discussed, high rates of psychiatric morbidity are experienced by clients with HIV infection (Khouzam et al 1998) and this may necessitate admission to mental health services.

Clark & Everall (1997) have recognised the contribution of liaison psychiatry in managing the care of people with HIV infection. Within the multidisciplinary team, the LMHN has a significant role in both educating and supporting mental health colleagues in hospital and community mental health services. This role can be divided into two broad spheres: education and consultation/liaison.

Education

Evidence exists to suggest nurses have a limited knowledge of HIV and display negative attitudes towards people with HIV infection (Tierney 1995). Mental health nurses are no exception to this. Many mental health nurses have limited knowledge of the physical or psychological impact of HIV, which may be due to their limited experience of working with HIV-positive clients and also exacerbated by their perception that HIV is purely a physical illness. The LMHN has a role in educating mental health colleagues about both physical and psychological aspects of HIV.

Mental health nurses need to understand the ways in which HIV infection is transmitted to protect clients, colleagues and themselves. Nurses need to recognise that sexual activity among clients in psychiatric units is fairly common and so are risk-taking behaviours (Herman et al 1994). Clients need to be protected from sexual exploitation, educated and supported in negotiating safer sex and have access to condoms. To protect themselves and colleagues, nurses need to ensure safe practice in injection technique and universal precautions (Department of Health 1998). This includes being particularly careful during violent incidents and being aware of procedures following accidental exposure to HIV or other bloodborne pathogens.

As well as caring for clients who are either recently diagnosed HIV positive or who may have been HIV positive for some time, mental health nurses have a role in supporting clients who request HIV testing. This requires an awareness of basic issues relating to antibody testing and confidentiality. Other issues that are particularly pertinent to mental health nurses are the use of the Mental Health Act 1983 in relation to HIV and drug interactions between psychiatric and HIV treatments.

In terms of health promotion, mental health nurses should be encouraged to incorporate HIV-related issues as part of their assessment of client needs, not just for those perceived to be 'at risk' but for all clients. This should include an assessment of risk factors, risk behaviours and any clinical evidence of HIV infection; at present it is not surprising that only a minority of HIV-positive clients are identified as such by psychiatric staff (Stefan & Catalan 1995).

Mental health professionals need to be aware of the huge range of HIV services available nationally and locally and how to access these in order to refer clients where appropriate and to foster collaborative working across medical and mental health services.

Consultation and liaison

It is neither feasible nor practicable for generic mental health nurses to become specialists in the care of people with HIV. The LMHN therefore has a vital role in supporting mental health colleagues involved in the care and management of clients with HIV. This consultation role may include offering advice and information on a range of care and treatment issues, accessing other disciplines who work specifically with HIV and providing clinical supervision on an individual or group basis. The LMHN may also become directly involved in the care of clients with HIV and therefore advice and information on referral procedures may be required. Whatever the role of the LMHN in relation to generic mental health colleagues, good liaison and communication skills are essential.

CONCLUSION

Working in the field of HIV is both complex and demanding, but an experience which can be highly rewarding as it challenges health-care professionals to utilise the breadth of their knowledge and skills. Clients with HIV have physical, psychological and social needs, with each of these domains clearly impacting on the others. The social context of HIV is particularly significant as the effects of stigma, prejudice and discrimination inevitably affect an individual's health and well-being. It is because of these complexities that working with individuals infected and affected by HIV is particularly suited to the specialty of liaison mental health nursing. Perhaps more than in any other field of contemporary health work, HIV care reinforces most strongly the foundations of nursing practice where, in contrast to other disciplines, there is 'less focus upon how people reached a particular point in their lives' and more upon 'how people move on from this point: how people change' (Barker 1999). This requires holistic assessment and a range of therapeutic interventions which have been highlighted and discussed.

The importance of multidisciplinary working and collaboration has been emphasised, as has the LMHN's role in offering consultation, education and supervision. There are many future challenges for nurses working in this field in maintaining awareness of HIV issues, from the prevention of HIV transmission to ensuring appropriate and high-quality community and residential care for clients with HIV-related brain impairment. However, perhaps the greatest challenge of all is to raise the profile of the psychological aspects of HIV and to ensure that the needs of this client group are recognised and responded to with innovative, sensitive and skilled liaison mental health nursing care.

QUESTIONS FOR DISCUSSION

◆ What skills do you need to develop in order to increase recognition of psychological needs within your assessment of clients affected by HIV?

◆ How can you develop collaborative working with other health professionals to ensure that people with HIV experiencing mental health problems receive appropriate and effective interventions?

◆ How might you seek to identify and reduce HIV risk behaviour in your area of nursing practice?

◆ What developments might your service require to enhance access and appropriateness of support for all individuals and groups affected by HIV?

ANNOTATED BIBLIOGRAPHY

Bor R, Miller R, Goldman E 1992 The theory and practice of HIV counselling: a systemic approach. Cassell, London

Green J, McCreaner A 1996 Counselling in HIV infection and AIDS, 2nd edn. Blackwell Science, Oxford

Winiarski M G 1991 HIV-related psychotherapy. Pergamon Press, Oxford

A selection of texts deriving from different approaches to the care and management of mental health problems in HIV.

Catalan J, Burgess A, Klimes I 1995 Psychological medicine of HIV infection. Oxford University Press, Oxford

Comprehensive and thorough description of current research and clinical practice on all aspects of psychological/psychiatric care for people with HIV.

Kalichman S 1998 Understanding AIDS: advances in research and treatment, 2nd edn. Braun-Brunfield, USA

Text offering comprehensive discussion of contemporary thinking on HIV and AIDS treatment and care.

Pratt R 1995 AIDS: a strategy for nursing care, 4th edn. Edward Arnold, London

Regularly updated and wide-ranging UK text on the nursing response to the HIV pandemic.

Journals/periodicals

AIDS Care: Psychological and Socio-medical Aspects of AIDS/HIV

Bi-monthly journal published by Carfax Publishing, PO Box 25, Abingdon, Oxfordshire, OX14 3UE

AIDS Treatment Update

Monthly newsletter published by National AIDS Manual, 16a Clapham Common Southside, London SW4 7AB Tel: 0207 627 3200

AIDS Letter

Bimonthly journal published by Royal Society of Medicine Press, 1 Wimpole Street, London W1M 8AE Tel: 0207 290 2900

REFERENCES

AIDS Letter 2000 Latest UK figures on AIDS. AIDS Letter 76:4–5

AIDS Manual 1999 HIV and AIDS treatment directory, 17th edn. NAM Publications, London

American Academy of Neurology AIDS Task Force 1991 Nomenclature and research definitions for neurologic manifestations of human immuno-deficiency virus type 1 (HIV 1) infection. Neurology 41:778–785

Anderson W, Weatherburn P, Keogh P, Henderson L 2000 Proceeding with care: phase 3 of an on-going study of the impact of combination therapies on the needs of people with HIV. Sigma Research, London

Antoni M H 1991 Psychosocial stressors and behavioural interventions in gay men with HIV infection. Int Rev Psychiatry 3:383–399

Asher R 1951 Munchausen's syndrome. Lancet i:339–341

Auerbach J, Oleson T, Solomon G 1992 A behavioural medicine intervention as an adjuvant treatment for HIV-related illness. Psychol Health 6:325–334

Barker P J 1999 The philosophy and practice of psychiatric nursing. Churchill Livingstone, London

Barroso J 1997 Reconstructing my life: becoming a long-term survivor of AIDS. Qual Health Res 7(1):57–74

Bor R, Miller R, Goldman E 1992 The theory and practice of HIV counselling: a systemic approach. Cassell, London

Catalan J 1993 HIV infection and mental health care: implications for services. World Health Organisation Regional Office for Europe, Copenhagen

Catalan J, Burgess A and Klimes I 1995 Psychological Medicine of HIV Infection. Oxford University Press, Oxford

Centers for Disease Control 1981 Pneumocystis pneumonia. Morbidity and Mortality Weekly Report 30:250–252

Clark B and Everall I 1997 What is the role of the liaison psychiatrist? Genitourin Med 73(6):568–570

Department of Health 1998 Recommendations of the Expert Advisory Group on AIDS and the Advisory Group on Hepatitis. Department of Health, London

Ellis D, Collis I and King M 1994 A controlled comparison of HIV and general medical referrals to a liaison psychiatry service. AIDS Care 6(1):69–76

Firn S 1992 Facing the challenge. Nurs Times 88(37):60–62

Gournay K, Sandford T, Johnson S, Thornicroft G 1997 Dual diagnosis of severe mental health problems and substance abuse/dependence: a major priority for mental health nursing. J Psychiatr Ment Health Nurs 4(2):89–95

Green J 1996 The worried well. In: Green J, McCreaner A (eds) Counselling in HIV infection and AIDS, 2nd edn. Blackwell Science, Oxford

Green J, McCreaner A 1996 Counselling in HIV infection and AIDS, 2nd edn. Blackwell Science, Oxford

Herek G M, Glunt E K 1988 An epidemic of stigma. Am Psychol 43:886–891

Herman R, Kaplan M, Satriano J, Cournos F, McKinnon K 1994 HIV prevention with people with serious mental illness: staff training and institutional attitudes. Psychosoc Rehabil J 17(4):97–103

Kavalier F 1989 Munchausen AIDS. Lancet i:852

Khouzam H, Donnelly N, Ibrahim N 1998 Psychiatric morbidity in HIV patients. Can J Psychiatry 43(1):51–56

King B H, Ford C V 1988 Pseudologia fantastica. Acta Psychiat Scand 77:1–6

Kurdek L, Siesky G 1990 The nature and correlates of psychological adjustment in gay men with AIDS-related conditions. J Appl Soc Psychol 20:846–860

Lennon M, Martin J, Dean L 1990 The influence of social support on AIDS-related grief among gay men. Soc Sci Med 4:447–484

MacDonald J, Wafer K 1989 Munchausen syndrome masquerading as AIDS-induced depression. Br J Psychiatry 154:420–421

Markowitz J C, Klerman G L, Perry S W, Clougherty K F, Josephs L S 1993 Interpersonal psychotherapy for depressed HIV-seropositive patients. In: Klerman G L, Weissman M M (eds) New applications of interpersonal psychotherapy. American Psychiatric Press, Washington DC

Miller D 1986 The worried well. In: Miller D, Weber J, Green J (eds) The management of HIV/AIDS patients. Macmillan, London

Muma R, Lyons B, Borucki M, Pollard R 1997 HIV manual for healthcare professionals, 2nd edn. Prentice Hall, London

Murphy M, Mulcahy F 1991 Feigned HIV disease. Int J STD AIDS 2:215–217

Nord D 1996 Issues and implications in the counseling of survivors of multiple AIDS-related loss. Death Studies 20(4):389–413

Otto-Salaj L, Heckman T, Stephenson L, Keely J 1998 Patterns, predictors and gender differences in HIV risk among severely mentally ill men and women. Community Ment Health J 34(2):175–190

Paradis B A 1992 Seeking intimacy and integration: gay men in the era of AIDS. Soc Work 38(6):260–274

Parmar M, Boag F, Jayasuriya P, Catalan J 1990 Feigned HIV disease. Int J STD AIDS 1:447–449

Price R W, Brew B J 1988 AIDS commentary: the AIDS dementia complex. J Infect Dis 158:1079–1083

Pugh K, O'Donnell I, Catalan J 1993 Suicide in HIV disease. AIDS Care 4:391–399

Remien R, Rabkin J, Williams J 1992 Coping strategies and health beliefs of AIDS long-term survivors. Psychol Health 6:335–345

Roberts D 1997 Liaison mental health nursing: origins, definition and prospects. J Adv Nurs 25(1):101–108

Schilts R 1987 And the band played on: politics, people and the AIDS epidemic. Penguin Books, Harmondsworth

Sherr L 1995 Grief and AIDS. John Wiley, Chichester

Simpson D, Knight K, Ray S 1993 Psychosocial correlates of AIDS – risk drug use and sexual behaviours. AIDS Educ Prev 5:121–130

Stefan M, Catalan J 1995 Psychiatric patients and HIV infection: a new population at risk? Br J Psychiatry 167(6):721–727

Sumpter J, Ryan C, Holmes-Smith S 1993 Mind, body and soul. Nurs Times 89(23):42–45

Sutton F, Smith C 1995 Advanced nursing practice: new ideas and new perspectives. J Adv Nurs 21:1037–1043

Thornton S, Catalan J 1993 Preventing the sexual spread of HIV infection – what have we learned? Int J STD AIDS 4:311–316

Tierney A 1995 HIV/AIDS: knowledge, attitudes and education of nurses – a review of the research. J Clin Nurs 4(1):13–21

Weiss A 1989 The AIDS bereaved: counselling strategies. In: Dilley J W, Pies C, Helquist M (eds) Face to face: a guide to AIDS counselling. AIDS Health Project, San Francisco

Weitz R 1990 Living with the stigma of AIDS. Qual Sociol 13(1):23–28

Willis J 1997 A positive contribution. Nurs Times 91(48):62–64

Winiarski M 1991 AIDS-related psychotherapy. Pergamon, New York

World Health Organisation 1990 Report of the Second Consultation on the Neuropsychiatric Aspects of HIV-1 infection. WHO, Geneva.

Wright J 1992 Developing a supportive role. Nurs Times 88(37):62–64

Wright J 1994 A shared understanding: developing a framework of mental health nursing care for people with HIV. Psychiatr Care 1(2):73–77

RESOURCES AND INFORMATION

AVERT (AIDS Education & Research Trust)
4 Brighton Road
Horsham RH13 5BA
Tel: 01403 210202

Body Positive
14 Greek Street
Soho
London W1V 5LE
Tel: 0207 287 8010

National AIDS Helpline
1st Floor
8 Mathew Street
Liverpool L2 6RE
Tel: 0800 567123 (24 hrs)

National AIDS Manual Publications
16a Clapham Common Southside
London SW4 7AB
Tel: 0207 627 3200
Includes AIDS Reference Manual, the UK AIDS Directory and the HIV & AIDS Treatments Directory

The Terrence Higgins Trust
52–54 Grays Inn Road
London WC1X 8JU
Tel: 0207 831 0330

Professional organisations

European Association of Nurses in AIDS Care (EANAC)
Steve Jamieson, Vice President
20 Cavendish Square
London W1M OAB
Tel: 0207 647 3431

HIV and Mental Health Nurses' Special Interest Group
Angela Lavery, Chair
Department of Liaison Psychiatry
Leeds General Infirmary
Great George Street
Leeds LS1 3EX
Tel: 0113 392 3139

RCN Mental Health Nursing Forum and Sexual Health Forum
20 Cavendish Square
London W1M OAB
Tel: 0207 647 3431

Section 3

Cognitive behavioural approaches

8

Cardiac rehabilitation: assessment and intervention strategies

Sarah Fisher   Robert Tunmore

KEY ISSUES

- Management of coronary heart disease
- Medication
- Lifestyle changes
- Relationship issues
- Psychological problems
- Cognitive behavioural interventions

INTRODUCTION

This chapter will look at liaison mental health nursing when mental health problems occur in conjunction with coronary heart disease (CHD). CHD represents the major cause of premature morbidity and mortality in the United Kingdom and is a key area for reduction in current health policy (Department of Health 1998a). Current treatment is still dominated by medical interventions, although there is evidence that emotional distress increases susceptibility to physical illness (Department of Health 1998a). Development of innovative services is needed to achieve the goals for CHD reduction described in *Our Healthier Nation* (Department of Health 1998a). Service development will need to focus on reducing inequalities in health, by targeting the various factors that can influence CHD development (Department of Health 1998b). This will require collaborative service design and delivery, so that care can be integrated across the health and social care sectors.

Liaison mental health nurses have a key role in defining such services by identifying areas of psychosocial need for clients with CHD.

High levels of anxiety have been identified among people following their experience of the first heart attack (Thompson 1989). Psychiatric complications including disorientation to place and time, perceptual illusions, delirium, hallucinations, paranoid ideation and agitation are reported in a third (32%) of patients following open heart surgery (Smith & Dimsdale, 1989). Being identified as hypertensive and being treated for hypertension may increase reports of psychosomatic symptoms, emotional problems, low mood, feelings of depression and general unhappiness. Depression and low mood are known to be among the side effects of medication used to treat hypertension and heart disease (Goldberg et al 1980).

Several important documents have emphasised the importance of addressing the physical health needs of people with long-term mental illness. The National Service Framework for Mental Health (Department of Health 1999) identifies how mental health problems can result from a wide range of adverse factors associated with physical illnesses and sets out standards for health improvement. The National Psychiatric Morbidity Survey showed high levels of physical ill health and higher rates of death amongst those with mental health problems compared to the rest of the population (Allebeck 1989, Harris & Barraclough 1998). The Mental Health Foundation (1997) highlight the important role of physical and spiritual factors in mental health and mental health problems and of tailoring programmes to meet individual circumstances and need.

Very high levels of morbidity from cardiovascular and respiratory disease and other serious physical illness have been identified among people with long-term mental illness (SNMAC 1999). Psychotropic medication, used to treat mental illness, often has physical side effects and may affect physical health. The Clinical Standards Advisory Group (1995) report that the standardised mortality rates for schizophrenia are 2.5 times those of the rest of the population. An incredible 45% of people with long-term conditions also have physical health problems, particularly cardiovascular and respiratory illnesses.

In order to achieve the standards set out in the National Service Framework for Mental Health, each primary care group will need the support of specialist mental health services to plan arrangements for physical health care. The primary care team will usually take responsibility for physical health care, but may be able to take on an extended role through liaison and consultation with mental health services in a holistic approach to the management of common mental health problems.

The primary care team and mental health services will need the necessary skills and organisational systems to provide the physical health care for people with severe mental illness. A multidisciplinary care plan will set out how and what will be provided – by the GP, social services and any other primary care support needed (see Chapter 4 for a discussion of liaison and consultation in primary care and community settings).

Co-morbidity of physical and psychological disorders is known to be prevalent, with up to 41% of those with a chronic medical condition also having a concurrent psychiatric condition, such as mood and anxiety disorders (Cohen & Rodriguez 1995). Studies of patients with known CHD show depression to be associated with increased CHD morbidity and mortality (Shapiro et al 1999). Despite this, psychosocial aspects of care are rarely addressed in physical illness. In addition, affective disturbances can have a major impact on development of physical disorders, by influencing various behavioural, cognitive and social pathways (Fig. 8.1). Mood and anxiety disorders have also been associated with poor health behaviours, such as increased smoking and reduced compliance with medication regimes. Such conditions, if undetected or ineffectively dealt with, can have a negative impact on the individual with CHD.

CORONARY HEART DISEASE: FACTS AND FIGURES

CHD accounts for 28% of deaths in those aged under 65. The most common manifestations of CHD are angina pectoris (heart muscle cramp) and myocardial infarction (MI; heart attack). Approximately 1.4 million people suffer from angina and another 300 000 will have a myocardial infarction annually, of which half will die. Many of these deaths occur without warning. Unsurprisingly, depressive illness is common after an acute cardiac event (De Bono 1998).

Mortality is higher in the north of England, Scotland and Northern Ireland and is inversely proportional to social class, with men in social classes IV and V being three times more likely to die than those in classes I and II. There has been a reduction in CHD mortality in the past decade but only in the higher socioeconomic groups, causing the health inequality gap to widen (BHF 1997). Those in the lower socioeconomic groups are still three times more likely to die from CHD than those in the higher groups.

Direct treatment costs are currently around £3.8 billion per annum (Department of Health 1998b) and represent a major drain on NHS finances. The majority of these costs are focused on acute treatment and intervention, with a very small proportion spent on prevention and rehabilitation.

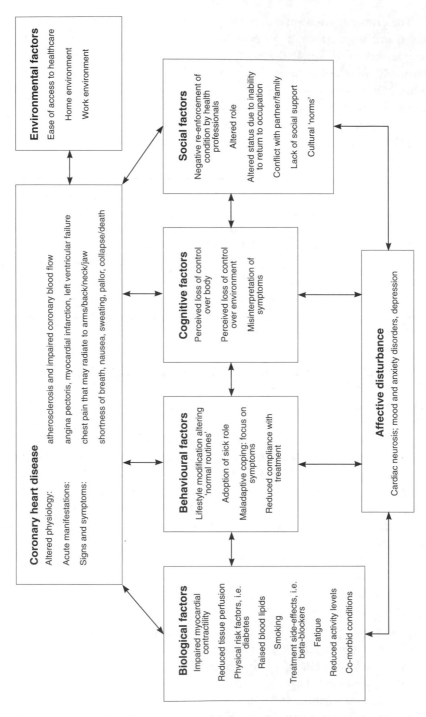

Fig 8.1 Factors influencing the development of affective disturbances in coronary heart disease.

CHD is a major cause of ill health and premature death in the UK causing higher mortality than many cancers, yet many health professionals still fail to recognise it as an essentially chronic and malignant condition. Consequently, treatment and resources are unequally distributed, with the focus on short-term 'curative' medical interventions at the expense of more long-term supportive aspects of care, such as helping people live with a chronic illness.

Key issues

Why has there been little input from health-care professionals who are formally trained in psychological care into the management of those with cardiovascular disorders? In other chronic, malignant diseases such as cancer, there is often a well-defined psychological support service, with specialist practitioners available to give psychosocial support or counselling for those who are going through a recognised life-threatening illness. Yet such services are not found routinely within cardiac care, despite it being the major cause of premature morbidity and mortality in the UK.

This may reflect the dominance of highly technological medical and nursing care, at the expense of more inclusive models of care, such as are seen in cancer. This seems to be in direct conflict with the data which support a high level of recordable psychiatric morbidity in cardiac patients. This should be rectified, to ensure that cardiac patients are not more disadvantaged than other groups of chronically ill patients.

Another possible reason for the lack of holistic services may be the degree of unpredictability of the clinical course of CHD and the non-specificity of common cardiac symptoms, making it difficult to plan and target specific interventions. Individuals with end-stage CHD do not have a clearly defined terminal phase of illness and so are rarely referred to palliative care teams for symptom control. They are more likely to be admitted to acute care settings where the emphasis is on cure rather than quality of life. Ultimately those with end-stage cardiac disease could undergo a 'disadvantaged death' (Harris 1990), compared to others with malignant diseases (NCHSPCS 1998).

Altered physiology

Atherosclerosis is the disease process underlying CHD. Fatty plaques form in the lining of the coronary arteries which supply the heart muscle, causing these vessels to become progressively narrower and, ultimately, to block. This is a slow process and symptoms do not usually start to appear until the mid 30s–40s for men and 50s–60s for women.

SIGNS AND SYMPTOMS

CHD can present as a variety of conditions (Table 8.1), the signs and symptoms of which can be very similar and can often only be diagnosed through clinical investigations. Symptoms can occur without warning and commonly include:

- ◆ chest discomfort or pain, related to increased physical effort or emotional stress
- ◆ breathlessness
- ◆ profuse sweating
- ◆ fainting
- ◆ collapse
- ◆ death

One of the difficulties in diagnosing CHD is the vagueness of the symptoms, which are not solely cardiospecific. People frequently fail to correctly identify their symptoms as cardiac in origin and so often delay seeking medical assistance. Symptoms may be interpreted in the context of prior illness experiences and it is not uncommon to find the symptoms of an acute MI attributed to a bad case of indigestion. The important differentiating factor for cardiac symptoms is they are commonly precipitated by physical activity or emotional stress and are rarely relieved by common analgesia or antacids (Table 8.2). Acute episodes of CHD often occur without any prior symptoms and are associated with a lot of psychological distress which is often given a low priority in the acute setting.

Table 8.1 Common manifestations of coronary heart disease

Angina pectoris
Chest pain/discomfort or breathlessness caused by narrowing of the coronary arteries supplying the heart muscle -a form of "heart muscle cramp". Symptoms can be mild or debilitating and are commonly related to physical exertion or emotional stress

Myocardial infarction
Death of heart muscle tissue, due to obstruction of a coronary artery by ruptured atherosclerotic plaque, which blocks blood vessel; This starves part of the heart muscle of oxygen and it dies. This is considered a medical emergency requiring prompt hospital treatment

Heart failure
The heart cannot pump effectively, often as a result of CHD or raised blood pressure. This results in a reduction in blood flow to all tissues of the body. The degree of pump dysfunction is a reliable predictor of prognosis. The poorer the pumping function of the left ventricle, the worse the prognosis and the higher the mortality. It can cause severe activity limitation, fatigue or symptoms of breathlessness/chest pain

---

Table 8.2 Characteristics of cardiac pain

Precipitating factors	Related to increased activity/stress. This increases the heart's demand for oxygen
Location	Central chest/epigastrium Usually diffuse rather than localised in one area Client will often make fist and move it over the area
Radiation/spread ['referred' pain]	Arms (one or both) Neck Between shoulder blades Jaw [NB some individuals will only have referred pain]
Description of symptoms	"Crushing, heaviness, tightness, constricting" "A band across chest"
Frequency and duration	Amount of episodes in day/week/month How long each episode lasts
Intensity	Symptoms may be mild or debilitating
Relieving factors	Rest may relieve some symptoms GTN spray or sub-lingual tablets commonly used Relief within 5–10 minutes

Table 8.3 Common non-cardiac causes of chest pain

Cause	Location	Characteristics	Relieving factors
Oesophageal spasm or hiatus hernia	Central May radiate to throat or left arm Can be accompanied by weakness and sweating	Precipitated by specific foods Occurs after eating Related to lying down after meal	Sitting/standing Antacids Sublingual GTN and Nifedipine
Biliary	Focused in right upper quadrant epigastrium	Occurs after rich, fatty foods Steady in nature Lasts several hours	Not relieved by GTN
Musculoskeletal	Upper chest discomfort [v. common]	Well localised Tender to touch May worsen on movement	Anti-inflammatories local heat application

Gastric discomfort is also common, which may explain why many individuals misinterpret cardiac symptoms as indigestion (Table 8.3), e.g. oesophageal spasm responds to sublingual nifedipine and GTN. This can cause confusion to both health professional and client, as both drugs are considered to be solely 'cardiac'. In fact, both drugs are also very effective in alleviating oesophageal spasm, hence their use (Table 8.4). However, this needs to be explained clearly to the client, otherwise they may erroneously assume that they have a 'heart problem' when they do not!

Table 8.4 Overview of common cardiac medication groups and some side effects

Drug group	Indications	Action	Common side effects	Contraindications
Beta-Blockers, i.e. atenolol metoprolol	Angina Hypertension Myocardial infarction Heart failure	Reduces force of heart's contraction Slows heart rate Lowers blood pressure	Fatigue, lethargy cold hands/feet Male impotence – erectile problems	*Absolute* Severe depression Asthma *Relative* Visual hallucinations Fatigue Psychotropic drugs Vivid dreaming
Calcium Channel Blockers, i.e. verapamil amlodipine nifedipine diltiazem	Angina Hypertension Fast rhythm Disturbances	Slow heart rate Lowers blood pressure	Constipation [verapamil] Heart failure Rhythm disturbances Flushing, ankle oedema and headache [nifedipine]	Certain slow rhythms Caution with beta-blockers and digoxin
Angiotensin Enzyme Converting Inhibitors, i.e. enalapril lisinopril captopril	Symptomatic heart failure Hypertension	Lower blood pressure	Dry cough Taste alterations Low blood pressure	Pregnancy
Aspirin	Used after MI to prevent arterial thrombus formation	Stops platelet adhesion (makes them less sticky, so less likely to clot)	GI effects, nausea, vomiting and dyspepsia and GI bleeds	Aspirin intolerance History of GI bleed
Nitrates, i.e. isosorbide mononitrate (long acting)	Long acting preparations used for angina	Vasodilation	Headaches [most common] – can limit compliance facial flushing Hypotension [most serious] syncope tachycardia	
Glyceryl trinitrate (GTN) (short acting)	Short acting preparations, i.e. GTN spray used as angina prophylaxis/ pain relief			

Table 8.4 Cont'd

Drug group	Indications	Action	Common side effects	Contraindications
Diuretics, i.e. frusemide bendrofluazide	Symptomatic heart failure raised blood pressure [bendrofluazide]	Reduces circulating volume	Low blood potassium levels tinnitus, rash low blood pressure	
Digoxin	Treatment of irregular heartbeat – atrial fibrillation	Slows heart rate and conduction of electrical impulses	Narrow range between toxicity and therapeutic	
		Strengthens force of levels	Causes rhythm disturbances	
			Toxicity common, causes: malaise, fatigue, confusion, coloured vision, anorexia, nausea, vomiting and diarrhoea	
			Distorted vision and colour perception	
			High levels – depression, hallucinations and delirium	
Lipid lowering agents, i.e. simvastatin pravastatin	Lower blood fats	Reduce total cholesterol and certain components	GI problems, flatulence, diarrhoea, constipation and nausea	

Perception of symptoms

For many people having an MI or being admitted to their local hospital with LVF or unstable angina is their first sign of CHD. On closer questioning, a history of progressive symptoms over several days or weeks gradually emerges, which the individual has put down to flu, indigestion or being under the weather. Many people do not know what the signs and symptoms of CHD are until they develop the condition.

Symptoms are often interpreted in the context of previous ill health experiences. The client should be encouraged to describe their symptoms in their own words, otherwise valuable information may be missed. They may often deny having any chest pain, but will discuss their 'asthma', 'flu' or 'stomach ulcer', which on closer questioning turns out to be cardiac in origin.

The Common Sense Model of Illness (Leventhal et al 1980) tries to identify how those suffering from acute MI utilise cognitive structures to influence their response to symptoms. It suggests that people have implicit beliefs about a disease and that these beliefs then influence their behaviour when seeking treatment (Johnson Zerwic et al 1997). Individuals who have an MI will seek treatment more quickly if their symptoms match their expectations of a heart attack (Johnson & King 1995).

Many have no further symptoms after the initial acute episode, but a size-able group is left with ongoing symptoms. Some will be left with residual angina which may manifest itself as chest discomfort or breathlessness. Such symptoms are usually related to activity and can range from quite mild to debilitating. Interestingly, severity of symptoms does not always correspond to severity of underlying disease. This group will need educating about what is now 'normal' for them and be given advice about when to seek further help and what type of help.

Increasing severity of symptoms is characterised by an increase in frequency, duration and perceived severity of symptoms, which usually occur with less provocation and require more analgesia than normal (Table 8.5). Such symptoms may alter over a period of days or weeks and the client

Table 8.5 Warning signs of increasing severity of symptoms

Increase in symptom	Frequency
	Duration
	Intensity
Symptoms precipitated by	Less activity than normal
Symptom relief	Rest requires more GTN than usual
	Relief not obtained: seek medical help immediately

should be encouraged to seek medical help promptly, usually from their GP. The GP should be bypassed in the case of severe unremitting symptoms and the individual should present to their local A&E unit instead. Severe, unrelieved chest pain of >15 minutes duration may herald the onset of an MI, which is a medical emergency requiring immediate hospital treatment to limit muscle damage and prevent death.

RISK FACTORS

Physical risk factors

A number of physical risk factors are associated with the development of atherosclerosis and yet they only account for approximately 50% of all CHD seen (Ridker 1998). Despite this, identification and modification of risk factors form the mainstay of CHD screening and prevention programmes and also cardiac rehabilitation programmes (CRP). There are two categories of risk factor (Table 8.6):

◆ modifiable – the effects of which can be reduced, e.g. smoking
◆ non-modifiable – these are fixed and cannot be altered, e.g. age

Psychosocial risk factors

There has been some research into possible psychosocial causes of CHD, in particular:

◆ the role of chronic stress
◆ degree of autonomy over one's environment

Table 8.6 Physical risk factors for coronary heart disease

Modifiable risk factors
Smoking
Raised blood lipids
Diabetes mellitus
Hypertension
Obesity
Sedentary lifestyle
Diet rich in unsaturated fats

Non-modifiable risk factors
Family history of CHD (1st degree relatives under the age of 60- siblings or parents)
Male sex
Increasing age

In times of stress or 'arousal' the body produces higher levels of hormones such as adrenaline and noradrenaline which prepare it for action, the so-called 'flight or fight' mechanism. This is a normal response to help an individual deal with a 'threatening' situation. However, long-term stress leads to chronic over-arousal which can lead to the development of CHD.

Findings from the Whitehall study also suggest that individuals who have low control over their working environment may be more prone to developing CHD compared to those who have a high degree of control or more autonomy (Marmot et al 1991). This is analogous to the theory of locus of control; those who have an external locus of control tend to deal with ill health poorly, adopting a reactive role to their circumstances, compared to those whose locus is internal, who deal with situations proactively and try to take control of their environment. Such findings may partly explain the higher incidence of CHD seen in lower socioeconomic groups, whose members may well have little control over their environment in terms of housing type and tenure and low levels of occupational autonomy.

Research into 'coronary-prone' behaviours has been inconclusive and contradictory. Possibly one of the most well-known areas of research has been that surrounding the Type A behaviour pattern (TABP). Early work suggested that individuals who exhibited competitive, impatient and hurried behaviour, so-called 'Type A behaviour', were more likely to suffer from CHD. Whilst there is a significant association between TABP and cardiovascular reactivity, epidemiological data are inconsistent and interest in this topic has lessened (Contrada et al 1997). Individuals who exhibit such behaviour before or at the time of MI are not at higher risk for recurrent morbidity and may have a lower risk than individuals who exhibit less aggressive behaviour (Cohen et al 1997). This may be related to the very strong internal locus of control exhibited by those with TABP. This work was also carried out amongst white men and there has been a lack of comparative work in women and different ethnic groups.

Loneliness and lack of a supportive social network have also been identified as risk factors for poor health. Social support networks may promote positive health practices, positive world views and resources for dealing with stressful situations for individual members. Integration into a social network provides individuals with higher self-esteem and allows them to feel more in control of environmental and behavioural changes (Fleury et al 1997), while strong emotional and social support networks may prevent illness and assist in recovery (House et al 1988). In the context of CHD, support from family and friends has been shown to positively influence behaviour change (Fleury et al 1997).

Negative mood states, as seen in anxiety and depression, can have a destructive effect on an individual's social support network. Members of a social group will avoid contact with a depressed or anxious individual, who

Table 8.7 Risk factors for suicide in coronary heart disease

Depression
High levels of agitation
Anxiety
Dependency
Dissatisfaction
Complaining behaviour
Lack of support from family
Lack of support from hospital
Lack of close and supportive relationship

may find their social support network falling away, which can then increase their risk for physical problems.

Common expressions of low mood states, often seen in CHD, can also help identify those who may be a suicide risk (Table 8.7).

MANAGEMENT OF CHD

Despite the chronic, progressive nature of CHD, both medical and nursing management are focused on acute treatment and interventions and can be broken down into several categories:

◆ medications for symptom control
◆ interventions to improve coronary blood supply
◆ lifestyle and behaviour modification
◆ psychological care

Medical interventions

Medication

Drug treatment is the mainstay of CHD management, with strong evidence to support use of medications such as aspirin and beta-blockers for reduction in further cardiovascular morbidity and mortality. The indications for such treatment are outside the focus of this chapter but a number of side effects are seen with the major medication categories which could affect compliance or give rise to psychological problems (Table 8.4). Many individuals who are prescribed such drugs may not be aware of these problems, assuming instead that there is something else wrong with them, which in turn can exacerbate any psychological distress further.

Many people with long-term illness – and that includes both physical illness and mental illness – have difficulties with medication. Those involved in the client's care need to be familiar with the client's medication history and their current prescription and be able to recognise and manage any side effects that the client may experience.

There may be a reluctance to take medication which may be due to, for example, a lack of understanding of how the medication works, a fear of unpleasant side effects or an inability to manage the prescribed medication. Clients and their carers need accurate, up-to-date information about medication, side effects and treatment and the approach to medication management needs to be collaborative and educational. It may be important to involve and educate carers and relatives in the use of medication as their attitudes may influence the success or otherwise of pharmacological interventions.

It is important to assess the balance between side effects and therapeutic effects of tests, investigations and medication. Medication may relieve symptoms but may also have distressing and disabling side effects. Long-term use of medication may reinforce the belief in abnormality, impairment or problem, i.e. that there must be a problem or abnormality if tablets are prescribed for it. Similarly, routine tests and investigations may reinforce notions that something is seriously wrong. Appropriate information and education about medication, tests and investigations are key components of treatment programmes and interventions.

Medication review

◆ Review medication with the prescribing physician and key carers.
◆ Review the client's self-medication of prescribed and non-prescribed medication.
◆ Encourage the client to monitor therapeutic or desired effects of medication and any side effects that they may experience.
◆ Monitor side effects and therapeutic effects related to changes in prescribed medication.

Interventions to improve coronary blood supply

An individual may undergo a number of investigations after suffering an acute coronary to identify whether they will require further treatment to 'unblock' their coronary arteries and improve their coronary circulation event (Table 8.8). Individuals who record a 'positive' exercise test will then undergo coronary angiography to determine how many of their coronary arteries are narrowed or blocked due to atherosclerosis. Those with a narrowing or stenosis in only one or two major vessels may be selected to undergo a PTCA, whilst those with several stenoses affecting three or more major vessels will undergo CABG. Both procedures will be carried out in a specialised cardiothoracic unit rather than a local district general hospital.

Table 8.8 Common investigations	
Electrocardiograph (ECG)	Electrodes are attached to body and picture of heart's electrical activity is obtained Gives information on heart rate, rhythm, size of heart chambers and evidence of ischaemia/infarction
Exercise ECG 'treadmill test' 'stress test'	ECG is recorded continuously whilst client walks on treadmill, that gets steeper and quicker. Blood pressure is also recorded – strenuous Used to differentiate cardiac/non-cardiac chest pain If pain is cardiac, ECG will show ischaemic changes during test, signs of insufficient blood supply to heart – a 'positive test'. Also used for risk stratification after MI – to identify those requiring further treatment
Creatine Kinase (CK)	Cardiac enzyme that is released when heart muscle is damaged, i.e. during MI. Amount of enzyme rise correlates with amount of muscle damage
Coronary angiogram 'cardiac catheterisation'	A tube is inserted into the femoral artery (via the groin) and fed into the aorta under X-ray. Dye is injected into the coronary arteries and into the chambers of the heart. This allows visualisation of the heart's blood vessels and shows up any narrowings or blockages. Information is also provided on the heart's pumping function
Echocardiogram 'echo'	Ultrasound investigation of the heart. Provides information about pumping action, valve motion and direction of blood flow
24-hour tape 'Holter monitoring'	Several electrodes are attached to the chest and a continuous ECG record of the heart rate and rhythm is obtained. Data is stored in a small tape recorder worn around the waist. Used to detect possible abnormal rhythms. Client documents any abnormal feelings and this is compared with tape

The two major forms of intervention are:

◆ *percutaneous coronary angioplasty (PTCA) and stent insertion* – involves insertion of a tube into the coronary artery and inflation of a balloon to 'open up' the narrowing and placement of a tube (stent) to keep the artery open. Carried out under local anaesthetic, with 2-day hospital stay
◆ *coronary artery bypass graft surgery (CABG)* – major surgery, involves bypassing the diseased artery with a vein graft (usually from the leg), to improve blood flow. Carried out under general anaesthetic, with 5-day hospital stay.

Lifestyle and behaviour modification

Acute care is characterised by high levels of surveillance and intervention which are gradually reduced throughout the inpatient phase until discharge.

Due to the severity of their condition, the individual is viewed as a collection of physical symptoms to be treated or manipulated, whilst the social and environmental context in which their illness occurs is often ignored or assigned a low priority.

The patient is encouraged to report any adverse signs to the nurse who will undertakes various investigations to ascertain the cause. Whilst this reflects the nursing and medical priority of the patient's physical condition, such constant emphasis on physical signs and symptoms may contribute to the anxiety and high levels of self-surveillance seen at discharge, the 'call-bell syndrome'. It can also serve to reinforce the seriousness of having a 'heart condition' for the patient.

This physical focus lessens during the inpatient phase as the patient stabilises and is transferred to a general care area, where there are lower levels of surveillance and intervention. However, this is not matched with a corresponding increase in psychosocial care to deal with anxieties and forthcoming discharge. Whilst the individual may be visited by the cardiac rehabilitation nurse during their inpatient stay, they are often too anxious to take in the information given and so may have anxieties about coping after discharge.

This is a normal pattern of care from the health professional's viewpoint but it can be very distressing for the client, who has been conditioned to report any ache or pain for investigation whilst an inpatient, so reinforcing the severity of their condition. They literally only need to press the call-bell and someone will come and offer reassurance and identify the cause of their symptoms. However, after discharge many individuals continue to monitor themselves for any signs of recurrence of their symptoms but have no-one to call on for reassurance.

This dependency on others can promote an external health locus, as the individual is not encouraged to make their own health choices but instead relies on the knowledgeable practitioner and so does not develop any strategies for identifying signs and symptoms and learning how to deal with them.

It is a paradox that acute care, whilst it serves to promote early assessment and intervention, does not promote recovery in the client and indeed may be to blame for the high anxiety levels seen.

Health professionals involved in the care of those with CHD come predominantly from acute medical/surgical backgrounds, with further training in acute cardiovascular disease management. The dominance of physical interventions and lack of psychological care which has been identified (Lewin 1995b) may merely reflect the dominant acute medical care paradigm.

Greater attention needs to be paid to the long-term psychological problems of anxiety and depression in those with CHD (Williamson 1997), as this area is often not assessed and may be a risk factor for early mortality. Those who are at risk of a major depressive order within 2 weeks of infarction have been shown to have a 6-month mortality rate 3.5 times that in those without depression (Shapiro et al 1999).

Lifestyle modification

Long-term modification of any health-damaging behaviours, e.g. cigarette smoking and poor diet, is required to minimise recurrence of further symptoms. The individual will also need encouragement to comply with drug therapy on a long-term basis, in order to reduce further morbidity. Extended compliance with behaviour change is critical for the success of secondary prevention of CHD and trying to identify how individuals make health-related decisions may prove useful in encouraging their compliance with behaviour change (Oldridge & Streiner 1990). This presents a number of challenges for the health professionals involved:

◆ identifying modifiable risk factors
◆ providing the client with information to make informed choices about their own health
◆ assisting the client to adopt health-promoting behaviours
◆ assisting the client to maintain their modified behaviours
◆ promoting compliance with medication regimens
◆ trying to avoid being prescriptive

Cognitive approaches encouraging the adoption of adaptive coping styles and strategies can improve the client's sense of control and mastery of their experience. Effects of planned lifestyle changes can be incorporated into programmes of cognitive behaviour therapy. Monitoring the effects of, for example, including or excluding certain foods, changing eating habits and modifying levels of activity introduce new approaches to lifestyle that complement any changes in physical health status. Simple changes may be identified along with the beneficial effect of the change, e.g., using low or non-fat substitutes for dairy produce, increasing the amount of fresh fruit and vegetables, reducing caffeine intake, trying a low-fat, low-salt diet.

People with newly diagnosed CHD are often ignorant of their personal risk (Johnson Zerwic et al 1997) and it will be necessary to carry out a risk factor assessment to identify each individual's risk factor profile. Assessment of an individual's perception of the causes of CHD is also valuable as it can provide a framework on which to base interventions. It is important to avoid blaming the client for their health behaviours; many express concern that they have 'failed' their risk factor assessment if multiple risk factors are identified and care must be taken to avoid this.

The nurse needs to explore the client's values, goals and, most importantly, their perceived ability to achieve those goals, before initiating any changes. Dissonance can occur between the health professional's view of recognised risk factors as being causal and the patient's view that psychosocial factors are the predominant cause (Fisher 1997, Murray 1989). It is important for health professionals to recognise the different emphasis placed on causes of CHD in order to plan their interventions to address the needs of the patients rather than a medically focused agenda.

Motivation will best be served by helping the client identify realistic and do-able goals, which will act as a positive reinforcement to maintain behaviour change. Exercise, relaxation and stress management have a beneficial effect on mental health. Practical actions that individuals can take include:

◆ using opportunities for relaxation and physical exercise
◆ taking alcohol in moderation – drinking sensibly and avoiding illegal drugs
◆ maintaining social contacts
◆ reducing smoking
◆ talking things over.

Introduce any such changes gradually. Follow short-term achievable and realistic goals to allow the client to take control of his or her life again and reduce any sense of being restricted and disabled by their illness. Clients who are not physically fit may experience muscle pain on taking up even gentle to moderate exercise. The beneficial effects of exercise on muscle tone, bowel function and general metabolism should be identified with the client.

Cardiac rehabilitation

Lifestyle modification programmes for individuals with CHD occur within the remit of cardiac rehabilitation programmes (CRP) which, although multidisciplinary in nature, are usually nurse-led. The aim of cardiac rehabilitation is to assist individuals to regain mastery of their lives after a cardiac event and reduce the risk of further CHD through risk factor identification and modification (Cay 1995). CRP are often hospital based and last between 6 and 8 weeks. Patients and their partners are invited to attend after discharge.

However, the majority of CRP are aimed at those who have sustained a first MI or who have had cardiac surgery. Those with long-standing conditions such as chronic angina or heart failure are not specifically catered for and so may not have access to specialist support services. Not all those who could benefit from CRP attend, such as women, older people, those from ethnic minorities and those from lower socioeconomic groups, despite their high morbidity and mortality. The majority of CRP are offered on a blanket basis, due to limited resources, and the programmes may not be suitable for many people. Increased age is associated with higher depression, lower quality of life, less social support and less attendance at formal cardiac rehabilitation (Conn et al 1991) whilst an investigation into quality of life post-MI suggested that women have a worse clinical, socioeconomic and psychosocial profile than men and are at higher risk of morbidity and mortality following infarction (Shumaker et al 1997). Women also report significantly higher frequencies of psychological and psychosomatic complaints, such as sleep disturbances a year postinfarction (Wiklund et al 1993).

There is extensive literature regarding the role of exercise in cardiac rehabilitation (Gulanick 1991, Hedbäck & Perk 1990), but few studies investigating the efficacy of psychosocial interventions, despite psychosocial outcomes being equally as important as physical outcomes (Conn et al 1991). Again this reflects the 'clinical gaze' of the health professionals most involved in CRP: general nurses and physiotherapists. Very few CRP have access to clinical psychologists or appropriately trained mental health professionals to meet these needs should they be identified. CRP can improve if there is a better understanding of the personal meanings that individuals give to their illness and if programmes then address these individual perceptions (Nolan & Nolan 1998). Nurses need to become more proactive and CRP need to be reconceptualised and develop more integrated psychological, social and spiritual interventions (Nolan & Nolan 1998), to address the individual's needs, abilities, risk factors and psychological status (Brennan 1997).

Evaluation of CRP is inconsistent; some claim they represent an efficient use of resources (Oldridge et al 1993), demonstrating improved psychosocial adjustment, fewer GP visits and improved compliance with treatment (Williamson 1997). Others suggest that there are no long-term benefits (Hampton & McWilliam 1992).

As CHD is a chronic condition, interventions must aim to produce long-term gains. The current focus on physical outcomes may reflect the pervading short-termism that has dominated British health care, coupled with the difficulty in assessment of psychosocial variables. It may be questionable to undertake a psychosocial assessment when there are no interventions in place for those identified as requiring them.

CHD has a multifactorial causation and many diverse health professionals could be involved in care delivery between the primary, secondary and tertiary care sectors. It may be impossible to identify which particular professional and which particular intervention has been the most effective. It would be more productive to develop a collaborative approach to care and focus on the overall outcomes rather than try and isolate the role of individual practitioners.

Psychological care

This dependency on others can promote an external health locus, as the individual is not encouraged to make their own health choices but instead relies on the knowledgeable practitioner and so does not develop any strategies for identifying signs and symptoms or learn how to deal with them.

Effective cardiac rehabilitation programmes intervene on multiple levels (psychological, social, occupational and physical) to assist the patient's psychosocial adjustment. Mental health promotion is a key component of rehabilitation programmes for patients recovering from a myocardial infarction. Programmes may include coping with stressful situations, anticipation of chest pain, emotional reactions such as anger, anxiety, depression, irritation and the importance of social networks, work and leisure activities and physical exercise (Fridlund et al 1992). Patel et al (1985) demonstrate the effectiveness of behavioural modification and the cognitive reappraisal techniques of cognitive therapy among patients with hypertension. Intervention significantly reduced the blood pressure level over a 4-year period. Wadden (1983) found relaxation training to be an effective treatment for some patients. Stress management and behavioural techniques, including breathing exercises, relaxation and meditation, appear to reduce heart disease and the complications of hypertension. These interventions may provide a cost-effective basis for primary prevention programmes to reduce risk factors for CHD.

Most people are able to adapt and adjust well, both physically and psychologically, following a heart attack. The psychological distress following a heart attack is usually relatively brief. The functional capacity pre- and post-resuscitation may be unchanged. However, for individuals with a history of emotional disturbance and mental illness, health adaptation and adjustment may be problematic. Common worries and anxiety at initial recovery include:

◆ anxiety about being left alone – fear of recurrence
◆ increased apprehension
◆ amnesia for the arrest

◆ emotional distress
◆ nightmares and disturbed sleep

The process of adjustment after a myocardial infarction is focused around the struggle to regain control, with four identifiable phases of adjustment (Johnson & Morse 1990):

1. defending oneself during the acute episode
2. coming to terms with perceived loss
3. learning to live again
4. establishing control

The month after discharge is often characterised by uncertainty, difficulties with coping and distress. Whilst the general practitioner is seen as the obvious source of support and information, many individuals have been dissatisfied by the response of their GPs. This raises questions about which health professionals are best placed to meet these needs (Thompson et al 1995). Major sources of anxiety at discharge are:

◆ loss of safe hospital environment
◆ having to fend for oneself
◆ fear of recurrence of symptoms/sudden death
◆ knowledge deficit about management of condition

In the first weeks after discharge, anxiety levels remain high and 'homecoming depression' is very common (Lewin 1995a). Individuals are very tearful and emotionally labile, demonstrating low mood and irritability. Partners and family members can find this time very stressful and feel that the individual is quite difficult to live with. The distress can be minimised prior to discharge by explaining and emphasising that these are normal reactions to what has been experienced as a life-threatening episode. During the inpatient phase, individuals become accustomed to constant surveillance, which can provide them with a sense of security. Any aches or pains they develop can be discussed with the health-care team and investigated further if necessary. Not surprisingly, discharge is highly stressful and is a time of great insecurity. The 'comfort zone' of the hospital is no longer present and the patient and their family group have to adjust to a normal life.

It is also worth emphasising that tiredness and lethargy after discharge are normal and to be expected. The heart is a muscle like any other and will need time to recover after an injury. However, unlike a broken leg for example, it cannot be immobilised for a period while it recovers!

Recovery and rehabilitation should involve balancing periods of rest with periods of activity, with the amount of activity being increased gradually over a period of several weeks (usually 6–8). The aim is for the client to return to what was normal for them prior to developing CHD, where possible.

It is not uncommon to meet individuals who are highly sensitive to their physical condition, spending much of their waking time being aware of how their heart is beating and acting in an overvigilant manner. Between 20% and 35% of individuals who survive an MI will have a formally diagnosable psychiatric condition one year later, which is a considerable number of people, even when preinfarct morbidity has been taken into account. However, only 21% of CRP have any psychology input (Lewin et al 1998). These individuals can be placed in two groups (Lewin 1995a):

1. those with mental health problems pre-MI
2. those who develop mental health problems as a direct result of the infarct, which acts as a 'trigger'

Another group at particular risk are those with a dual diagnosis of mental illness and substance misuse. Clients with long-term mental illness are at higher risk of coronary heart disease where substance abuse is involved. Alcohol misuse and use of illicit substances increase the likelihood of cardiac problems and long-term use can lead to physical illness (Table 8.9).

Table 8.9 Harmful effects of substance misuse on cardiac function and mental health

Marijuana	May increase heartbeat up to 50%. Increases blood pressure. Increased risk to those with hypertension and heart disease. Damage to pituitary gland affects blood pressure.
	Smoke from Marijuana yields more than double the tar from cigarette smoke – increases risk of other serious physical illness – lung cancer, infections and inflammation.
	Distorted perception and thinking Poor concentration Confusion Loss of motivation Mood swings Aggression and hostility Depression Anxiety and paranoia
Cocaine	Constricts heart's blood vessels, increasing blood pressure, heart rate, breathing and body temperature. Cocaine and crack use cause constriction of blood vessels throughout the body leading to increased risk of heart attack. Causes heart attack, heart failure, irregular heartbeat and sudden death. May lead to heart attacks in babies born to mothers who are users.

	Causes euphoria and depression Irritability, anxiety, panic, erratic behaviour, Delusions, hallucinations, suspicion and paranoia confusion, aggression, violence, suicidal behaviours
Alcohol	Increases blood pressure and risk of heart attack and strokes. Tachycardia Weakens heart muscle and affects ability to pump. Causes heart muscle enlargement, abnormal heart signs, and irregular heartbeat.
	Limits production of red and white blood cells Decreases production of blood clotting agents in the liver – may cause uncontrolled bleeding
	Loss of pain perception, disturbed visual and hearing ability, delayed reactions Mild euphoria, loss of inhibitions Impaired judgement, concentration and co-ordination, mood swings and emotional behaviour.
Amphetamines	Cardiac problems include increased blood pressure, tachycardia, arrhythmias, vasoconstriction, sweating – risk of heart attack and strokes
	Impaired judgement, high and low moods, depression, psychomotor agitation, paranoid and suicidal ideation
Inhalents/solvents	Increases blood pressure and risk of heart attack and stroke. Tachycardia, sweating, Cardiac arrhythmia may lead to coma, stupor or death Impaired judgement, euphoria.

DEPRESSION AND ANXIETY

Greater attention needs to be paid to the long-term psychological problems of anxiety and depression in those with CHD (Williamson 1997), as this area is often not assessed and may be a risk factor for early mortality.

Depression and cardiovascular disease

Musselman et al (1998) review the literature on depression and cardiac problems and conclude that depression can be a major risk factor for both the development of cardiovascular disease and for death after a myocardial infarction. It is also associated with other chronic physical illnesses. Those who are at risk of a major depressive order within 2 weeks of infarction have been shown to have a 6-month mortality rate 3.5 times that in those without depression (Shapiro et al 1999).

The strong association between depression and suicide highlights the need for specific and thorough assessment of cardiac patients. Farberow et al (1966) match characteristics from case records of suicide with non-suicide controls among patients with respiratory and cardiac disease. An increased risk of suicide appears to be linked to higher levels of agitation, depression and anxiety. High dependency combined with dissatisfaction, complaining behaviour and a lack of support from family and hospital are other risk factors. The importance of a close and supportive relationship in suicide prevention is emphasised (Badger 1990).

Depression can be treated by structured psychological therapies, such as cognitive behaviour (Parry & Richardson 1996, Roth & Fonagy, 1996). Cognitive therapy may also reduce relapse rates (NHS 1993, Thase et al 1997). The combination of antidepressants and psychotherapy is often an effective means of treating depression among people with cardiac problems.

The cognitive model of depression

Beck's cognitive model of depression describes how people make assumptions about themselves, the world and the future based on their own experience. These assumptions shape the individual's perception and behaviour. They are important in helping the individual to make predictions about the future and to make sense of their experience and originate in childhood development. However, some assumptions the individual makes about his or her experience and behaviour may hinder coping and adaptation to certain life events. These assumptions are dysfunctional in the sense that they are often resistant to change.

These dysfunctional assumptions lead to 'automatic negative thoughts'. These are thoughts that are experienced automatically in the sense that they 'appear' in consciousness without being part of any rational thought process. They are believed – not questioned or challenged but accepted as if they were real, inevitable and unavoidable. People with cardiac problems may experience automatic negative thoughts including:

◆ If I cannot do XYZ what is the point? Life is not worth living.
◆ I'll never be able to do things as well as I did before the heart attack, anything else is second best.
◆ It's my own fault, now I am being punished.
◆ I'm a worthless person – I deserve this to happen to me.
◆ There isn't anything else, I'm just waiting to die.
◆ It's too late to do anything about it now – the damage is done.
◆ I'm just not up to it now so I'll leave it until another time.
◆ I won't enjoy anything again.

◆ I may have another heart attack at any time – I cannot plan anything. What is the point in trying?

These automatic negative thoughts affect the individual's perception of events, experiences and behaviour and can lead to other symptoms of depression.

◆ *Behavioural problems* – avoidance, withdrawal, inactivity
◆ *Physical problems* – loss of appetite, disturbed sleep, muscular tension, aches and pains
◆ *Motivation problems* – loss of interest, general inertia
◆ *Emotional problems* – guilt, anxiety
◆ *Cognition problems* – poor concentration, memory loss, difficulty making decisions

These cognitive distortions develop into a vicious circle, where the person has a negative view of themselves, the world and the future. Cognitive behaviour therapy sets out to break this negative cycle by teaching clients to identify, question and challenge automatic negative thoughts.

Anxiety and cardiovascular disease

Panic attacks, phobias or persistent generalised anxiety can have severe disabling effects on a person's ability to work, form relationships, raise children and participate fully in life. GPs often see anxiety, mixed anxiety and depressive disorders, which may be associated with high levels of disability (Meltzer et al 1995).

Anxiety disorders respond to cognitive behavioural therapy with sustained recovery following psychological treatment. Anxiety among people with coronary heart disease is often characterised by an increased focus of attention on physical health:

◆ increased physiological arousal – heightened awareness of physical characteristics, symptoms and sensations
◆ preoccupation with physical health problems
◆ reassurance and avoidance behaviours

Increased physiological arousal

Many clients find that they are more aware of body sensations. Normal changes in body sensations, which usually go unrecognised, may become a strong focus of attention. For example, having experienced breathlessness during a heart attack, a client may be more aware of their breathing patterns. Changes may be interpreted as signs of pathology, increasing the client's worry and anxiety. Focusing on the sensation may bring about physiological

Table 8.10 Common effects of anxiety	
Physical sensations in anxiety states	**Psychological effects**
Palpitations	Difficulty making decisions
Sweating	Poor concentration
Dry mouth	Restlessness
Dizziness	
Nausea	
Diarrhoea	
Flushes and chills	
Frequency of micturition	
Difficulty swallowing	
Tiredness	
Sleep disturbance	
Blurred vision	

changes leading to further discomfort and disability. Selective attention may reinforce negative beliefs about physical health problems.

The source of anxiety may be internal or external. *Internal* sources of anxiety involve the misinterpretation and misconception of normal body function and harmless sensations as threatening. The physiological effects of anxiety (Table 8.10) may be misinterpreted as evidence to support the beliefs of physical abnormality. Catastrophic interpretation of altered bodily sensations is associated with beliefs that sensations related to normal body function – palpitations, sweating, breathlessness, dizziness and the like – are signs of serious impairment. For example, the client who awakes at night sweating interprets this in terms of a problem with circulation and the onset of another heart attack. This leads to further anxiety and increased physiological arousal, increasing pulse rate and further sweating which reinforce the belief in the threat. Increased awareness of physical sensations is often associated with heightened arousal.

External sources of anxiety involve misunderstandings and misinterpretation of information leading to distorted, exaggerated and unrealistic beliefs. External sources may relate to medical information from professionals and other people, overheard conversations, newspaper articles, television and radio programmes. Anticipatory anxiety may be experienced in relation to planned investigations and procedures. Sometimes quite innocuous circumstances, information and sensations can lead to anxiety.

Preoccupation with physical health problems

A preoccupation with physical health is part of normal adjustment following a cardiac event. Physical sensations may be realistic evidence of altered body function and illness. However, these sensations may be interpreted as more dangerous than they actually are. The threat experienced may be out of proportion to the stimulus or trigger. Health education, focusing on the expected and anticipated physiological changes following a cardiac episode, may be reinforced with the client's self-monitoring of physiological measures. Increased familiarity with normal body function and expected changes along with an improved understanding of the nature and effects of anxiety may help the client experience a greater sense of control over any symptoms they experience.

Assurance and avoidance behaviours

Preoccupation with aspects of physical health can lead to clients seeking reassurance about symptoms and sensations. Constant or continued reassurance-seeking behaviour may lead to the development of response patterns from others with the focus of attention on the client's worries. Where reassurance is given relief is likely to be short term and the client may experience problems with long-term preoccupation. Repeated reassurance may become counterproductive if the client focuses on the reassurance itself as evidence of a worsening condition (Table 8.11). Reassurance-seeking behaviours may include repeated and excessive use of nurse call-bells or panic buttons in a

Table 8.11 Common negative thoughts in cardiac patients

Situation	Body sensations	Interpretation	Rational response
Lying awake at night Counting every heart beat	Palpitations pounding heartbeat, dizziness, light-headedness	'Something is wrong with my heart'	Worrying about the palpitations makes me more anxious The palpitations have increased because I am anxious.
		'I'm having a heart attack'	
	Breathlessness, tight chest Difficulty breathing	'I'm going to die'	The palpitations are caused by my anxiety – I am not having a heart attack.
	Sweating, trembling		She is concerned about me because I am ill.
The doctor asked how I am getting on	Tension in back and neck Palpitations	'They are always asking how I am – they must be expecting something awful to happen'	There is nothing unusual about this I trust her to tell me if something is wrong She has always been open and honest with me It is just me getting worried again

hospital ward. Preoccupation with physical health may be accompanied by checking behaviours related to bodily signs and symptoms. Catastrophic thoughts can lead to avoidance behaviour. For example, a client who interprets palpitations and dizziness as evidence of another episode of angina or a heart attack may avoid activities that they believe increase pressure on the heart, for example sexual activity, exercise or exertion.

Sometimes the client may feel they are wasting the time of doctors and nurses and that they are a burden. Rather than providing reassurance – that they are not wasting time and they are not a burden – provide an alternative explanation based on the cognitive behavioural model. The low mood, negative thoughts and anxiety associated with their physical illness often lead to thoughts and interpretations like these. The goal of intervention is to identify and challenge such thoughts.

Treatment goals

Psychological treatment aims to provide satisfactory realistic alternative explanations and interpretations of sensations and symptoms that are less anxiety provoking. Taking a step-by-step approach, gradual improvements over a longer period of time help the client to gain control of their life and improve their quality of life. Realistic and achievable short-term goals that the clients sees as beneficial can be set to help reduce the psychological distress associated with physical health and the prevention of further deterioration and distress. Following the initial assessment a series of sessions can be planned to address some of the client's problems. A contract may be drawn up between the nurse and the client which:

◆ provides a structured framework for interventions
◆ provides a time span for resolution of problems
◆ helps to contain anxiety
◆ leads to opportunities for alternative adaptive coping styles and strategies
◆ acknowledges the therapeutic relationship between client and nurse.

Cognitive behavioural interventions depend on a specific focused and detailed assessment of the problem which should be undertaken in the broader context of an assessment of the client's health and social functioning (Table 8.12). Problem identification involves a detailed description of the problem and the nature and degree of disability relating to the problem.

Problem identification

◆ The situation
◆ Physical reaction/sensation

Table 8.12 Initial assessment	
Biological factors	Symptoms
Behavioural factors	Medication
Cognitive factors	Weight and blood pressure
Social factors	Diet
	Exercise
	Lifestyle
	Social functioning
	Risk and need
	Regular screening for physical health problems

◆ Client's experience of symptoms
◆ Cognitions, thoughts and beliefs, perception of events
◆ Impact on life, outlook on life

Behaviour

◆ List types of situation where the problem is most severe/likely to occur.
◆ List situations and activities that are avoided because of the problem.
◆ Identify factors that make the problem better or worse.
◆ Other people's reactions, behaviours, attitudes to the client and their problem.
◆ Beliefs about the cause of the problem.
◆ Previous ways of dealing with the problem.
◆ Previous experience of illness – self and others.
◆ Personal strengths for dealing with the problem.

Interventions

Information about anxiety and depression

Clients and carers should be provided with information about the nature of anxiety including the common symptoms, causes and effects. The common effects of anxiety are identified as normal bodily responses to anxiety. This may itself alter the perception of the problem and help the client to understand the cognitive behavioural models of anxiety.

Medical information and understanding

Routinely check clients' understanding of information in relation to:

◆ what they have been told by medical and nursing staff, relatives, friends and peers

◆ what they have read or heard about their treatment via TV and radio programmes, Internet, newspapers and magazines
◆ treatment sessions and progress
◆ misunderstandings and gaps in knowledge.

Encourage the client to discuss their understanding of information and the implications for them. Identify relevant information and provide appropriately, in terms of amount, timing and stage of illness. Coordinate information with other members of the multidisciplinary team with regular updates and progress reviews, involving them in the delivery of care wherever appropriate, e.g. provision of useful information. Interventions should be tailored to the client's specific needs.

Self-monitoring of physical sensations

Understanding and being able to carry out some simple physiological observations helps the client and their carer to identify normal patterns and responses. Self-monitoring of physical sensations may include the following.

◆ *Blood pressure* – the client may be taught to monitor their own blood pressure and learn about their normal patterns.
◆ *Pulse* – the client can learn how to check their own pulse (and those of others) and identify normal patterns of variation throughout the day and following different activities.
◆ *Sleep* – keep a record of sleeping and waking hours.
◆ *Medication* – some sensations may be due to the side effects of medication and vary with the dose and times of administration.
◆ *Respiratory rates* – understand the range of normal breathing patterns and factors that change their breathing rate.

The client should also be helped to identify 'normal' physiological responses from abnormal ones, that could indicate a severity of their heart condition (see Tables 8.2, 8.3 and 8.5). This is an important part of client education. All too frequently the client is given information about the warning signs of abnormal cardiac function but the manifestations of anxiety, which are very common and similar, are not mentioned.

Distraction techniques

These techniques may help the client to gain a sense of control over the physiological changes characteristic of anxiety states. If there is a preoccupation with physical sensations and an internal source of anxiety, distraction techniques encouraging the senses to focus on external surroundings and the environment may be of benefit. These exercises may, with practice, distract the client from worrying about internal physical sensations.

Describe the surroundings For example, the client may ask themselves:

◆ What can you see around you? Describe the largest object. Describe the smallest object
◆ What can you smell? Describe the smell, pleasant or unpleasant
◆ What can you hear? How near or distant are the sounds? How many can you hear?
◆ What can you touch? How do your clothes feel? Describe the texture of the nearest surface.

Describe an object Focus on a single object and use all their senses to describe it – size, shape, colour, texture, position smell, sounds, etc.

Mental exercises The idea of this is to become absorbed and occupied by a distracting activity. For example:

◆ count backwards from 1000 in 7s
◆ go through the alphabet and identify the title of a popular song for each letter.

Absorbing activities These can be used as a means of effectively blocking unpleasant thoughts and ruminations. They require different levels of concentration and the client may need to practise using them in a planned and systematic way. Examples include:

◆ gentle exercise – walking, light gardening
◆ crosswords and other word games
◆ jigsaw puzzles
◆ creative activities – painting, writing, modelling
◆ housework – hoovering, dusting, ironing.

Identifying and challenging automatic negative thoughts

Describe the cognitive behavioural approach and discuss this with the client in relation to their own personal experience, encouraging them to identify the links between their own symptoms and body sensations, thoughts, beliefs and behaviours (Fig. 8.2). Changing or modifying beliefs involves helping the client to identify automatic negative thoughts and evidence that supports and challenges them. It involves keeping a record of activities, sensations, thoughts, feelings, mood, and behaviour.

Help the client to focus on the observations, then their interpretation of these observations and alternative interpretations of these observations. Self-monitoring helps to elicit the client's beliefs and automatic negative thoughts and can identify ways to test different interpretations, collecting evidence through checking information from a range of different sources against the client's own observations. For example:

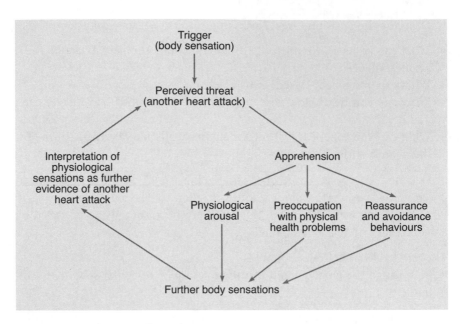

Fig 8.2 The physiological effects of anxiety.

◆ At the moment how strong is your belief you will have another heart attack? 0–100%
◆ Does the strength of your belief vary in different situations?
◆ Does it vary over time?

This can then be reviewed with the client to see how they account for any differences.

Often negative automatic thoughts underpin avoidance behaviours. Psychological therapy draws out the relationship between the client's perception and anticipation of negative outcomes and their behaviour. The following approach may help to address avoidance behaviour.

◆ What is the worst that could happen if you didn't manage to avoid the situation?
◆ What are the alternatives?
◆ How strongly do you believe that the worst would have happened?
◆ How likely are the other outcomes?
◆ Can you identify the disadvantages and advantages to thinking in this way?

Interventions need to be adapted and tailored to meet individual need. They will be dependent on the client's experience and practical ability to follow through therapy sessions with homework tasks. The involvement of the client's partner is an important component of psychological therapy and of the client's continued psychological support and adjustment.

SEXUAL ACTIVITY IN CARDIAC CLIENTS

It is common for individuals to report a reduced interest in sex after an acute coronary event. Discussion of sexual matters often occurs indirectly, if at all, and is rarely mentioned by medical staff. It traditionally falls within the remit of the cardiac rehabilitation nurses, who have little professional training for counselling clients on such matters. Many individuals feel embarrassed discussing their sexual lives and this area needs to be approached sensitively by nurses (Table 8.13). It is a topic that is often left until the end of a consultation.

Lack of information about sexual activity can be frustrating and can lead to insecurity, confusion and depression as clients will often rely on myths and misinformation (Steinke & Patterson-Midgley 1992). There is a tendency to overestimate the amount of physical exertion involved with sexual intercourse (Table 8.14). Fatigue and fear of chest pain are most commonly cited, with some men also reporting erectile problems, which may

Table 8.13 Common question asked by patients and their partners about sexual activity

Will I be able to have sex again?
When could sexual activity resume?
What type of sexual activity could be undertaken?
How could symptoms be prevented?
Will sexual activity cause recurrence of symptoms?

Table 8.14 Practical information about resuming sexual activity

Sexual activity can be resumed – usually 2 weeks after discharge or when two flights of stairs can be climbed without symptoms occurring
Be aware of 'performance anxiety' – acknowledge such feelings are normal for both participants
Avoid strenuous positions – adopt a passive role, engage in foreplay
Ensure a comfortable setting
Avoid alcohol or heavy food intake prior to sex
Avoid 'playing away from home'
Explain possible effects of medication on sexual function, i.e. beta-blockers
Take anti-anginal medication before sex as a preventative measure
Inform health professional if anginal symptoms occur during sex

be psychosomatic or caused by medication such as beta-blockers. Whilst 'performance anxiety' is to be expected in the aftermath of a cardiac event, the nurse will encounter some individuals with long-standing sexual difficulties and others for whom the cardiac event may act as a trigger in identifying any underlying sexual/relationship problems.

Fear of death, rather than physical limitations, prevents many individuals from resuming an active sex life (Piper 1992) although sudden death precipitated by sexual intercourse has been shown to be associated with extramarital activity, rather than sex with a regular partner (Mackay 1978). Recent research into sexual activity in men and mortality has shown an inverse association between death from CHD and orgasmic frequency (Davey Smith et al 1997). There is a lack of corresponding research in women, with most studies investigating their roles as spouses of males with CHD.

THE PARTNER'S NEEDS

The needs of partners are often overlooked, although they are also known to have high psychological morbidity (Dickerson 1998) and to need rehabilitation (Cay 1995, Thompson et al 1995). Partners have been found to display more mood disturbance and less satisfaction with marriage and family and to have lower levels of support than the client (Rankin 1992).

Male patients whose wives have been involved in a rehabilitation programme adjust more successfully than those who have not (Cay 1995). Unfortunately there are no data regarding male partners of female patients or same-sex couples. Help is required the most at the time of hospitalisation and when the patient returns home (Dickerson 1998), with partners requiring meaningful information to help them cope with uncertainty.

Many partners of clients with cardiac problems report feelings of conflict (Table 8.15). They are more vigilant of their partner, sometime overprotective, 'wrapping then in cotton wool' or waking in the night to see if their partner is

Table 8.15 Concerns expressed by partners of cardiac patients

Conflicting emotions: relief, anger, low mood
Not wanting to leave partner alone in house in case of recurrence
Waking at night and checking to see if partner is still breathing
Concern that partner has `changed'
Conflict re role changes in relationship
Feeling taken for granted
Blaming self for partner's mood changes
Worry that partner will die suddenly
Not wanting to leave partner unsupervised

still breathing. This may be coupled with feelings of anger and resentment over their partner's behaviour. Individuals with CHD may also have a range of feelings, from being anxious and not wanting to be left on their own at home to wanting to be left alone and finding their family's concern stifling.

Such situations can lead to the build-up of stress between patient and partner, which may not be brought out into the open. The partner may also feel they are to blame for the patient's labile mood and the patient may actually allow them to feel this. The partner may be reluctant to discuss any problems for fear of confrontation or exacerbating cardiac symptoms. CHD may be perceived as a major threat to patterns of dependency and roles in the relationship. Therapy should draw out changes in their relationship and their association with the cardiac event as well as the effect of significant events on the current illness. Clients may be asked, for example, 'How have your feelings for each other changed since the heart attack?'.

Common relationship problems include:

◆ frequent arguments
◆ resentment
◆ anger
◆ blame
◆ criticism
◆ depression and anxiety
◆ loss of satisfaction
◆ decrease/absence of sexual relations
◆ lack of affection
◆ infidelity
◆ sexual dysfunction

Hospitalisation can amplify any preexisting tensions in a relationship and the quality of the relationship is an important determinant in psychological recovery from the cardiac event. Consequently, the relationship with the partner needs to be investigated. It is again important to stress that many of the feelings experienced by both partners are normal and to encourage open discourse between both. Structured cognitive behaviour therapy sessions may involve both partners although it may be appropriate to conduct individual sessions with each partner. These should address individual concerns and expectations of therapy and also any confidential information the individual wishes to disclose or would prefer not to disclose to their partner. Psychological assessment during the first few sessions leads to the formulation of the couple's situation, an overview of their problems and needs.

Initial assessment and formulation should include (where appropriate):

◆ reason for referral for psychological therapy
◆ presenting problem

- changes in relationship and role
- previous patterns of relating
- family history of illness, causes of death among parents/siblings
- strengths and weaknesses, concerns
- agreement of plan, goals and activities
- agenda setting and task identification
- contract/agreement for specific number of sessions

Ongoing psychological therapy with couples may focus on:

- communication skills training
- expression of feelings
- problem solving
- conflict resolution
- anticipation of difficult situations
- dealing with small setbacks

Working with couples may be more difficult where there are unrecognised problems, a denial of problems or different expectations of therapy. However, in general the client with cardiac problems and their partner will receive greater long-term benefits, with less likelihood of any relapse of psychological problems, if they are able to address their concerns together in a supportive and safe environment.

THE ROLE OF LIAISON MENTAL HEALTH NURSES

There is a large body of literature around the psychology of recovery from a MI and yet little has been incorporated into practice (Lewin 1995a). There are three areas to consider:

1. assisting individuals to cope with the 'normal' psychosocial reactions to CHD
2. assisting them in the process of adjustment and possible behaviour change
3. identifying those who are at risk of developing psychological morbidity and intervening appropriately.

Such assessments should be undertaken by suitably qualified health professionals. Liaison mental health nurses are ideally placed to do this and could ensure that individuals with problems are referred to the appropriate services.

Involvement of liaison nurses could help redress the current imbalance between physical and psychological care and improve the mental health of individuals with CHD. The liaison nurse could have an important role to play in helping the patient to avoid undue illness behaviour, characterised by high anxiety levels, avoidance of activity or exertion and a dependent attitude. Individuals who develop a more positive view of their health status tend to have more favourable rehabilitative outcomes.

Between 6 and 12 weeks is the most suitable time to assess the long-term outcomes of psychiatric morbidity (Lewin 1995b) as the majority of patients will attend the hospital for routine follow-up at this time, presenting an ideal opportunity to undertake a formal assessment. Alternatively, it could be carried out as part of the cardiac rehabilitation programme but there are problems here in that not all eligible patients attend, especially women, older patients and members of ethnic groups, all of whom are at high risk.

CONCLUSION

Promoting wellness requires development of intervention strategies tailored to individual needs and goals. Whilst care is usually focused around modification of risk factors and compliance with medical treatment, lack of adherence to such regimes is a common problem. This could be a result of the physical treatment focus at the expense of investigating how best an individual may be motivated to change their health behaviours. Human behaviour is very complex and successful interventions are those which work on a variety of different levels, i.e. behavioural, social, psychological as well as physical.

QUESTIONS FOR DISCUSSION

◆ What can liaison mental health nursing bring to cardiac care?

◆ Are there any potential barriers to liaison mental health involvement?

◆ What interventions could be provided?

◆ How could the effectiveness of liaison mental health nursing be demonstrated in cardiac care?

REFERENCES

Allebeck P 1989 Schizophrenia: a life-shortening disease. Schizophr Bull 15:81–89
Badger T A 1990 Men with cardiovascular disease and their spouses: coping, health and marital adjustment. Arch Psychiatr Nurs 4(5):319–324
Brennan A 1997 Efficacy of cardiac rehabilitation 1: a critique of the research. Br J Nurs 6(12):697–702
British Heart Foundation 1997 Coronary heart disease statistics – mortality. http://www.dphpc.ox.ac.uk/bhfhprg/97stats/MORTALIT.HTM [19/03/99]

Cay E L 1995 Goals of rehabilitation. In: Jones D, West W (eds) Cardiac rehabilitation. BMJ Books, London, p31

Clinical Standards Advisory Group 1995 Schizophrenia. HMSO, London

Cohen L, Ardjoen R, Sewpersad K 1997 Type A behaviour pattern as a risk factor after myocardial infarction: a review. Psychology and Health 12:619–632

Cohen S, Rodriguez M 1995 Pathways linking affective disturbances and physical disorders. Health Psychol 14(5):374–380

Conn V, Taylor S, Abele P 1991 Myocardial infarction survivors: age and gender differences in physical health, psychosocial state and regimen adherence. J Adv Nurs 16:1026–1034

Contrada R, Czarnecki E, Li-Chern Pan R 1997 Health-damaging personality traits and verbal-autonomic dissociation: the role of self-control and environmental control. Health Psychol 16(5):451–457

Davey Smith G, Frankel S, Yarnell J 1997 Sex and death: are they related? Findings from the Caerphilly cohort study. BMJ 315:1641–1644

De Bono D 1998 Models of cardiac rehabilitation. BMJ 316:1329–1330

Department of Health 1998a Our healthier nation. A contract for health. HMSO, London

Department of Health 1998b National Service Framework on Coronary Heart Disease – emerging findings report. HMSO, London

Department of Health 1999 National Service Framework for Mental Health. HMSO, London

Dickerson S 1998 Cardiac partners' help-seeking experiences. Clin Nurs Res 7(1):6–28

Farberow N L, McKelligott J W, Cohen S, Darbonne A 1966 Suicide among patients with cardiorespiratory illness. JAMA 195(6):422–428

Fisher S 1997 Evaluation of a community based cardiac liaison nurse service. Br J Community Health Nurs 2(4):184–190

Fleury J, Thomas T, Ratledge K 1997 Promoting wellness in individuals with coronary heart disease. J Cardiovasc Nurs 11(3):26–42

Fridlund B, Pihlgren C, Wannestig L A 1992 Supportive-educative caring rehabilitation programme: improvements of physical health after myocardial infarction. J Clin Nurs 1:141–146

Goldberg E L, Comstock G W, Graves C G 1980 Psychosocial factors and blood pressure. Psychol Med 10:243–255

Gulanick M 1991 Is phase 2 cardiac rehabilitation necessary for early recovery of patients with cardiac disease? A randomized, controlled study. Heart Lung 20(1):9–15

Hampton J, McWilliam A 1992 Purchasing care for patients with acute myocardial infarction. Qual Health Care 1:68–73

Harris E C, Barraclough B 1998 Excess mortality of mental disorder. Br J Psychiatry 173:11–53

Harris L 1990 Disadvantaged dying. Nurs Times 86(22):27–29

Hedbäck B, Perk J 1990 Can high-risk patients after myocardial infarction participate in comprehensive cardiac rehabilitation? Scand J Rehabil Med 22:15–20

House J, Landis K, Umbertson D 1988 Social relationships in health. Science 241:540–545

Johnson J, King K 1995 Influence of expectations about symptoms on delay in seeking treatment during a myocardial infarction. Am J Crit Care 4:29–35

Johnson J, Morse J 1990 Regaining control: the process of adjustment after myocardial infarction. Heart Lung 19(2):126–135

Johnson Zerwic J, King K, Saidel Wlasowicz G 1997 Perceptions of patients with cardiovascular disease about the causes of coronary artery disease. Heart Lung 26(2):92–98

Leventhal H, Meyer D, Nerenz D 1980 The common-sense representations of illness danger. In: Rachman S (ed) Contributions to medical psychology and health. Pergamon, New York

Lewin B 1995a Cardiac disorders. In: Broome A, Llewellyn S (eds) Health psychology: processes and applications, 2nd edn. Chapman and Hall, London

Lewin B 1995b Psychological factors in cardiac rehabilitation. In: Jones D, West R (eds) Cardiac rehabilitation. BMJ Books, London

Lewin R, Ingleton R, Newens A, Thompson D 1998 Adherence to cardiac rehabilitation guidelines: a survey of rehabilitation programmes in the United Kingdom. BMJ 316:1354–1355

Mackay F 1978 Sexuality and heart disease. In: Comfort A (ed) Sexual consequences or disability. George F Stickley Company, Philadelphia

Marmot MG, Smith GD, Stansfeld S Patel et al 1991 Health inequalities among British civil servants: the Whitehall II study. Lancet 338(8758): 58–59

Meltzer H, Gil B, Petticrew, M, Hinds K 1995 The prevalence of psychiatric morbidity among adults living in private households. HMSO, London

Mental Health Foundation 1997 Knowing our own minds: a survey of how people in emotional distress take control of their lives. Mental Health Foundation, London

Murray P 1989 Rehabilitation information and health beliefs in the post-coronary patient: do we meet their information needs? J Adv Nurs 14:686–693

Musselman D L, Evans D L, Nemeroff C B 1998 The relationship of depression to cardiovascular disease. Arch Gen Psychiatry 55:580–592

National Council for Hospice and Specialist Palliative Care Services (NCHSPCS) and Scottish Partnership Agency for Palliative and Cancer Care 1998 Reaching out: specialist palliative care for adults with non-malignant disease. Occasional paper 14.

NHS Centre for Reviews and Dissemination 1993 The treatment of depression in primary care. NHS Centre, York

Nolan M, Nolan J 1998 Rehabilitation: scope for improvement in current practice. Br J Nurs 7(9):522–526

Oldridge N, Streiner D 1990 The health belief model: predicting compliance and dropout in cardiac rehabilitation. Med Sci Sports Exercise 22(5):678–683

Oldridge N, Furlong W, Feeny W et al 1993 Economic evaluation of cardiac rehabilitation soon after acute myocardial infarction. Am J Cardiol 72:154–161

Parry G, Richardson A 1996 NHS Executive review of psychotherapies: a review of strategic policy. HMSO, London

Patel C, Marmot M G, Terry D J, Carruthers M, Hunt B, Patel M 1985 Trial of relaxation in reducing coronary risk: four year follow up. BMJ 290(6475):1103–1106

Piper KM 1992 When can I do 'it' again nurse? Sexual counselling after a heart attack. Professional Nurse 8(2): 168–172

Rankin S 1992 Psychosocial adjustments of coronary artery disease patients and their partners: nursing implications. Nurs Clin North Am 27(1).271–284

Ridker P 1998 Inflammation, infection, and cardiovascular risk. How good is the clinical evidence? Circulation 97:1671–1674

Roth A, Fonagy P 1996 What works for whom? Guilford Press, New York

Shapiro P, Lespérance F, Frasure-Smith N et al 1999 An open-label preliminary trial of sertraline for treatment of major depression after acute myocardial infarction (the SADHAT Trial). Am Heart J 137(6):1100–1106

Shumaker S, Brooks M M, Schron E B et al 1997 Gender differences in health-related quality of life among post myocardial infarction patients; brief report. CAST Investigators. Womens Health 3(1):53–60

Smith L W, Dimsdale J E 1989 Postcardiotomy delirium. conclusions after 25 years? Am J Psychiatry 146(4):452–458

Standing Nursing and Midwifery Committee (SNMAC) 1999 Practice guidance: the nurses contribution to assertive community treatment. SNMAC, Department of Health, London

Steinke E, Patterson-Midgley P 1996 Sexual counseling of MI patients: nurses' comfort, responsibility and practice. Dimens Crit Care Nurs 15(4):216–223

Thase M E et al 1997 Treatment of major depression with psychotherapy or psychotherapy-pharmacotherapy combinations. Arch Gen Psychiatry 54:1009–1015

Thompson D R 1989 A randomized controlled trial of in-hospital nursing support for first time myocardial infarction patients and their partners: effects on anxiety and depression. Adv J Nurs 14:291–297

Thompson D, Ersser S, Webster R 1995 The experiences of patients and their partners 1 month after a heart attack. J Adv Nurs 22:707–714

Wadden T 1983 Predicting treatment response to relaxation therapy for essential hypertension. J Nerv Ment Dis 171(11):683–689

Wiklund I, Herlitz J, Johansson S, Bengston A, Karlson B, Persson N 1993 Subjective symptoms and well-being differ in women and men after myocardial infarction. Eur Heart J 14(10):1315–1319

Williamson G 1997 Why should acute trusts be interested in cardiac rehabilitation? Br J Nurs 6(190):1111–1130

RESOURCES

British Association for Cardiac Rehabilitation
c/o Action Heart
Wellesley House
117 Wellington Road
Dudley DY1 1UB
Provides information for all those directly involved with cardiac rehabilitation.

British Heart Foundation
14 Fitzhardinge Street
London W1 4DH
Website: *http://www.bhf.org.uk/*
Major cardiac research charity. Provides resources and information for those involved in cardiac care delivery.

Government Information Service
Website: *http://www.open.gov.uk/*
Government, NHS and related links. Information on government health policy and strategies.

9

Chronic fatigue syndrome: a cognitive behavioural approach

Alicia Deale   Trudie Chalder

INTRODUCTION

Chronic fatigue syndrome (CFS) is characterised by severe, disabling fatigue that can persist for many years. The precise causes are unknown and it is widely regarded as a heterogeneous condition of multifactorial aetiology (Wilson et al 1994b). People who receive a diagnosis of CFS may be referred to specialists in the general hospital for advice. A psychiatric referral is often made when investigations fail to find any abnormalities or when concomitant emotional distress or affective disorder is noted. Although seldom welcomed by the client, such a referral may prove fruitful, as members of the liaison psychiatry team are well placed to deliver an effective, evidence-based treatment programme.

This chapter will provide an overview of CFS, a cognitive behavioural model for understanding the condition and practical guidance about assessment and management.

WHAT IS CHRONIC FATIGUE SYNDROME?

Debilitating fatigue of uncertain origin is not a new problem. It is widely documented in the medical literature of the 19th century (Abbey & Garfinkel 1991, Shorter 1993, Wessely 1990) and can be found in various forms throughout the 20th century (Wessely 1991). Fatigue syndromes attracted public or professional interest during the 1980s, when 'Yuppie flu' or 'ME' rapidly became a media issue (Abbey 1993, Aronowitz 1992). This has resulted in a dramatic rise in the numbers of people thought to be suffering from CFS.

There are a number of alternative names for CFS, including myalgic encephalomyelitis (ME) and postviral fatigue syndrome (PVFS). Chronic fatigue syndrome is generally preferred by clinicians as it is short, accurate and makes no assumptions about cause.

Clinical presentation

Clients with CFS complain of intense fatigue, exacerbated by minor exertion. Symptoms include physical exhaustion, loss of energy, difficulty in thinking clearly, poor concentration and memory, word-finding difficulties and slips of the tongue. The fatigue is described as qualitatively different from the type of tiredness experienced when well. It follows a persistent or relapsing course, fluctuates in severity and is seldom entirely absent.

Sleep disturbance is common, including hypersomnia, irregular sleep patterns and sleeping during the day. A variety of additional symptoms may be present, such as muscle and joint pain, headaches, gastrointestinal symptoms and flu-like symptoms. Disability can vary considerably; a few patients are able to continue working, while others will be confined to bed or to a wheelchair.

Psychological distress is marked and many people diagnosed with CFS also meet criteria for a psychiatric diagnosis (Wessely 1997). Depression is thought to be present in between a third and three quarters of cases (David 1991). The rates of depression, anxiety and somatisation disorders in CFS exceed rates found in the general population and in control groups of patients with comparable medical illnesses (Johnson et al 1996, Katon et al 1991, Pepper et al 1993, Wessely & Powell 1989).

There is some evidence that people with CFS seen in primary care differ from those seen in hospital settings (Euba et al 1995). Primary care subjects tend to be less disabled, less distressed and have a better prognosis. CFS patients seen in hospital settings tend to have an overrepresentation of females, Caucasians, professionals and higher social classes. Disability is marked, levels of psychological distress are high and many patients also fulfil criteria for psychiatric disorder. Most believe they have a physical illness

Case Study 9.1 Clinical presentation

Teresa was a 33-year-old single teacher, referred for cognitive behavioural therapy by her GP. She had a 2-year history of persistent physical and mental fatigue, accompanied by myalgia, headaches, chest pain, poor concentration and word-finding difficulties. All these symptoms were made worse by any exertion. Her mood was depressed and she felt pessimistic about recovery. She had given up work and all daily activities were restricted. At night, her sleep was fitful and broken, so she tended to sleep in the mornings and catnap during the day. She usually rested in bed until 11 am and spent most of her time sitting at home, sometimes reading or listening to music but usually resting on the sofa. Her main exercise was walking to local newsagents. Occasionally she had a 'good' day, when she would try to do as much as possible, spending hours working in the garden, seeing friends or shopping. She always 'paid for it later' with increased exhaustion and rest.

Her illness had begun after a prolonged bout of flu, which she felt she had never recovered from. Physical examination and routine investigations were all normal, and she had been diagnosed with ME at a private clinic. Her GP prescribed some antidepressants, but she stopped taking them after a month due to side effects.

Teresa read widely about ME. She believed that the flu had damaged her entire system and that some sort of virus was still present in her body. She thought she had pushed herself too much in the past and that she should manage the illness by resting and conserving energy. She was also following an anti-candida diet and taking vitamin supplements. She felt she had no control over symptoms, feared doing anything that might make the symptoms worse and felt frustrated and demoralised.

caused by a virus, best managed by rest (Clements et al 1997, Powell et al 1990, Ray et al 1995, Sharpe et al 1992, Vercoulen et al 1994, Wilson et al 1994a). Such beliefs may make sense of the sufferer's experience but are rarely accurate or helpful.

Case definitions for chronic fatigue syndrome

There are no distinctive physical signs and no diagnostic tests for CFS and the central complaint of fatigue is subjective, not amenable to objective measures or tests (Klonoff 1992, Shafran 1991, Swanink et al 1995). To compound matters, the range of accompanying symptoms reported by sufferers is largely non-specific and often overlaps with symptoms found in affective and anxiety disorders. Although difficulties in diagnosis and classification continue, they can be minimised if clearly defined operational criteria are used.

Five case definitions have been proposed, from America (Fukuda et al 1994, Holmes et al 1988, Schluederberg et al 1992), Australia (Lloyd et al 1988) and the UK (Sharpe et al 1991). All define CFS as a main complaint of disabling fatigue, unexplained by current medical or psychiatric illness. All allow for the presence of other symptoms, including sleep disturbance, mood disorder and muscle pain.

The UK criteria (Sharpe et al 1991) require patients to have severe, disabling fatigue of definite onset affecting physical and mental functioning, with a minimum duration of 6 months, leading to substantial impairment of premorbid activity levels. This is broader than the American and Australian criteria and therefore more easily applied. It is the only definition to require mental fatigue (defined as 'a subjective sensation characterised by lack of motivation and alertness') as well as physical fatigue (defined as 'lack of energy or strength, often felt in the muscles'). Depression and anxiety may coexist with CFS but the presence of a major mental illness such as schizophrenia would be considered an exclusion criterion.

The term 'idiopathic chronic fatigue' refers to clinically evaluated unexplained fatigue that fails to meet the criteria for CFS. It is more common and less severe than CFS (Fukuda et al 1994).

Fatigue: category or continuum?

Operational case definitions are essential in research and diagnosis but in practice there is little reason to suppose that CFS is a discrete entity. It can be viewed as lying on a continuum, with fatigue as a symptom at one end of the spectrum and CFS at the other. Current case definitions act as arbitrary cut-offs at a point where there is no natural division (Wessely 1997). The label 'chronic fatigue syndrome' is probably best seen as a clinical description of a cluster of symptoms, behaviours and beliefs rather than a discrete diagnosis (Demitrack & Greden 1991, Swartz 1988, Wilson et al 1994b).

Prevalence

Fatigue is common, chronic fatigue syndrome less so. A British community survey found that 38% of respondents reported substantial fatigue (Cox et al 1987). Idiopathic chronic fatigue is also common, affecting between 10% and 20% of GP attenders (Buchwald et al 1987, David et al 1990). CFS seems to be rarer, affecting approximately 1% of GP attenders and 0.2% of the community (Steele et al 1998, Wessely 1997) although rates vary according to the diagnostic criteria used.

Prognosis

The prognosis in CFS is poor, particularly for adult patients seen in hospital clinics (Joyce et al 1997). Less than 10% make a full recovery and about

10–20% of patients appear to worsen over time. The remainder make some improvements but often remain functionally impaired, unable to work or undertake any significant social or physical activity (Hill et al 1999, Tirelli et al 1994, Vercoulen et al 1996a, Wilson et al 1994a).

TREATMENTS FOR CFS

A variety of novel treatments for CFS has been proposed, including antiviral drugs, immunological therapy, interferon, porcine liver extract, evening prim-rose oil, ascorbic acid, zinc and vitamin B12. Few such agents have been adequately investigated and many claims are made on the basis of uncontrolled evaluations. Controlled trials have reported a marked placebo effect and/or refuted or failed to replicate earlier claims of efficacy. To date, there is little evidence that novel pharmacological agents have much to offer in the management of CFS (Wessely 1997, Wilson et al 1994b).

Complementary medicine offers numerous treatments for CFS and is widely used (Ax et al 1997). Although some patients report transient benefits, few alternative therapies have been systematically evaluated. Results of those which have been evaluated are discouraging (Dowson 1993, Peters et al 1996).

There has been much interest in the role of antidepressants in CFS, both in the treatment of depression and as broad-spectrum agents acting on pain, sleep and energy. Uncontrolled studies and single case reports suggest that antidepressants may improve some affective and somatic symptoms but not functional impairment. Tricyclic antidepressants are widely reported in uncontrolled case series but have not been subjected to any controlled evaluations. Two controlled trials found an SSRI (fluoxetine) to have little or no effect (Vercoulen et al 1996b, Wearden et al 1998) but old and new MAOIs appear more promising (Natalson et al 1996, White & Cleary 1997).

WHAT CAUSES CFS?

The aetiology of CFS has been a source of controversy and debate for many years. Viral models of CFS are popular, possibly because most CFS sufferers associate the onset of fatigue with a virus (Clements et al 1997). However, there is no conclusive evidence of a viral or infective aetiology for CFS and no evidence that common viruses cause CFS (Wessely et al 1995). Some serious infections (such as glandular fever, hepatitis and meningitis) may cause delayed recovery and persistent fatigue but this is relatively infrequent (Berelowitz et al 1995, Hotopf et al 1996, White et al 1995). Viral infection may contribute to the onset of CFS in predisposed individuals (Hotopf & Wessely 1994) but cannot adequately explain the chronicity of fatigue and disability which characterises CFS.

Some immunological abnormalities have been detected in some patients but these are generally minor, appear unrelated to any clinical features of the condition (Peakman et al 1997) and are probably not the cause of symptoms (Buchwald & Komaroff 1991). The immunological changes in CFS are also present in depressed patients and often accompany stress in healthy adults: the changes may be transient and unrelated to any disease process (Glaser & Glaser 1998, Strober 1994, Whiteside & Friberg 1998).

Although CFS is sometimes attributed to neuromuscular disease, studies show that muscle strength, endurance and fatiguability are normal in most CFS patients (Gibson et al 1993, Kent-Braun et al 1993, Lloyd et al 1988, 1991, Riley et al 1990, Sisto et al 1996). The available evidence suggests that muscle weakness or pain in CFS arises from inactivity rather than myopathy (Edwards et al 1993, Wessely 1997). Also, many of the symptoms associated with CFS (such as poor concentration, short-term memory difficulties and making frequent slips of the tongue) cannot be explained by muscular disease.

The high rate of psychiatric disorder noted in CFS patients and the overlap between symptoms of CFS and depression have led some observers to propose a psychiatric aetiology, such as misdiagnosed depression or anxiety (Greenberg 1990) or a somatised expression of major depression (Manu et al 1988). This may be true for some cases but many patients who fulfil criteria for CFS do not meet criteria for any psychiatric diagnosis. Also, the presence of psychiatric disorder alone is insufficient evidence for a psychiatric aetiology: it may simply be a result of overlapping case definitions. Genetic studies suggest that fatigue is aetiologically independent of depression or anxiety (Hickie et al 1999). The relationship between CFS and psychiatric disorder is complex and neither condition can fully explain the other (Demitrack 1988).

It is possible that CFS and psychiatric disorders involve a shared disturbance of brain function (Wessely 1997). There is some evidence pointing to abnormal functioning of the hypothalamic-pituitary-adrenal axis (Cleare et al 1995, Demitrack et al 1991, Scott & Dinan 1999, Scott et al 1999). This could account for some of the major symptoms of CFS, including postexertional fatigue, myalgia, arthralgia, mood and sleep disturbances (Bearn et al 1995, Demitrack et al 1991). However, such neuroendocrine changes may be a consequence rather than a cause of behavioural changes in CFS: for example, a similar pattern of neuroendocrine changes can be recreated in healthy nightshift workers (Leese et al 1996).

It has been suggested that autonomic dysfunction contributes to CFS (Bou-Holaigah et al 1995, Rowe & Calkins 1998). However, it is difficult to judge the prevalence of autonomic dysfunction in CFS patients and the

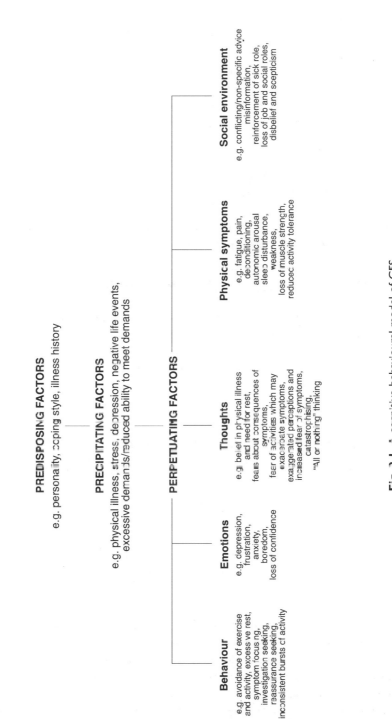

PREDISPOSING FACTORS

e.g. personality, coping style, illness history

PRECIPITATING FACTORS

e.g. physical illness, stress, depression, negative life events,
excessive demands/reduced ability to meet demands

PERPETUATING FACTORS

Behaviour

e.g. avoidance of exercise
and activity, excessive rest,
symptom focusing,
investigation seeking,
reassurance seeking,
inconsistent bursts of activity

Emotions

e.g. depression,
frustration,
anxiety,
boredom,
loss of confidence

Thoughts

e.g. belief in physical illness
and need for rest,
fears about consequences of
symptoms,
fear of activities which may
exacerbate symptoms,
exaggerated perceptions and
increased fear of symptoms,
catastrophising,
"all or nothing" thinking

Physical symptoms

e.g. fatigue, pain,
deconditioning,
autonomic arousal
sleep disturbance,
weakness,
loss of muscle strength,
reduced activity tolerance

Social environment

e.g. conflicting/non-specific advice
misinformation,
reinforcement of sick role,
loss of job and social roles,
disbelief and scepticism

Fig. 9.1 A cognitive behavioural model of CFS.

symptoms of neurally mediated hypotension and orthostatic intolerance may be a consequence rather than a cause of physical inactivity or cardiovascular deconditioning (Jain & DeLisa 1998).

A small number of studies have used neuroimaging techniques and some (but not all) show changes in CFS patients compared to controls, but variations in the inclusion criteria, methods used and results obtained prevent any firm conclusions being drawn (Cope & David 1996).

In summary, specific factors (such as EBV infection or depression) may explain a subset of cases, but it is unlikely that any single cause can adequately explain all or even the majority of cases of CFS. The available evidence points to a heterogenous condition of multifactorial aetiology (Wilson et al 1994b). It is likely that a complex interaction of physiological, cognitive, behavioural and affective factors is responsible for the development and maintenance of fatigue and disability.

A COGNITIVE BEHAVIOURAL MODEL OF CFS

Cognitive behavioural models of CFS draw a distinction between predisposing, precipitating and perpetuating factors (Fig. 9.1). It is suggested that the factors that trigger fatigue are not the same as those that maintain it. Fatigue may be precipitated by a virus, depression and/or stress but is maintained by potentially treatable factors, chiefly maladaptive beliefs and behaviours (Chalder et al 1996b, Surawy et al 1995, Wessely et al 1991).

Predisposing and precipitating factors

Premorbid personality may be a risk factor for CFS, particularly perfectionism, 'action proneness' and achievement orientation (Magnusson et al 1996, Surawy et al 1995, Van Houdenhove et al 1995, Ware & Kleinman 1992). However, recent studies suggest that the role of personality may have been overemphasised and that the characteristics described could be a response to chronic illness rather than having any aetiological significance (Blenkiron et al 1999, Buckley et al 1999, Wood & Wessely 1999). Vulnerability to depressive disorder, preexisting or concurrent depression may increase the risk of prolonged fatigue.

Individuals who were exceptionally physically fit prior to onset may be at increased risk of a delayed recovery (MacDonald et al 1996, Wessely et al 1991). They are likely to undergo rapid physical deconditioning after relatively brief periods of inactivity, resulting in unexpectedly severe symptoms when activity is resumed.

Stress is often noted prior to onset of CFS (Salit 1997). Negative life events, chronic difficulties and stress may contribute to the severity of chronic fatigue. In a primary care study, an increased number of negative life events, lack of social support, prior psychological distress and the presence of infection were all independently associated with fatigue (Chalder 1998, unpublished PhD thesis).

Initially, fatigue occurs as a normal response to an acute trigger, such as an infection and/or stress. An adaptive response would be to rest and reduce activity initially followed by gradual increases in activity, calibrated against fatigue symptoms. Most individuals will thereby make a normal recovery. A minority will fear any fresh exposure to fatigue and associated symptoms and will therefore continue to avoid or restrict activities which may make them feel worse, relying instead upon prolonged rest and avoidance of activity. Avoidance is driven by a number of perpetuating factors, including illness beliefs, misleading advice and/or circumstances in which an individual's personal coping resources are depleted.

Perpetuating factors

Beliefs and expectations

Beliefs and expectations are important, because they influence behaviour and mood. These may include beliefs about:

◆ the nature of the condition (e.g. that fatigue is caused by a physical illness such as a persistent viral infection or that recovery is not under personal control)
◆ the meaning of symptoms (e.g. that muscle pain indicates muscle damage or symptoms make activity impossible)
◆ the consequences of activity (e.g. activity will make symptoms worse).

Such beliefs are associated with perpetuation of disability and symptoms in chronic illness (Sensky 1990). In CFS, several longitudinal and naturalistic studies have found an association between physical illness attributions and poor outcome (Chalder et al 1996a, Sharpe et al 1992, Vercoulen et al 1996a, Wilson et al 1994a). Catastrophic beliefs about the consequences of increasing activity have also been associated with worse disability and fatigue (Petrie et al 1995). It seems plausible that patients who believe they have a physical illness caused by an ongoing disease will fear exacerbating symptoms. They are likely to be highly motivated to avoid or reduce activity (resulting in diminished fitness and worse symptoms). Fear of activity may also be influenced by unexpectedly severe or prolonged fatigue at onset or attempts to do 'too much too soon'. Memories of severe fatigue following such activity can sensitise patients, confirm illness beliefs and reinforce avoidance (Wessely et al 1991).

Physical factors and psychological effects of inactivity

Physical factors likely to perpetuate fatigue and disability include immuno-logical and neuroendocrine changes. Deconditioning and inactivity are also very important.

Even in healthy adults, inactivity can cause fatigue (Hughes et al 1984, Montgomery 1983). The long-term consequences of inactivity are deleterious. It can cause physical deconditioning, loss of mobility, muscle pain, weakness, wasting, impaired cardiovascular response to exertion, reduced activity tolerance, postural hypotension, dizziness and impaired thermoregulation (Greenleaf & Kozlowski 1982, Saltin et al 1968). Such changes have been produced in healthy adults forced to sit in a chair for one week (Lamb et al 1965). Inactivity can also affect mental performance; healthy adults immobilised for a week have impaired recall and verbal fluency (Zubeck & Wilgosh 1963).

Inactivity has adverse psychological and cognitive consequences. These include a reduced sense of control, heightened expectation that activity will increase symptoms, reinforcement of invalid status, symptom focusing and exaggerated symptom perception (Lethem et al 1983). Inactivity is demo-tivating, reduces the desire to undertake exertion (Zorbas & Matveyev 1986) and may increase the risk of depression (Farmer et al 1988). In studies of CFS sufferers, avoiding exercise or activity and accommodating to illness were associated with greater disability (Antoni et al 1994, Ray et al 1995, Sharpe et al 1992).

Inconsistent activity: 'boom and bust'

Although by definition CFS is distinguished by the prolonged rest and avoidance of activity, clinical observations show that avoidance is often only partial; periods of inactivity are often interspersed with bursts of excessive activity (Deale & David 1994, Surawy et al 1995). These bursts are often a response to an apparent reduction in symptoms, frustration, boredom, social demands, performance expectations, achievement orientation or attempts to regain premorbid performance levels (Deale & David 1994, Surawy et al 1995). They are usually excessive in proportion to the physical debilitation of sufferers and therefore are exhausting and unsustain-able. The resulting exacerbation of symptoms can reinforce illness beliefs and reliance on rest. Partial avoidance or inconsistent activity may have some adaptive function in preventing extremes of disability associated with total avoidance but it also inhibits sustained recovery (Deale & Wessely 1994).

Altered sleep

Alterations in sleep routine such as sleeping for longer at night or sleeping during the day, can increase physical symptoms and lethargy. Healthy adults who increased or reduced their sleep time by 2 hours at night over one week reported feeling unrefreshed and physically weak, with muscle pain and poor concentration (Neyta & Horne 1990).

Symptom focusing

People who are fearful of symptoms are likely to focus attention on them (Ray et al 1995, Vercoulen et al 1996b). Increased attention intensifies the awareness, perception and experience of symptoms (Warwick & Salkovskis 1990) which can confirm illness beliefs and reinforce avoidance and illness behaviour (Deale & Wessely 1994). A cross-sectional study of CFS subjects found that focusing on symptoms was associated with increased fatigue, 'giving up' and withdrawal of effort from dealing with the illness (Ray et al 1995).

Depression

Depression is associated with poor outcome in several longitudinal studies (Bombardier & Buchwald 1995, Clark et al 1995, Sharpe et al 1992, Wilson et al 1994a). If not present at onset, depression may develop as a reaction to illness, the limitations it imposes, the potency, uncontrollability and aversive nature of its symptoms.

Depression reduces motivation to resume activity, thereby reinforcing avoidance (Wessely & Powell 1989). It can also account for symptom persistence; symptoms common to CFS (such as fatigue, functional impairment, sleep disturbance and myalgia) can all be features of depressive disorders (Wessely & Powell 1989).

Social environment

Symptoms that occur in the absence of disease are often attributed to psychological causes. This is popularly interpreted as meaning that symptoms are imaginary, 'all in the mind' or indicative of personal weakness or malingering (Abbey & Garfinkel 1991, Greenberg 1990, Ware 1992). In contrast, a 'physical' disease label legitimises illness, validates the reality of symptoms and explains disability to friends, family and employers. CFS sufferers can feel they have to prove their personal worth, but also the 'reality' of their illness

Case Study 9.2 Predisposing, precipitating and perpetuating factors

Teresa described herself as having always been very fit and healthy, with no serious illnesses in the past. She had led a busy active life: she worked full-time, was involved with a local charity and had a wide circle of friends.

Immediately prior to onset, she was exceptionally busy at work and increased her level of exercise in order to unwind. She went for a 10-mile run daily, cycled at weekends and was 'the fittest she had ever been'. She then caught flu but tried to ignore it. After struggling on for a week she collapsed and spent 2 weeks in bed. She then tried to return to work and resumed her normal activities despite still feeling unwell. To her surprise, there was a sharp increase in fatigue and flu-like symptoms, which caused her great anxiety. She was forced to go on sick leave again, became increasingly exhausted and her GP arranged a series of tests, without giving her any real explanation. She became very worried about the cause of her symptoms while waiting for the tests and was unable to sleep. She oscillated between resting completely and trying to exercise her way out of the illness. Each attempt was followed by further fatigue, which heightened her anxiety and convinced her that there was something seriously wrong.

When the results of tests were inconclusive, her GP diagnosed depression. She felt that her physical symptoms were being ignored and approached a private clinic for further investigations. There, she was diagnosed with ME and advised to rest and follow an anti-candida diet. Initially, she was relieved at being given a name for her illness and advice as to its management. She rested diligently but as time went on, she became increasingly worried at the lack of improvement. She was unable to return to work and became increasingly socially isolated.

An alternative model of Teresa's illness is that while a viral illness precipitated fatigue, a combination of predisposing and perpetuating factors prevented a normal recovery. The initial flu-like illness may have been more severe because of the demands being made of her at the time. Her level of physical fitness may have produced rapid physical deconditioning during the fortnight of bedrest. Although resting may have brought some short-term symptom relief, she then tried to do 'too much too soon', resulting in an increase in symptoms. The uncertainty while awaiting a diagnosis exacerbated this. When she followed the advice to rest, her activity tolerance was undermined further, producing more symptoms at progressively lower levels of exertion. Her occasional bursts of activity were unsustainable because they were too demanding, unplanned and inconsistent. They exacerbated her symptoms and prevented her making a phased return to normal activities. The depression that had arisen since onset had undoubtedly increased both the severity of fatigue and associated symptoms.

(Ware 1992). They may stress the 'physical' nature of their complaint and press physicians for a physical diagnosis or further investigations. This may strengthen physical illness attributions. It can also lead to treatable factors (such as maladaptive beliefs and behaviours, depression, sleep disturbance) being minimised or overlooked by sufferers.

Fear of fatigue and reliance on rest may also be reinforced by contradictory, inaccurate or non-specific information and advice given to CFS patients through the media or from health professionals, family and friends (Ax et al 1997, Chalder et al 1996b, Fitzgibbon et al 1997).

The social environment may become a source of reinforcement for illness. Although CFS can disrupt social relationships, some people find that marital or family relationships actually improve. Others may find that loss of occupational and social roles make it difficult to give up the 'sick role', especially if employers or the benefits system are unable to allow a staged return to work (Sharpe & Chalder 1994).

COGNITIVE BEHAVIOURAL THERAPY FOR CFS

Cognitive behavioural models suggest that a range of different factors combine to precipitate and perpetuate fatigue. This distinction between precipitating and perpetuating factors is important, as it points towards positive treatment interventions. In general terms, it is suggested that individuals unwittingly perpetuate fatigue and disability through excessive rest and/or inconsistent bursts of activity. This behaviour is often symptom driven and influenced by idiosyncratic illness beliefs. Cognitive behaviour therapy seeks to unlock this cycle of fatigue and disability by altering the interaction of symptoms, behaviour and beliefs.

Treatment is a collaborative process. Treatment goals are jointly agreed between therapist and client, progress is constantly reviewed and clients are encouraged to take an increasingly active part in planning and implementing their treatment programme.

The process of rehabilitation requires time, patience and, above all, persistence on the part of both therapist and client. Typically, a course of treatment will involve 12–15 sessions, at fortnightly intervals. When these sessions come to an end, clients are expected to continue following a self-directed programme for at least another year, with progress monitored at regular follow-up sessions. Box 9.1 outlines the three phases of treatment.

Phase 1: Assessment and engagement

The initial sessions form the groundwork of treatment. It is wise to spread the assessment/engagement phase of treatment over two or three sessions, lasting 1–2 hours. The aims are:

◆ to form a therapeutic alliance with the client
◆ to make a careful individual assessment in order to identify specific perpetuating factors
◆ to give the client a rationale for treatment.

> **Box 9.1** Treatment outline
>
> **Phase 1: Assessment and engagement**
> Detailed assessment of current difficulties and history
> Establish a therapeutic alliance
> Treatment rationale
> Self-monitoring diaries
> Clinical measures
> Involve relative or friend
>
> **Phase 2: Active treatment**
> Establish programme of scheduled, consistent activity and planned rest
> Graded increases in activity and reductions in rest
> Establish sleep routine
> Address illness beliefs through discussion and cognitive restructuring
>
> **Phase 3: Preparation for discharge and follow-up**
> Client takes lead in planning treatment programme
> Client draws up discharge plan of short, medium, long-term goals
> Rehearse strategies for dealing with setbacks
> Long phased follow-up with booster sessions

Engaging clients in therapy

Forming a good therapeutic alliance is essential. Most clients believe they have a physical illness and may feel stigmatised by or hostile to a referral to a department of liaison psychiatry, particularly if the reasons for such a referral have not been clearly explained. Some will view their referral as a thinly veiled message that their condition is 'psychological' (and therefore not 'real') after all. The behaviour of some clients may be influenced by earlier unsatisfactory encounters with health-care professionals in which they felt their condition was demeaned, disbelieved or dismissed. Clients may also view treatment with trepidation; they may believe it to be a rigid exercise programme, which will worsen their condition, or they may feel that a 'psychological' treatment is inappropriate for a 'physical' illness.

In order to overcome these difficulties, it is important that the clinician puts aside sufficient time for the initial sessions (1.5–2 hours). It is important to give the client time to 'tell their story', so that they feel listened to and taken seriously. The clinician should be explicit in conveying empathy and belief in the reality of physical symptoms. It is important to seek the client's own views on the nature and cause of their illness and to treat them with respect (regardless of whether the clinician actually agrees with them). It is also useful to ask the client for their views on the referral. Ventilating previous dissatisfaction is important and can be facilitated by asking whether the client has had experiences of being disbelieved or dismissed and whether they have been given much advice on the management of their illness.

The clinician should be sensitive in use of language. If the client calls their condition 'ME', the clinician should avoid alienating them by using the term 'CFS' rigidly or without explanation. If the client calls their condition an 'illness', the clinician should be careful to avoiding referring to it as a 'problem'. The clinician should avoid using psychiatric jargon or implying that physical complaints are psychogenic in origin. Most importantly, the clinician should avoid using the term 'psychological' – it is a broad, non-specific term, which is likely to be misinterpreted and to provoke conflict. You should avoid becoming enmeshed in a dichotomous 'physical' versus 'psychological' debate and seek to broaden rather than challenge or confront the client's beliefs. It is more helpful to steer the discussion towards considering how the illness can best be managed.

Assessment

A careful assessment is part of the process of building a therapeutic alliance. The main purpose of the assessment is to establish a detailed, individualised understanding of the client's illness in order to devise a treatment programme and deliver a treatment rationale.

As in any assessment, it is important to set the scene by explaining the purpose and likely duration of the assessment. A useful engagement strategy is to tell the client that if the interview becomes too tiring, they can stop at any time. It is also helpful to ask the client if they have any questions or comments they would like to make before the assessment begins. This can be an opportunity to 'clear the air' and address any misconceptions that may otherwise cloud the assessment.

The clinician may begin by asking the client to describe their main symptoms. Somatic symptoms are likely to be uppermost in the client's mind and this opening demonstrates that the clinician is interested in them and takes them seriously. Details about the nature of symptoms, variations and fluctuations should then be clarified. The clinician should obtain a clear description of the fatigue, both physical (exhaustion, lack of energy, exacerbated by minor exertion) and mental (poor memory and concentration, word-finding difficulties, slips of the tongue). The presence of other symptoms (such as muscle pain, headaches and sore throats) should also be determined.

The clinician can then move on to enquire about the effect of symptoms on the patient's daily life. It is useful to ask about restrictions, avoidances and modifications to activities in the areas of work, social and private leisure, home management (shopping, cooking, housework, gardening), child care and physical activity/exercise. The quality and quantity of rest and sleep should be described. Much of this information can be elicited by asking the patient to describe a typical day.

The clinician can then move on to taking a history of the illness. In order to build up as full a picture as possible of potential precipitating factors, the clinician should ask not only how the illness started but what were the circumstances leading up to onset. The course of the illness since onset should be described: this should include fluctuations in the course of symptoms, periods when the illness has been significantly worse or significantly better and a description of previous investigations and treatments.

It is important to enquire about the client's understanding of their illness. This includes asking them what they believe caused their illness and why they think it has persisted for so long. They will have given much thought to different ways of coping with their illness and it is important to ask them for their views on what has helped their symptoms and what has made them worse.

A description of the client's current situation is important. This includes details of the involvement, beliefs and attitudes of the family and significant others, concurrent treatment or investigations, disability benefits and employment status. It is also important to ask the patient what they would like to do when they recover from the illness.

Having built up a picture of the illness and its impact on the client, it is easier to move on to a mental state examination, using a non-threatening question such as 'How has all this affected your mood?'. It is important to identify depression or anxiety as such disorders, if severe, may require treatment in their own right.

After gathering these details of the main problem and its impact on daily life, the clinician should take a general background family and personal history, including a past medical and psychiatric history and details of premorbid personality and lifestyle. Throughout the assessment, the clinician should summarise and feed back what the client has said. This helps ensure that the information being recorded is accurate, helps the client to feel understood and listened to and is part of the process of developing a shared understanding of the illness.

Offering a treatment rationale

Having completed the assessment, the clinician can offer the client a cognitive behavioural formulation of their illness. Using information gathered during the assessment process, the clinician should give an explanation for the onset (emphasising a multifactorial origin) and the maintenance of symptoms and disability. Those factors that the patient believes have caused the illness should be incorporated into this model wherever possible.

When being given a formulation, clients are told that an 'organic' trigger to symptoms is not precluded, but that successful rehabilitation depends upon dealing with maintaining factors, such as excessive rest (which is useful in response to acute illness but detrimental in the longer term), an altered sleep pattern, a 'boom and bust' approach to activity, low mood.

It is explained that the aim of treatment is to increase activities without exacerbating fatigue and that increased activity will improve strength and stamina, which in turn will reduce the severity of fatigue and associated symptoms. The main components of treatment should be described. These will include some or all of the following.

◆ A programme of consistent, planned activity and rest.
◆ Graded increases in activity will be made as the patient becomes more confident, always set at a jointly agreed, manageable level.
◆ Establishing a sleep routine.
◆ Specific beliefs or fears that may be contributing to the client's difficulties are addressed directly, through discussion and cognitive restructuring.
◆ Other interventions (such as strategies for alleviating depression or reducing perfectionism), depending on the individual perpetuating factors identified for each client.

When giving a formulation and treatment rationale, the clinician should invite discussion and questions. Scepticism or at least lack of enthusiasm is to be expected; few clients are 'converted' immediately. However, provided they understand what treatment entails and agree to at least try it, treatment can proceed.

Acceptance of the rationale may waver during treatment (often in parallel with fluctuations in symptoms) and it is important for the clinician and client to review and repeat the treatment rationale frequently.

Self-monitoring diaries

Self-monitoring diaries are an essential adjunct to assessment. In order to obtain a detailed picture of activity, rest and sleep, clients are asked to keep an hour-by-hour account for 2 weeks. The diaries provide more detailed information than can be obtained from interviewing alone. They are a basis for setting the initial treatment programme and can be used throughout treatment to monitor progress.

Box 9.2 Recommended investigations in CFS

Routine: full blood count, erythrocyte sedimentation rate, liver function tests, urea and electrolytes, thyroid function tests, urinalysis for protein and sugar

If indicated by history: EBV serology, chest X-ray, rheumatoid factor and ANF, serological testing for Q fever, toxoplasmosis, HIV

Not useful: enteroviral serology, neuroimaging

Measurement

Measurement is an important part of treatment. It can be difficult to assess progress over a long period, particularly when the pace of improvement is gradual and symptoms fluctuate. Clinical outcome measures given at regular intervals provide valuable feedback to client and therapist. They also serve to keep the treatment focused and goal directed.

One of the most useful measures is an individualised problem and goal rating (Marks 1986). The therapist and client jointly agree on a definition of the main problem to be treated (for example, 'persistent physical and mental fatigue that fluctuates in severity and is accompanied by headache, muscle pain and weakness'). The client then rates how severe the problem is on a scale of 0 (does not upset me or interfere with normal activities) to 8 (very severely upsetting, continuously interferes with normal activities). Clients are then asked to identify between two and four long-term goals. These should be activities that they wish to achieve and which would represent a substantial improvement in functioning and fatigue (for example, 'to go swimming for half an hour twice a week' or 'to work part time, for 3 hours 5 days a week'). Progress towards these long-term goals is rated on a scale of 0 (complete success) to 8 (no success at all). Agreeing long-term goals helps the client and clinician to know that they are working towards the same end.

It is also useful to have a measure of functional impairment, such as the Work and Social Adjustment Scale (Marks 1986); a measure of fatigue, such at the Fatigue Questionnaire (Chalder et al 1993); and a measure of mood, such as the Hospital Anxiety and Depression Scale (Zigmond & Snaith 1983). Clinical global improvement measures can provide a helpful summary of overall progress.

Investigations and treatment

Research suggests that in anyone with fatigue lasting more than 6 months, physical investigation is largely unhelpful (Kroenke et al 1988, Ridsdale et al 1993, Valdini et al 1989). There is no diagnostic test for CFS and the principal symptom of fatigue is a factor in many illnesses. There is scope for diagnostic confusion, but in practice making a diagnosis of CFS is usually simple, provided a careful history is taken and some simple tests (Box 9.2) arranged (Wessely 1997). Provided these have been carried out, the clinician should resist the temptation to overinvestigate which serves no purpose other than to strengthen physical illness attributions and generate fear and uncertainty. An agreement should be reached early on to call a halt to further tests.

The client may be receiving a variety of other treatments. It is generally desirable to suspend these as competing therapies and models may be incompatible and confusing to the client. It also makes it impossible to know which treatment is responsible for change.

Phase 2: Active treatment

Treatment sessions generally take up to 1 hour. Throughout, it is helpful to begin each session by reminding the client how long the session will take and agreeing an agenda, so that you can both make best use of the time available. At each treatment session, short-term targets are agreed, which the client will work on at home. Treatment sessions normally begin with a review of the client's activity diaries and progress with the agreed targets. As much as possible, potential difficulties should be anticipated (it is always useful to ask clients whether they foresee any difficulties in carrying out their programme over the coming weeks) and problem-solving strategies should be devised. Discussion in sessions often involves exploring issues that may be preventing the client from making changes. The session ends with agreeing new short-term targets.

Activity scheduling and graded activity

The key element of treatment is to help clients resume normal activities and reduce reliance on rest without exacerbating fatigue. Although the deleterious effects of inactivity are well known, simply asking clients to 'do more' is insufficient. Many clients will have already tried to 'do more' with disastrous results. It is therefore important to begin by emphasising the need for planned rest and consistent rather than variable activity: a middle way between doing too much and doing too little. This is reassuring to clients and ensures that initial targets will be manageable and achievable.

At the first treatment session, the client's self-monitoring diaries are reviewed carefully in order to ensure that initial targets are set at an appropriate level. A structured programme is devised, planned so that the same amount of activity and the same amount of rest is undertaken consistently every day, regardless of fluctuations in symptoms. Initial targets should be modest and small enough to be sustained despite fluctuations in symptoms. At first, there may be no actual increase in activity. Instead, in the interests of establishing structure and consistency, clients may be asked to do less rather than more or to reschedule their activity so that they do less than they would normally do on a 'good' day but slightly more than they would normally do on a 'bad' day. For example, rather than going for a 45-minute walk once a week, a client might be asked to carry out three 5-minute walks every day. Activity and rest are divided into small, manageable portions spread across the day. It is very important that targets are clear and specific, stating what is to done, where, when and how often.

Careful attention should be given to planned rest. Initially, the optimal amount of rest can be calculated by totalling the amount of rest taken over a week or a fortnight, averaging it out to give a daily total and dividing the total into even chunks across the day. What constitutes 'rest' may vary from one person to another and it is important to specify what a rest should be (for instance, sitting watching the television for 20 minutes maybe restful for some but not others). Relaxation techniques can play a part for those people who find it difficult to 'switch off' during rests. It is also important that both client and clinician are clear in distinguishing periods of rest from 'light pottering' and specific activity targets.

Once an initial programme is established, the amount of activity (both duration and type) can be gradually increased and rest reduced. Adjustments to the programme should be made gradually, as sudden or extreme changes are likely to precipitate unacceptably high levels of fatigue. Activity can be increased when fatigue levels have either reduced or remained stable and manageable for 4–6 days.

Targets typically involve a variety of specific tasks, encompassing work, social and leisure activities together with rest. Some light exercise is important – short walks are ideal. As the treatment progresses, it is often useful to make the walks rather more brisk or to introduce cycling or swimming. However, there should also be a range of targets reflecting normal or desired activities of daily living, which are either restricted or absent from the client's current behavioural repertoire. It is important to make sure that the programme contains some activities that are enjoyable and interesting. Tasks that require mental effort (such as reading or studying) can be included, but improvements in concentration will often develop naturally, following improvements in physical functioning.

Words of warning

◆ It is most important that clients persevere with their targets; many will wish to reduce them on a bad day or (more commonly) exceed them on a good day. The clinician should warn clients against doing this, as it will undermine efforts to build a stable foundation from which activity can be systematically increased.

◆ It is normal for fatigue levels to rise whenever activity is increased. This should be explained and clients told that as long as the planned increase has been set at a low enough level, the initial rise in symptoms will be manageable and will subside as tolerance develops.

◆ Clients should be told that they will not feel any great changes in fatigue for some time. Fatigue and associated symptoms tend to fluctuate, even well into recovery, and it can take months for the overall levels to diminish. The most marked reductions in fatigue usually take place between discharge and final follow-up. It is important to emphasise that the main goal of treatment is to stick to the programme, not to overcome all the symptoms at once.

Establishing a sleep routine

Many people with CFS have chaotic sleep habits and almost all will require a sleep routine. Many spend long periods of time in bed and this should be gradually reduced. Daytime sleep should be phased out. Rising at a specific time each morning is important; for people who tend to sleep long into the day, the wake-up time can be gradually brought forward (for example, rising at 11am instead of 11.30 for 2 weeks, then 10.30, 10, etc. until the target time is reached). People who have trouble getting off to sleep or who wake for long periods in the night will require a set rising time and a ban on daytime sleep. They may also need advice on sleep hygiene and stimulus control techniques (see Lacks 1987).

Modifying negative thoughts

Negative thoughts, illness beliefs and fears about the consequences of activity can interfere with graded increases in activity. Many clients will have read and consulted widely on their condition and misleading or incorrect information may have shaped their beliefs about the illness. It is therefore important to try to elicit and discuss misinformation from the outset of treatment. The physiological consequences of inactivity should be described and clients should be reassured about the safety of exercise and of the proposed treatment programme.

Illness beliefs, negative thoughts and fears often decrease as clients become more active and more confident. Graded increases in activity are a potent means of gently testing out beliefs such as 'exercise is harmful', 'rest is the best treatment for my condition' and 'the symptoms are controlling me'. However, it is sometimes helpful to use a more structured cognitive approach (Beck et al 1979). The aim here is to help the client identify thinking patterns which may be impeding their recovery and find different ways of viewing the situation which may be more helpful and less distressing.

Clients are asked to write down what is going though their mind when their symptoms worsen, when they are having difficulty with their programme or when their mood drops. They record their thoughts in a structured diary, rating how strongly they believe it. In discussion and as homework, they then practise generating alternative, less catastrophic interpretations of events. For example, a classic negative thought 'I am still feeling really exhausted, this treatment isn't working' might be replaced by an alternative 'I do still feel exhausted at times, but I'm able to do a lot more than I was 2 months ago and I'm no more tired now than I was then'. The aim is not to simply substitute a positive for a negative or find the 'right' answer, but to learn how to question unhelpful thoughts in order to find different ways of looking at the situation which helps the client to feel better and move forward.

Phase 3: Preparation for discharge and follow-up

As treatment proceeds, clients take increasing responsibility for their treatment programme. This is an important part of preparing people for discharge. During the final sessions, clients are usually asked to draw up a discharge plan. This consists of short, medium and long-term goals to guide them through the coming months. Their progress towards achieving these goals is then reviewed in follow-up sessions. Clients should be prepared for their symptoms to feel worse again from time to time (for instance, if they get a cold or a viral infection or if they are very busy) and strategies for dealing with setbacks should be rehearsed. The golden rule is not to panic and not to abandon the principles of treatment. It is often helpful to ask clients to write down a list of what they have learnt in treatment, which specific techniques they have found useful and what things they would like to remember during setbacks.

Follow-up is an important part of treatment. By the time regular sessions end, most clients will have made some improvements and be in a position to continue with a self-directed treatment programme. A long, phased follow-up with 'booster' sessions is therefore essential in order to ensure progress continues and troubleshoot any difficulties. In our department, clients are normally followed up at 3 months, 6 months and 1 year post-treatment, with additional sessions arranged if required.

Special issues in treatment

Adjunctive interventions

CFS is a heterogeneous condition and the specific combination of perpetuating factors may differ from one client to the next. Treatment should not be delivered in a textbook fashion; rather, the specific interventions used should be selected according to the individual problem formulation devised for each client. Thus for some clients, treatment may include training in problem-solving strategies or exposure therapy for agoraphobia or social anxiety. The principles of cognitive behavioural therapy can be combined with other interventions. These may include physiotherapy (for patients who are severely disabled), relaxation (for improving sleep and rest, alleviating stress

---

Case Study 9.3 Treatment

Initially Teresa was not enthusiastic about treatment, as she felt that she had already tried unsuccessfully to increase activity. She agreed that it might be helpful to have some guidance in building up activity in a more graded way. She decided to give it a try and completed some self-monitoring diaries for a fortnight. When she reviewed these with the therapist, she realised that there was often considerable variation in activity levels; on two occasions she walked for 2 miles and on others she was unable to walk for more than 5 minutes. She found it difficult to regulate her activity and tended to be overly ambitious; after doing too much gardening one day she had stabbing pains in her arm muscles and had to spend a day in bed.

The initial programme was based on what Teresa felt she could manage on a bad day: a 10-minute walk twice daily and 15 minutes of gardening twice daily. Specific times at which these activities were to be carried out were agreed. Five 30-minute rest periods were planned at 9am, 11am, 1.30pm, 4pm and 7pm. Outside the rest and activity times she would be reading, listening to music or 'pottering'. She was asked to establish a set wake-up time each morning (8.30am) and to stop sleeping during the day. Ways of 'winding down' for the night were discussed. Teresa achieved these targets on all but one occasion, when visitors arrived. She spent time with them, missed her planned rests and activities and was left exhausted by the talking. After talking it over with her therapist, she decided that if visitors called in future she would still go for walks and take her planned rests in another room.

At the next treatment session, she reported that although she had carried out all her targets, the fatigue and muscle pain became much worse. She was worried that the programme was too demanding, that overexertion had activated a virus and that she would have to resign herself to living within limits. Her diaries showed that she had started joining up her two gardening sessions, because she felt frustrated at only doing 15 minutes at a time. Her therapist suggested that making too large an increase in activity all at once might have caused the dramatic increase in symptoms. A more successful approach would have been to increase the total amount of time slightly but keep it divided into manageable sections, such as two 20-minute sessions daily.

Case Study 9.3 Cont'd

By mid-treatment, Teresa was finding the treatment easier to follow, her fatigue ratings had stabilised at a managable level and she was sleeping better. The graded increases in activites continued, in a step-by-step fashion, a greater variety of activities was introduced and the length of rest periods was slowly reduced. Increasingly, Teresa took the lead in planning her own treatment programme and the focus of sessions turned to preparation for discharge. The need for a balance of activity and rest was discussed, especially in the context of her activity-prone lifestyle prior to onset. Teresa set some short, medium and long-terms goals for follow-up. These included returning to part-time work, increasing her exercise and doing more social activities. She broke these targets down into smaller goals and decided to set a specific time each week when she would review progress.

By the end of treatment, Teresa's daily schedule included a 20–30-minute walk, a 20-minute cycle ride and 1 hour of gardening daily. She rested for 20 minutes mid morning and mid afternoon and for 40 minutes at lunchtime. She went out socially twice a week and had joined a local choir. She was about to begin some voluntary work for 2 hours one morning a week She rated herself as very much improved and although she still felt tired, the severity and intensity of fatigue and associated symptoms had reduced considerably. She felt physically stronger, her concentration and memory had improved, her sleep was refreshing and rarely disturbed and she felt far more positive and optimistic about the future. Teresa continued to follow a self-directed treatment programme during follow-up. One year after treatment ended, she was working as a teacher again 4 days a week. She went out socially, swam and cycled regularly. She had joined the Ramblers Association, which she very much enjoyed. Although she still suffered from excessive fatigue occasionally, it was not handicapping and she felt able to manage it appropriately.

and pain management) and counselling (provided it is not focused solely on accepting disability).

The role of antidepressants in the management of CFS should not be overlooked. When clinical depression is found in conjunction with CFS, it should be treated. Even in the absence of clinical depression, antidepressants can improve fatigue, pain and sleep. When starting antidepressant treatment, clients should be told about potential side effects, so that these are anticipated and not confused with a 'relapse' of the condition. Older tricyclic antidepressants can be poorly tolerated (Lynch et al 1991) and therefore are often given at lower doses than in routine psychiatric practice (Gantz & Holmes 1989).

Work and disability benefits

Few clients will be in employment when they begin treatment and those who are working may well have reduced their hours. Before preparing clients for a return to work, it is important to ascertain whether a job exists for them to return to and whether they actually want to return to their old (or any) job. The practicalities of making a phased return to work should be explored. In some cases, work will have contributed to the onset of CFS and some clients will want to pursue a career change or alter their working practices. Planning for this should be incorporated into treatment.

Difficulties can arise if the client is on sick leave, with pressure to get well fairly quickly in order to return to work. In our experience, having such deadlines (whether real or imagined) can militate against a graded activity programme, as clients try to 'run before they can walk'. It is worth finding out how real the deadline is and negotiating with the employer to defer making a decision and/or for a phased return to work.

Some clients receive disability benefits and payments that are contingent upon them remaining unwell. Gradual recovery can cause a period of financial instability, as clients may be well enough to disbar them from receiving payments but not well enough to support themselves with a permanent earned income. It may be necessary to negotiate some period of overlap between work and payments – 'therapeutic earnings', voluntary work or part-time study are possibilities.

Applying for medical retirement or a new disability benefit during treatment can pose a problem. Applying for medical retirement was associated with unimproved outcome in a randomised controlled trial of cognitive behavioural therapy for CFS (Deale et al 1997) and changing or leaving employment was associated with poor outcome in an earlier longitudinal study (Sharpe et al 1991) During treatment, it seems understandable that the uncertainty and stress of having to prove oneself ill in pursuit of a claim might militate against improvement. Decisions should be made on a case-by-case basis, but it may be worth considering deferring treatment until such claims are settled, as medical retirement or disability claims settled before treatment begins appear to have little effect on outcome.

The therapist may be asked to comment on benefits or insurance claims. Benefit systems and insurance agencies can be sceptical about CFS. In our experience, we generally support the client in claims for benefit as much as is possible. Claims for medical retirement on the grounds of permanent ill health may be more problematic; the therapist may feel that such a claim cannot be supported until all reasonable efforts at rehabilitation have been tried. On the other hand, attempting a programme of cognitive behaviour therapy in such circumstances is fraught with difficulties.

Psychosocial problems

Social, psychological or relationship difficulties often emerge during treatment. For instance, a relationship that functioned while the client was ill may show signs of strain as the client begins to improve. Such problems can prevent further progress and it is important that they are incorporated into treatment, using a problem-solving approach. However, it is not always possible to address them fully within the time available and additional sessions or referral onwards once treatment ends may be appropriate. The clinician should not lose sight of the main purpose of treatment, which is rehabilitation. Addressing new problems while staying focused on rehabilitation can be a difficult balancing act but being distracted from the principal task is likely to lead to treatment failure. Conversely, improvements in one area of a patient's life will usually generalise to other areas.

The role of families

Relatives and friends can act as 'co-therapists' in CBT (Hawton et al 1989, Marks 1987). This role can be especially helpful in the management of CFS as significant others may unwittingly reinforce maladaptive beliefs and inadvertently encourage disability.

It is often useful to involve relatives in the assessment phase of treatment, provided the client agrees. They may be invited to sit in on all or part of the initial sessions or be invited to a special session. It is important to enquire into the relative's views as to the cause and management of the condition and to give them a rationale for treatment directly, rather than asking the client to relay it to them.

Once treatment is under way, relatives should be encouraged to give clients appropriate praise and encouragement for progress made and to support clients in the efforts being made towards achieving goals, even if they have not yet been reached. They can be especially helpful in ensuring clients do not exceed their programme during a good patch.

If relatives have any worries about treatment or feel it may be harmful, they are advised to ask the client whether they can contact the therapist or come to a treatment session. The therapist may need to advise relatives on what to do if they feel the client is not carrying out their treatment properly. In general, relatives are advised to avoid *telling* clients what to do, as this often leads to arguments and resentment. They are reminded that difficulties with the programme will be discussed during each treatment session. It is suggested that if relatives are worried, it is probably best to ask the client directly, in a supportive and non-judgemental manner, whether there are any problems with the programme and whether they would like to discuss it. If the answer is no, relatives are advised not to persist but simply to ensure that the client knows they are there if needed.

Does it work?

There are a number of uncontrolled studies reporting CBT to be effective in the management of CFS (Butler et al 1991, Cox & Findley 1994, Essame et al 1998, Vereker 1992). An early randomised controlled trial from Australia found CBT to be no better that high-quality medical care (Lloyd et al 1993). However, their therapy was brief, consisting of only six sessions in total. In the UK, a more intensive cognitive behaviour therapy has been evaluated in randomised controlled trials from Oxford (Sharpe et al 1996) and London (Deale et al 1997). Both studies found that CBT was safe, acceptable to clients and more effective than either standard medical care or relaxation therapy. In both studies, around 70% of subjects who received CBT showed significant and similar improvements in functional impairment and fatigue, with improvements increasing during follow-up. Although between one-quarter and one-third of patients made slight or no improvements, no negative effects were associated with CBT.

There have been two randomised controlled trials of graded exercise. In one, graded exercise was effective in CFS patients who had no psychiatric disorder or sleep disturbance (Fulcher & White 1997). Significant improvements were noted in fatigue and functional impairment. The second trial found that exercise (with either fluoxetine or placebo) produced more modest benefits in a more representative group of CFS patients (Wearden et al 1998). The exercise was less carefully graded than in the earlier trial and produced a higher drop-out rate. Nevertheless, these trials suggest that carefully graded exercise is safe and produces benefits that are not simply physiological.

Outcome in the two CBT trials and the first graded exercise trial were strikingly similar. About 70% of subjects in the intervention groups rated themselves as very much improved and 65% were working or studying at the end of follow-up. There are clear differences in the interventions evaluated in the three trials. Cognitive interventions were strongly emphasised in the Oxford CBT study, less so in the London CBT study and not at all in the graded exercise study. All three studies involved graded increases in activity, which suggests that behavioural change is the key component of treatment. This does not mean that cognitive variables should be ignored: discussion of patients' fears, expectations and beliefs is an integral part of good behavioural analysis and implementation. Attention to cognitive variables may enhance the acceptability of treatment and produce greater improvements in mood. However, it does appear that an intervention which helps CFS sufferers to make gradual increases in activity levels will lead to improved outcome, whether this is achieved through graded exercise or CBT, through the manipulation of behaviour, changing of beliefs or fostering a sense of control.

In the London and Oxford studies, improvements in the CBT group continued during follow-up, after treatment ended. This is in keeping with the emphasis in therapy on homework practice and self-directed treatment. In our experience, progress is often slow during the initial stages of treatment. This can be demoralising for both the therapist and client, so it is important to be aware that many people only begin to make substantial improvements towards the end of treatment, which increase during follow-up. The pace of progress is often increased when clients are able to sustain more aerobic or demanding exercise (such as brisk walking, cycling or swimming), but it takes time and practice to reach this stage.

CBT can lead to improved functioning and fatigue in about two-thirds of sufferers. It is also cost effective (Best 1996). However, CBT is not a 'cure' for CFS and it does not remove all symptoms and restrictions. It is more helpful to see CBT as means of producing earlier improvement than would be found in an untreated population (Bonner et al 1994). At present, little is known about factors that influence treatment outcome. Poor outcome may be influenced by treatment-resistant depression, strongly held beliefs about the need to avoid exercise and rest more, the beliefs of family members (particularly in children and adolescents) and taking medical retirement during treatment (Butler et al 1991, Deale et al 1997, 1998, Essame et al 1998, Vereker 1992). In our experience, treatment may be more difficult in cases where clients cannot identify clear or specific goals they wish to work towards (although this is rare) and when clients suffer from severe pain in addition to fatigue.

CONCLUSION

Cognitive behaviour therapy is a practical, evidence-based approach to managing clients who present with chronic fatigue syndrome. The principles of treatment are those used in the management of medically unexplained symptoms in general (Sharpe et al 1992). Although the principles of treatment are simple, the therapist must apply them carefully, tailoring treatment to the individual client.

Guidelines for practice

Form a therapeutic alliance.

◆ Listen to the patient.
◆ Take symptoms seriously and show that you believe them to be genuine and distressing.

- Avoid a physical versus psychological debate.
- Be sensitive in language used.
- Try to broaden (rather than confront) illness beliefs.

Make a careful assessment and identify individual perpetuating factors.

- Enquire about symptoms, level of disability and restrictions, amount of rest, sleep patterns, coping strategies and patient's own beliefs.
- Enquire about previous encounters with health-care professionals and previous experiences of treatment.
- Identify any psychiatric disorder.

Give a clear rationale for treatment.

- Shift the agenda away from what may have started the illness towards identifying and modifying obstacles to recovery.
- Give the patient a model for understanding their illness which distinguishes between precipitating and perpetuating factors.
- Give practical examples of how individual perpetuating factors will be treated.
- Be prepared to repeat it as often as necessary throughout treatment.

Treatment should be pragmatic, individualised and carefully graded.

- Adopt a problem-solving approach.
- Tackle perpetuating factors one at a time, beginning with the area of greatest dysfunction.
- Be flexible; tailor treatment to the needs of the individual patients and draw upon a variety of treatment techniques.
- Treat depression if it is present.
- Work towards clearly specified, jointly agreed goals.
- Provide regular appointments, monitoring and support.
- Persevere and persist: the process of change takes time.

QUESTIONS FOR DISCUSSION

- What specific difficulties in engaging clients would you expect to encounter in your service?

- How would you respond to a client who wants more investigations because they feel that something important has been missed?

- How would you deliver treatment to a client who spends most of their time in a wheelchair?

ANNOTATED BIBLIOGRAPHY

Sharpe M, Chalder T, Palmer I, Wessely S 1997 Chronic fatigue syndrome: a practical guide to assessment and management. Gen Hosp Psychiatry 19:185–187

A practical, evidence-based guide to the general principles of assessment and management illustrated with case examples.

Wilson A, Hickie I, Lloyd A, Wakefield D 1994 The treatment of chronic fatigue syndrome: science and speculation. Am J Med 96:544–549

Outlines the methodological problems of treatment outcome studies in CFS and gives guidelines for good clinical care.

Essame C, Phelan S, Aggett P, White P 1998 Pilot study of a multi-disciplinary inpatient rehabilitation of severely incapacitated patients with chronic fatigue syndrome. J Chronic Fatigue Syndrome 4:51–60

Marlin R, Anchel H, Gibson J, Goldberg W, Swinton M 1998 An evaluation of a multidisciplinary intervention for chronic fatigue syndrome with long-term follow-up, and a comparison with untreated controls. Am J Med 105(3A):s110–115

These papers are examples of the application of a cognitive behavioural approach in very different treatment settings. The first describes a multidisciplinary approach to inpatient treatment of severe CFS; the second describes treatment of CFS in the home environment.

Wessely S, Hotopf M, Sharpe M 1998 Chronic fatigue and its syndromes. Oxford University Press, New York

A lengthy 'state of the art' overview detailing the nature and history of fatigue, chronic fatigue and CFS. Comprehensive overview of the various aetiological theories and treatment approaches.

Chalder T 1995 Coping with chronic fatigue. Sheldon Press, London

A self-help book offering practical advice on managing fatigue.

REFERENCES

Abbey S 1993 Somatisation and illness attribution. In: Kleinman A, Straus S (eds) Chronic fatigue syndrome: Ciba Foundation symposium. Wiley Interscience, Chichester, pp 238–252

Abbey S, Garfinkel P 1991 Neurasthenia and chronic fatigue syndrome: the role of culture in the making of a diagnosis. Am J Psychiatry 148:1638–1646

Antoni M, Brickman A, Lutgendorf S et al 1994 Psychosocial correlates of illness burden in chronic fatigue syndrome. Clin Infect Dis 18(sl):S73–78

Aronowitz R 1992 From myalgic encephalitis to yuppie flu: a history of chronic fatigue syndromes. In: Rosenberg C, Golden J (eds) Framing disease. Rutgers University Press, New Jersey

Ax S, Gregg V, Jones D 1997 Chronic fatigue syndrome: sufferers' evaluation of medical support. J R Soc Med 90:250–254

Bearn J, Allain T, Coskeran P et al 1995 Neuroendocrine responses to D-fenfluramine and insulin induced hypoglycaemia in chronic fatigue syndrome. Biol Psychiatry 37:245–252

Beck A, Rush A, Shaw B, Emery G 1979 Cognitive therapy of depression. Guilford Press, New York

Berelowitz G, Burgess A, Thanabalasingham T, Murray-Lyon I, Wright D 1995 Post-hepatitis syndrome revisited. J Viral Hepat 2:133–138

Best L 1996 Cognitive behaviour therapy in the management of chronic fatigue syndrome. Wessex Institute of Public Health Medicine, Southampton

Blenkiron P, Edwards R, Lynch S 1999 Associations between perfectionism, mood and fatigue in chronic fatigue syndrome: a pilot study. J Nerv Ment Dis 187(9):566–570

Bombardier C, Buchwald D 1995 Outcome and prognosis of patients with chronic fatigue versus chronic fatigue syndrome in a primary care practice. Arch Intern Med 153:2759–2765

Bonner D, Ron M, Chalder T, Butler S, Wessely S 1994 Chronic fatigue syndrome: a follow up study. J Neurol Neurosurg Psychiatry 57:617–621

Bou-Holaigah I, Rowe P, Kan J, Calkins H 1995 The relationship between neurally mediated hypotension and the chronic fatigue syndrome. JAMA 274:961–967

Buchwald D, Komaroff A 1991 Review of laboratory findings for patients with chronic fatigue syndrome. Rev Infect Dis 13(sl):s12–18

Buchwald D, Sullivan J, Komaroff A 1987 Frequency of 'chronic active Epstein Barr virus infection' in a general medical practice. JAMA 257.2303–2307

Buckley L, MacHale S, Cavanagh J, Sharpe M, Deary I, Lawrie S 1999 Personality dimensions in chronic fatigue syndrome and depression. J Psychosom Res 46(4):395–400

Butler S, Chalder T, Ron M, Wessely S 1991 Cognitive behaviour therapy in the chronic fatigue syndrome. J Neurol Neurosurg Psychiatry 54:153–158

Chalder T, Berelowitz G, Hirsch S, Pawlikowska T, Wallace P, Wessely S, Wright D 1993 Development of a fatigue scale. J Psychosom Res 37:147–153

Chalder T, Power M, Wessely S 1996a Chronic fatigue in the community: a question of attribution. Psychol Med 26:791–800

Chalder T, Butler S, Wessely S 1996b In-patient treatment of chronic fatigue syndrome. Behav Psychother 24:351–366

Clark M, Katon W, Russo J et al 1995 Chronic fatigue: risk factors for symptom persistence in a 2.5 year follow up study. Am J Med 98:187–195

Cleare A, Bearn J, Allain T, Wessely S, McGregor A, O'Keane V 1995 Contrasting neuroendocrine responses in depression and chronic fatigue syndrome. J Affect Disord 35:283–289

Clements A, Sharpe M, Simpkin S, Borril J, Hawton K 1997 Chronic fatigue syndrome: a qualitative investigation of patients' beliefs about the illness. J Psychosom Res 42:615–624

Cope H, David A 1996 Neuroimaging in chronic fatigue syndrome. J Neurol Neurosurg Psychiatry 60:471–473

Cox B, Blaxter M, Buckle A et al 1987 The health and lifestyle survey. Health Promotion Trust, London

Cox D, Findley L 1994 Is chronic fatigue syndrome treatable in an NHS environment? Clin Rehabil 8:76–80

David A 1991 Post viral fatigue syndrome and psychiatry. Br Med Bull 47:966–988

David A, McDonald E, Mann A, Pelosi A, Stephens D, Ledger D, Rathbone R 1990 Tired, weak or in need of rest: fatigue among general practice attenders. BMJ 301:1199–1202

Deale A, David A 1994 Chronic fatigue syndrome: evaluation and management. J Neuropsychiatry 6:189–194

Deale A, Wessely S 1994 A cognitive behavioural approach to chronic fatigue syndrome. Therapist 2:11–14

Deale A, Chalder T, Marks I, Wessely S 1997 A randomised controlled trial of cognitive behaviour therapy for chronic fatigue syndrome. Am J Psychiatry 154:408–414

Deale A, Chalder T, Wessely S 1998 Illness beliefs and treatment outcome in chronic fatigue syndrome. J Psychoso Res 45:77–83

Demitrack M 1998 Neuroendocrine aspects of chronic fatigue syndrome: a commentary. Am J Med 105(3A):s11–14

Demitrack M, Greden J 1991 Chronic fatigue syndrome: the need for an integrative approach. Biol Psychiatry 30:747–752

Demitrack M, Dale J, Straus S et al 1991 Evidence for impaired activation of the hypothalamic-pituitary axis in patients with chronic fatigue syndrome. J Clin Endocrinol Metab 73:1224–1234

Dowson D 1993 The treatment of chronic fatigue syndrome by complementary medicine. Complement Ther Med 1:9–13

Edwards R, Gibson H, Clague J, Helliwell T 1993 Muscle physiology and histopathology in chronic fatigue syndrome. In: A Kleinman A, Straus S (eds) Chronic fatigue syndrome (Ciba Foundation symposium). John Wiley, Chichester

Essame C, Phelan S, Aggett P, White P 1998 Pilot study of a multi-disciplinary inpatient rehabilitation of severely incapacitated patients with chronic fatigue syndrome. J Chronic Fatigue Syndr 4:51–60

Euba R, Chalder T, Deale A, Wessely S 1995 A comparison of the characteristics of chronic fatigue syndrome in primary and tertiary care. Br J Psychiatry 168:121–126

Farmer M, Locke B, Moscicki E, Dannenberg A, Larson D, Radloff L 1988 Physical activity and depressive symptoms: the NHANES 1 epidemiologic follow up study. Am J Epidemiol 128:1340–1351

Fitzgibbon E J, Murphy D, O'Shea K, Kelleher C 1997 Chronic debilitating fatigue in Irish general practice: a survey of general practitioners experience. Br J Gen Pract 47:618–622

Fukuda K, Straus S, Hickie I et al 1994 Chronic fatigue syndrome: a comprehensive approach to its definition and study. Ann Intern Med 121:953–959

Fulcher K, White P 1997 Randomised controlled trial of graded exercise in patients with the chronic fatigue syndrome. BMJ 314:1647–1652

Gantz N, Holmes G 1989 Treatment of patients with chronic fatigue syndrome. Drugs 38:855–862

Gibson H, Carroll N, Clague J, Edwards R 1993 Exercise performance and fatiguability in patients with chronic fatigue syndrome. J Neurol Neurosurg Psychiatry 56:993–998

Glaser R, Glaser J 1998 Stress-associated immune modulation: relevance to viral infections and chronic fatigue syndrome. Am J Psychiatry 105(3A):s35–42

Greenberg D 1990 Neurasthenia in the 1980's: chronic mononucleosis, chronic fatigue syndrome and anxiety and depressive disorders. Psychosomatics 31:129–137

Greenleaf J, Kozlowski S 1982 Physiological consequences of reduced physical activity during bedrest. Exercise Sports Sci Rev 10:84–119

Hawton K, Salkovskis P, Kirk J, Clark D (eds) 1989 Cognitive behaviour therapy for psychiatric problems: a practical guide. Oxford University Press, Oxford

Hickie I, Kirk K, Martin N 1999 Unique genetic and environmental determinants of prolonged fatigue: a twin study. Psychol Med 29(2):259–268

Hill N, Teirsky L, Scavalla V, Laveietes M, Natalson B 1999 Natural history of severe chronic fatigue syndrome. Arch Phys Med Rehabil 80(9):1090–1094

Holmes G, Kaplan J, Gantz N et al 1988 Chronic fatigue syndrome: a working definition. Ann Intern Med 108:387–389

Hotopf M, Wessely S 1994 Viruses, neurosis and fatigue. Journal of Psychosom Res 38:499–514

Hotopf M, Noah N, Wessely S 1996 Chronic fatigue and minor psychiatric morbidity after viral meningitis: a controlled study. J Neurol Neurosurg Psychiatry 60:504–509

Hughes J, Crow R, Jacobs D, Mittelmark M, Leon A 1984 Physical activity, smoking and exercise induced fatigue. J Behav Med 7:217–230

Jain S, DeLisa J 1998 Chronic fatigue syndrome: a literature review from a psychiatric perspective. Am J Phys Med Rehabil 77(2):160–167

Johnson S, DeLuca J, Natalson B 1996 Depression in fatiguing illness: comparing patients with chronic fatigue syndrome, multiple sclerosis and depression. J Affect Disord 38:21–30

Joyce J, Hotopf M, Wessely S 1997 The prognosis of chronic fatigue and chronic fatigue syndrome: a systematic review. Q J Med 90:223–233

Katon W, Buchwald D, Simon G, Russo J, Mease P 1991 Psychiatric illness in patients with chronic fatigue and rheumatoid arthritis. J Gen Intern Med 6:277–285

Kent-Braun J, Sharma K, Weiner M, Massie B, Miller R 1993 Central basis of muscle fatigue in chronic fatigue syndrome. Neurology 43:125–131

Klonoff D 1992 Chronic fatigue syndrome. Clin Infect Dis 15:812–823

Kroenke K, Wood D, Mangelsdorff D, Meier N, Powell J 1988 Chronic fatigue in primary care: prevalence, patient characteristics and outcome. JAMA 260:929–934

Lacks P 1987 Behavioural treatment of persistent insomnia. Pergamon Press, New York

Lamb I, Stevens P, Johnson R 1965 Hypokinesia secondary to chair rest from 4 to 10 days. Aerospace Med 36:755–763

Leese G, Chattington P, Fraser W 1996 Short term night-shift working mimics the pituitary adrenocortical dysfunction of chronic fatigue syndrome. J Clin Endocrinol Metab 81:1867–1870

Lethem J, Slade P, Troup J, Bentley G 1983 Outline of a fear-avoidance model of exaggerated pain perception I & II. Behav Res Ther 21:401–416

Lloyd A, Wakefield A, Boughton C, Dwyer J 1988 What is myalgic encephalomyelitis? Lancet i:1286–1287

Lloyd A, Gandevia S, Hales J 1991 Muscle performance, voluntary activation, twitch properties and perceived effort in normal subjects and patients with the chronic fatigue syndrome. Brain 114:85–98

Lloyd A, Hickie I, Brockman A 1993 Immunologic and psychologic therapy for patients with chronic fatigue syndrome: a double blind, placebo controlled trial. Am J Med 94:197–203

Lynch S, Seth R, Montgomery S 1991 Antidepressant therapy in the chronic fatigue syndrome. Br J Gen Pract 41:339–342

MacDonald K, Osterholm M, LeDell K et al 1996 A case control study to assess possible triggers and cofactors in chronic fatigue syndrome. Am J Psychiatry 100:548–554

Magnusson A, Nias D, White P 1996 Is perfectionism associated with fatigue? J Psychosomat Res 41:377–384

Manu P, Matthews D, Lane T, Tennen H, Hesselbrook V, Mendola R, Affleck G 1988 The mental health of patients with a chief complaint of chronic fatigue: a prospective evaluation and follow-up. Arch Intern Med 148.2213–2217

Marks I 1986 Behavioural psychotherapy. Maudsley pocket book of clinical management. Wright, Bristol

Marks I 1987 Fears, phobias and rituals: panic, anxiety and their disorders. Oxford University Press, Oxford

Montgomery G 1983 Uncommon tiredness among college undergraduates. J Consult Clin Psychol 51:517–525

Natalson B, Chen J, Pareja J, Ellis S, Policastro T, Findley T 1996 Randomised, double blind controlled placebo phase in trial of low dose phenelzine in the chronic fatigue syndrome. Psychopharmacology 124:226–230

Neyta N, Horne J 1990 Effects of sleep extension and reduction on mood in health adults. Human Psychopharmacol 6:173–188

Peakman M, Deale A, Field R, Mahalingham M, Wessely S 1997 Clinical improvement in chronic fatigue syndrome is not associated with lymphocyte subsets of function or activation. Clin Immunol Immunopathol 82:83–91

Pepper C, Krupp L, Friedberg F, Doscher C, Coyle P 1993 A comparison of neuropsychiatric characteristics in chronic fatigue syndrome, multiple sclerosis and major depression. J Neuropsychiatry Clin Neurosci 5:200–205

Peters D, Lewis P, Chaitow L, Watson C 1996 Chronic fatigue. Complement Ther Med 4:31–38

Petrie K, Moss-Morris R, Weinman J 1995 The impact of catastrophic beliefs on functioning in chronic fatigue syndrome. J Psychosom Res 39:31–37

Powell R, Dolan R, Wessely S 1990 Attributions and self esteem in depression and chronic fatigue syndromes. J Psychosom Res 34:665–673

Ray C, Jeffries S, Weir W 1995 Coping with chronic fatigue: illness responses and their relationship with fatigue, functional impairment and emotional status. Psychol Med 25:937–945

Ridsdale L, Evans A, Jerrett W, Mandalia S, Osler K, Vora H 1993 Patients with fatigue in general practice: a prospective study. BMJ 307:103–106

Riley M, O'Brien C, McCluskey D, Bell N, Nicholls D 1990 Aerobic work capacity in patients with chronic fatigue syndrome. BMJ 307:103–106

Rowe P, Calkins H 1998 Neurally mediated hypotension and chronic fatigue syndrome. Am J Med 105(3A):s15–21

Salit I 1997 Precipitating factors for the chronic fatigue syndrome. J Psychiatr Res 31(1):59–65

Saltin B, Blomquist G, Mitchell J 1968 Response to exercise after bed rest and training: a longitudinal study of adaptive changes in oxygen transport and body composition. Circulation 38 (s7):s1–55

Schluederberg A, Straus S E, Peterson P 1992 Chronic fatigue syndrome research: definition and medical outcome assessment. Ann Intern Med 117:325–331

Scott L, Dinan T 1999 The neuroendocrinology of chronic fatigue syndrome: focus on the hypothalamic-pituitary-adrenal axis. Funct Neurol 14(1):3–11

Scott L, Teh J, Reznek R, Martin A, Sohaib A, Dinan T 1999 Small adrenal glands in chronic fatigue syndrome: a preliminary computer tomography study. Psychoneuroendocrinology 24(7):759–768

Sensky T 1990 Patients' reactions to illness. BMJ 300:622–623

Shafran S 1991 The chronic fatigue syndrome. Am J Med 90:730–739

Sharpe M, Chalder T 1994 Management of the chronic fatigue syndrome. In: Illis L (ed) Neurological rehabilitation. Blackwell Science, Oxford

Sharpe M, Archard L, Banatvala J et al 1991 Chronic fatigue syndrome: guidelines for research. J R Soc Med 84:118–121

Sharpe M, Hawton K, Seagroatt V, Pasvol G 1992 Follow-up of patients presenting with fatigue to an infectious diseases clinic. BMJ 305:147–152

Sharpe M, Hawton K, Simkin S et al 1996 Cognitive behaviour therapy for the chronic fatigue syndrome: a randomised controlled trial. BMJ 312:22–26

Shorter E 1993 Chronic fatigue: a historical perspective. In: Kleinman A, Straus S (eds) Chronic fatigue syndrome. Wiley Interscience, Chichester

Sisto S, MaMance J, Cordero D et al 1996 Metabolic and cardiovascular effects of a progressive exercise test in patients with chronic fatigue syndrome. Am J Med 100:634–640

Steele L, Dobbins J, Fukuda K, Reynes M, Randall B, Koppelman M, Reeves W 1998 The epidemiology of chronic fatigue syndrome in San Francisco. Am J Med 105 (3A):s83–90

Strober W 1994 Immunological function in chronic fatigue syndrome. In: Straus S (ed) Chronic fatigue syndrome. Dekker, New York

Surawy C, Hackman A, Hawton K, Sharpe M 1995 Chronic fatigue syndrome: a cognitive approach. Behav Res Ther 33:534–544

Swanink C, Vercoulen J, Bleijenberg G, Fennis J, Galama J, Van der Meer J 1995 Chronic fatigue syndrome: a clinical and laboratory study with a well matched control group. J Intern Med 237:499–506

Swartz M 1988 The chronic fatigue syndrome: one entity or many? N Engl J Med 319:1726–1728

Tirelli U, Marotta G, Improta S, Pinto A 1994 Immunological abnormalities in patients with chronic fatigue syndrome. Scand J Immunol 40:601–608

Valdini A, Steinhardt S, Feldman E 1989 Usefulness of a standard battery of laboratory tests in investigating chronic fatigue in adults. Fam Pract 6:286–291

Van Houdenhove B, Onghena P, Neerinkx E, Hellin J 1995 Does high 'action proneness' make people more vulnerable to chronic fatigue syndrome? A controlled psychometric study. J Psychosom Res 39:633–640

Vercoulen J, Swanink C, Fennis J, Galama J, Van der Meer J, Bleijenberg G 1994 Dimensional assessment of chronic fatigue syndrome. J Psychosom Res 38:383–392

Vercoulen J, Swanink C, Fennis J, Galama J, Van der Meer J, Bleijenberg G 1996a Prognosis in chronic fatigue syndrome (CFS): a prospective study. J Neurol Neurosurg Psychiatry 60:489–494

Vercoulen J, Swanink C, Zitman F et al 1996b Randomised double blind placebo controlled study of fluoxetine in chronic fatigue syndrome. Lancet 347:858–861

Vereker M 1992 Chronic fatigue syndrome: a joint paediatric-psychiatric approach. Arch Dis Child 67:550–555

Ware N 1992 Suffering and the social construction of illness: the delegitimation of illness experience in chronic fatigue syndrome. Med Anthropol Q December:347–361

Ware N, Kleinman A 1992 Culture and somatic experience – the course of illness in neurasthenia and chronic fatigue syndrome. Psychosom Med 54:546–560

Warwick H, Salkovskis P 1990 Hypochondriasis. In: Scott C, Williams J, Beck A (eds) Cognitive therapy: a clinical casebook. Croom Helm, London

Wearden A, Morriss R, Mullis R et al 1998 A randomised, double-blind, placebo-controlled trial of fluoxetine and graded exercise for chronic fatigue syndrome. Br J Psychiatry 172:485–490

Wessely S 1990 Old wine in new bottles: neurasthenia and ME. Psychol Med 20:35–53

Wessely S 1991 The history of the post viral fatigue syndrome. Br Med Bull 47:919–941

Wessely S 1997 Chronic fatigue syndrome. In: Weller M, Van Kammen D (eds) Advances in clinical psychiatry. W B Saunders, London

Wessely S, Powell R 1989 Fatigue syndromes: a comparison of chronic 'postviral' fatigue with neuromuscular and affective disorders. J Neurol Neurosurg Psychiatry 52:940–948

Wessely S, Butler S, Chalder T, David A 1991 The cognitive behavioural management of post-viral fatigue syndrome. In: Jenkins R, Mowbray J (eds) Post viral fatigue syndrome. John Wiley, Chichester

Wessely S, Chalder T, Hirsch S, Pawlikowska T, Wallace P, Wright D 1995 Post infectious fatigue: a prospective study in primary care. Lancet 345:1333–1338

White P, Cleary K 1997 An open study of the efficacy and adverse effects of moclobemide in patients with chronic fatigue syndrome. Int Clin Psychopharmacol 12:47–52

White P, Thomas J, Amess J et al 1995 The existence of a fatigue syndrome after glandular fever. Psychol Med 25:907–916

Whiteside T, Friberg D 1998 Natural killer cells and natural killer cell activity in chronic fatigue syndrome. Am J Med 105(3A):s28–34

Wilson A, Hickie I, Lloyd A, Hadzi-Pavlovic D, Boughton C, Dwyer J, Wakefield D 1994a Longitudinal study of outcome of chronic fatigue syndrome. BMJ 308:756–759

Wilson A, Hickie I, Lloyd A, Wakefield D 1994b The treatment of chronic fatigue syndrome: science and speculation. Am J Med 96:544–549

Wood B, Wessely S 1999 Personality and social attitudes in chronic fatigue syndrome. J Psychiatr Res 47(4):385–397

Zigmond A, Snaith P 1983 The Hospital Anxiety and Depression Scale. Acta Psychiat Scand 67:361–370

Zorbas Y, Matveyev L 1986 Man's desirability in performing physical exercises under hypokinesia. Int J Rehabil 9:170–174

Zubeck J, Wilgosh L 1963 Prolonged immobility of the body: changes in performance and in the electroencephalograms. Science 140:306–308

10

Psychological approaches to body image disturbance

Rob Newell

KEY ISSUES

◆ Understanding of body image is essential to health care

◆ Body image is related to self-image, self-esteem and self-concept

◆ Disfigured people experience stigma in social situations

◆ Facilities to address the psychological needs of disfigured people are limited

◆ Some of these psychological difficulties are phobic in nature

◆ A cognitive behavioural model of psychological difficulties in disfigurement may be of value

◆ Continuing research and development of treatment approaches are needed

INTRODUCTION

An understanding of body image is essential to health care across a wide range of settings. People can experience threats to the integrity of their body image through trauma (for example, road traffic accident, assault, fire, chemical burns), surgery for benign or maligant disease, skin complaints, deformity from birth or through the normal actions of the ageing process. Threats to body image are associated with psychological distress (Malt & Ugland 1989) and this may be especially so when disfigurement results, particularly to the face (Williams & Griffiths 1991). Moreover, there are disorders of body image which are primarily psychological in nature (most notably anorexia nervosa and body dysmorphic disorder). These difficulties can themselves give rise to physical consequences, for example through fasting or seeking plastic surgery, and also have established co-morbidity with other psychological disorders (Fairburn & Cooper 1989, Veale et al 1996). It is likely that health-care practitioners will come into contact with people who are experiencing threats to their body image at frequent intervals throughout their clinical practice. However, despite the work of several important theorists (Dropkin 1989, Price 1990a,b, Rumsey 1983), relatively little empirical work has been undertaken.

In this chapter, we will explore the concept of body image, the ways in which it may become disturbed, some consequences of this disturbance and the possible remedies which health-care practitioners may use to address the difficulties of people suffering the consequences of disturbed body image. A number of models of body image disturbance will be introduced and discussed. For the bulk of the chapter, examples will be drawn from the area of facial disfigurement, an area of difficulty whose consequences are recognised as potentially catastrophic to the sufferer. Whilst some important work has been undertaken from the psychiatric field, this will be examined only in so far as it illuminates more general aspects of body image and its disturbance. Moreover, in the interests of space, related issues such as self-esteem will not be covered, although it is recognised that such concepts are linked with that of body image (Dewing 1989). Similarly, possible interactions between body image and such issues as concern over being diagnosed as suffering from a life-threatening illness (as in disfigurement following surgery for cancer) will not be examined, although they clearly contribute to psychological distress following surgery and the ways in which they interact with threats to body image are currently not established.

THE CONCEPT OF BODY IMAGE

Body image is central to the consideration of disfigurement and disability. It appears that preferences for non-disfigured and non-disabled individuals are learnt early in life and demonstrable across a wide range of situations (Rumsey et al 1986a, Sigelman & Singleton 1986).

Numerous commentators agree that the term 'body image' has often been used in a loose, ill-defined way (Brown et al 1990, Cumming 1988, Lacey & Birchnell 1986), although it is generally agreed that the term is separate from, although related to, such concepts as self-image, self-esteem and self-concept (Dewing 1989). Schilder's (1935) definition of body image as 'the picture of our body which we form in our mind, that is to say the way in which our body appears to ourselves' has been followed by most later writers. Schilder often uses the term 'body image' interchangeably to apply to *physical* perception of the body and *psychological* attitudes to it. Schilder is usually credited with the incorporation of psychological and sociological elements into the idea of body image. In particular, he notes that body image is subject to continuous change, both as a consequence of developmental changes in response to short-term alterations such as changes of mood or even changes of clothing or the use of instruments such as tools. We can easily verify these latter assertions by noting how we may feel less attractive when we feel unhappy or noticing how a much-loved piece of jewellery or a musical instrument feels 'like part of us'.

'Body schema' is most often currently used to refer to the perceptual elements of body image, whilst 'body image' often includes both these elements and evaluative components (e.g. Cumming 1988, Slade 1988). Cumming (1988) has pointed out that, for practical purposes, the distinction between body schema and body image refers to whether we are considering body image in a neurological or psychological sense. In the first instance, we are talking of perceptual facts whilst in the second, we are describing subjective experiences, although this is an incomplete distinction.

Schilder (1935) views bodily sensations, psychological body image and the ego as being intimately related, a view consistent with the Freudian formulation of the ego as principally deriving from bodily phenomena, as described by Bronheim et al (1991). Schilder, however, goes beyond this view of body image as an internally driven phenomenon by stating that body image is essentially a *public* phenomenon. Body image is continuously constructed, destroyed and reconstructed through a process of reciprocal interaction with the body images of those with whom we come into contact (Schilder 1935, p 241). This involves, in part, imitation of others, whose body images come to be incorporated within our own.

MODELS OF BODY IMAGE

In health care, perhaps the clearest and most comprehensive account of body image comes from Price (1990a,b), who regards body image as consisting of three related components: body reality, body ideal and body presentation (Fig. 10.1).

Body reality refers to the body as it is constructed and includes both external elements such as height and weight and internal elements such as organs of the body and functions such as digestion or fluid balance. Since awareness of characteristics of the body (for example, proprioception) is a bodily function, it is, by inference, part of body reality in Price's model. This reality is changeable throughout the life cycle and in immediate response to our

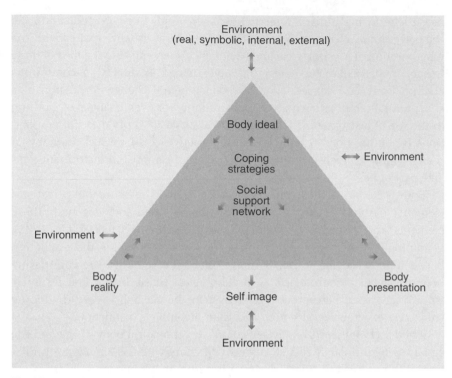

Fig 10.1 Price's model of body image (adapted from Price 1990a)

interactions with the environment, including the results of insults to the body through disease or trauma. Body reality is not consequent upon our attitudes to it, but consists of physical attributes of the body.

By contrast, *body ideal* is attitudinal and represents the way we would wish the body to be. Price sees this ideal as being gained through a process of identification with the body ideals of others, as revealed to us through our interactions with the rest of society. Our body ideal reflects a set of internalised societal norms of how society as a whole thinks we should look and the way in which it thinks our bodies should function. Newell (1991) has noted the behavioural view of how individuals might acquire such ideas through the process of differential reinforcement of behaviours which reflect attitudes consistent with the prevailing norms of body image. According to this argument, body ideal is a largely learned phenomenon, contingent upon societal definitions of the ideal.

Body presentation refers to how we present all aspects of our bodily appearance, including dress, grooming and behaviour. It is, to a marked extent, under the conscious control of the individual who may, within limits, alter the presentation of the body reality in the direction of conformity with the ideal.

To these three linked elements, Price (1990a) has added several contributing components which influence them (see Fig. 10.1). *Coping strategies* direct
how individuals will respond to threats to body image integrity in the context
of their *social support network*, which forms part of a more general *influence
of environment*. Price also emphasises the related nature of body image and
self-image.

Price (1990a,b) sees the three elements of body image as existing in a state
of tension or balance which together make up a satisfactory body image
which humans strive to maintain. Increased tension between body reality and
body ideal (for example, as a result of disfigurement) may lead the individual
to attempt to decrease that tension by altering body presentation to compen-
sate for the deficiency in body reality or to change their own attitudes as to
what constitutes their body ideal, invoking particular coping strategies and
social supports in order to help make these compensatory changes.

Price's (1990a,b) model is important because it is one of very few such
models to go beyond simple statement of the distinction between perceptual
and evaluative aspects of body image. Moreover, it has a high profile amongst
British nurses and is explicitly tied to clinical practice, from whose observations it is drawn and to which its implications are linked in the form of recommendations for nursing activity. Finally, it has been influential in increasing
nurses' awareness of body image issues and stimulating debate.

However, in spite of these strengths, Price's model possesses a number of
shortcomings. Although the description of the various components of body
image is comprehensive, the way in which these elements influence each
other and the putative consequences if one or more of the elements are
disturbed are not clearly described. We do not know, for example, whether
changes in one aspect of body image cause changes in another, are consequent upon such changes or independent of them. Indeed, it may prove difficult even to ask such questions in ways which operationalise the various
elements of Price's model to a sufficient degree to make specific predictions
which can then be tested. The general construction of the model is somewhat
circular, so that prediction of possible responses which might result from
its assumptions is difficult. This difficulty is compounded by the lack of a
sufficiently clear definition within the model of what constitutes a 'satisfactory body image'. Perhaps because of this, there have been no systematised
empirical investigations of Price's model. Price provides numerous clinical
examples of disturbance in body image, its effect in terms of the three
elements and of how the elements relate to a model of care. However, these
are largely anecdotal and we have no sense of whether they are in any
way typical. As Gournay et al (1997) have remarked, Price's model of body
image remains a set of untested assumptions and is, in consequence, purely
speculative.

Dropkin (1989) has presented an important alternative account of body image disturbance and adaptation. Dropkin's model draws considerably on Lazarus's (1966) cognitive transactional formulation of stress and coping, which sees coping as a series of cognitive and behavioural attempts to deal with threats to the person. Whilst Lazarus's model appears cognitively led, Dropkin (1989) describes coping responses according to the three systems: 'neurocognitive, affective and physiological responses... which may be observed in the behavioural response dimension' and is thus similar to Lang's (1971) three systems model.

Dropkin's model was developed principally in the context of postoperative recovery following head and neck surgery for cancer. The surgical procedure for removal of cancer is seen as the stressor to which adaptation is required. The person's cognitive appraisal of this threat leads to affective, physiological and behavioural responses. These responses are seen as indicative of adaptation or what Dropkin describes as body image reintegration, when they involve 'confrontation, compliance and redefinition' (redefinition of the person's value system towards an appreciation that change in appearance or function does not change the nature of the person). Self-care, grooming and socialisation are viewed as key elements of this process. However, the role of health-care staff in facilitating these behaviours and attitudinal changes is not described in detail. Dropkin has extensively investigated the postoperative behaviours of head and neck patients, using this stress-coping model (Dropkin & Scott 1983, Scott et al 1980).

Dropkin's model has considerable attraction from the viewpoint of the cognitive behavioural approach to disturbed body image to be described later in this chapter. Her model shares a similar general view of human behaviour and experience with the three systems model often practised in cognitive behavioural therapy (CBT). More critically, it emphasises the importance of behavioural confrontation and, to a lesser extent, attitude change. The first of these, in particular, is seen as important in cognitive behavioural approaches. However, Dropkin's approach has a number of limitations. Her investigations are almost exclusively in the important but specialised and complex field of cancer surgery. In such settings, patients may have to adapt to many stressors other than those involving body image. For example, the patient may face difficulties of bodily functioning, may have to adapt to diagnosis of life-threatening illness or to face the continuing danger of recurrence. In such settings, investigating the contribution of body image to a patient's difficulties is particularly difficult. Second, Dropkin is concerned primarily with short-term adjustment during the postoperative period and longer term difficulties or adaptation may be very different. Finally, the precise process by which self-care and socialisation tasks lead to adaptation is not described and adequate investigation of cause and effect relationship between these tasks and psychosocial adjustment has not been undertaken.

We noted earlier that psychiatry has contributed to our understanding of eating disorders. Slade (1994) describes an account of body image development and disturbance which, whilst prinicipally based on an examination of eating disorders, is capable of extension to a broader range of disturbances of body image. Slade (1994) notes the convergence of approaches to body image disturbance from observations of perceptual defects in neurological disorders, the body image distortion in eating and weight disorders and the 'delusional misperception' of body dysmorphic disorder (BDD), where sufferers strongly believe a particular bodily attribute is offensive. He suggests that these influences have led to the idea that body image disorder is primarily a perceptual problem. He regards this emphasis as misplaced and argues that even the measurement of perceptual phenomena (such as body size in anorexia nervosa) involves participants in judgements which rely to a marked extent on attitude, affect and cognition.

Slade argues that mental representation of, for example, body size is not fixed but fluctuates within a limited range (body image band). Under normal circumstances that representation will be in the middle of the band but emotional and attitudinal bias, such as strong concern about body size in anorexia nervosa, will result in judgments of size at the limits of the range. The most frequent description of anorexia nervosa sufferers is that they have a fixed distorted body image of delusional proportions (Bruch 1962), but Slade suggests instead that their body image is uncertain, unstable and weak. This, he suggests, is translated into overly cautious estimates of body characteristics. We might wish to extend this view to apply to BDD sufferers who, it might be suggested, have a similarly unstable image of a particular bodily attribute or function which is likewise overemphasised in situations of stress such as social interaction.

Slade's (1994) model consists of seven components, which all influence the 'loose mental representation of the body' he says best describes body image. A history of sensory input to the body regarding its form, size, shape and appearance gives a general mental representation of the body. Cultural and social norms about the body inform both attitudes to weight and shape and the general body image, whilst individual attitudes both input directly to body image and affect cognitive and affective variables. Biological variables also impact on body image. Individual psychopathology such as anorexia nervosa both influences body image disturbance and is influenced by factors such as cultural norms and cognitive and affective variables whilst, in eating disorders, a history of weight change is construed as leading to a broadening of the body image band and thus a loosening of the body image (Fig. 10.2).

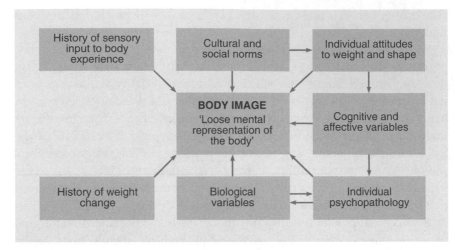

Fig 10.2 Slade's model of body image disturbance (adapted from Slade 1994)

Like Price's (1990a,b) model, Slade's view of body image has not been subjected to empirical testing. However, Slade has drawn considerably on empirical evidence from both clinical and experimental studies of eating disorders in its construction. Moreover, it is closely related to a fear and avoidance model of pain perception (Lethem et al 1983, Slade et al 1983) which has proved valuable in the examination and treatment of pain (Rose et al 1992). However, Slade's (1994) model is narrow in focus in two senses. First, it is essentially a model of bodily perception. Attitudes and other elements of appraisal or satisfaction are essentially important because of the role they play in determining that perception. Second, since Slade's approach is based on the pathology of eating disorders, extrapolations to other disorders of body image must be made with caution. Generalisations to individuals without disturbed body image should be even more cautious.

MEASUREMENT OF BODY IMAGE

Measurement of body image began with quite general approaches but has usually reflected the division between perceptual and attitudinal/affective components. According to McCrea et al's (1982) review, the great breadth of sources from which investigation of body image has occurred has led to a tendency towards vague, equivocal definitions of the concept and to a proliferation of different measurement approaches.

Secord (1953) constructed the earliest systematised scale to examine elements of body image. This scale was derived from the procedures of analytical psychology and consisted of a series of 75 homonyms with either body or non-body meanings which were presented to subjects. As well as being important in its own right as an early attempt to systematise examination of attitudes to the body, this scale was the forerunner of the Body Cathexis Scale (Secord & Jourard 1953) which became a widely used tool in the investigation of body image. The Body Cathexis Scale investigated only cathexis (the level of feeling of satisfaction or dissatisfaction with bodily parts or processes) and consisted of five point scales related to 46 body parts or functions, indicating different levels of satisfaction. The authors hypothesised that bodily feelings would be similar to feelings about the self, a prediction which was confirmed, suggesting a relationship between body image and self-esteem.

Bruchon-Schweitzer (1987), noting that the Body Cathexis Scale measured only one dimension of body image (satisfaction), proposed that body image was multidimensional and devised a body image questionnaire of 19 items. Four stable factors were found within the scale: accessibility/closeness; satisfaction/dissatisfaction; activity/passivity; relaxation/tension. The identification of these component factors of body image enables investigators to move away from a global examination of the body image towards more precise specification of both elements of body image and their possible relationships with other variables. For example, the Bruchon-Schweitzer study found a positive correlation between body satisfaction and extroversion on the Eysenck Personality Inventory (EPI) and negative correlations between body activity and relaxation and EPI neuroticism scales.

The multidimensional nature of body image has also been explored by Cash (1989) and Brown et al (1990). Cash et al's (1986) Body Self Relations Questionnaire (BSRQ) takes into account cognitive and behavioural factors as well as the affective component examined by the Body Cathexis Scale, in order to reflect the concept of an *attitude* towards the body more accurately, and consists of 54 items. The scale was factor analysed to yield seven factors, leading the authors to conclude that separate dimensions of body image experience existed and that investigators should both beware of the 'uniformity myth' of the body image construct and distinguish between perceptual and attitudinal modalities. Since the conclusions of Cash and his co-workers regarding dimensions of body image are based upon the general population rather than clinical population subjects, their general applicability is considerably increased.

The Cash (1989) paper also demonstrates that, whilst assessment of body image attitudes may be divided into examination of the whole body and of individual body parts, the individual elements do not contribute *equally* to overall evaluation of the body. Specifically, weight, upper torso, face, mid torso, lower torso and muscle tone (in descending order of importance) predicted overall appearance satisfaction and self-rated attractiveness in men, with only height satisfaction making no predictive contribution. In women, weight, upper torso, mid torso, lower torso and face predicted the general measures, with height and muscle tone making no contribution. Cash concluded that body part satisfaction and global satisfaction converge and that most body parts make a unique and additive contribution to the general appraisal of the body, but these contributions are not equal.

DISFIGUREMENT AND SOCIAL INTERACTIONS

The importance of social interaction as part of the construction of body image is noted by all the writers whose models of body image have been described earlier in this chapter. This section outlines some important studies of social interaction as they relate to disfigurement. The social difficulties experienced by disfigured people are a major source of complaints by them and a number of studies demonstrate that the stigmatisation recounted by disfigured people is generally observed in both laboratory and field studies, although the quality of such studies is variable.

One fascinating account, whilst purely anecdotal, gives an insight into the social world of the disfigured person. Carlisle (1991), a member of the staff of *Nursing Times*, donned make-up to simulate a scar, entered a variety of social situations and reported the responses of others to her. Unfortunately, there is considerable opportunity for bias in her report, which reads as an object lesson in the inappropriate use of an assumed causative factor to explain observations. For example, the presence of a scar is recounted by the author as a cause of both staring *and* looking away and of offering both more *and* less help. Whilst these differing responses might both be generated by the presence of a scar, considerable experimental control would be needed in order to exclude the effects of expectation on the part of the author.

The difficulty involved in accepting subjective accounts of the motivations of others is further demonstrated by Kleck & Strenta (1980), who showed that subjects believed reactions were being made to their simulated disfigurement even after this had been secretly removed. However, we should be cautious in extrapolating this conclusion to include genuinely disfigured or otherwise stigmatised people, since the subjects in this study were not, in fact, members of such a group and so should not be considered as likely to respond in the same way. Moreover, these subjects had had their attention called to the presence of the disfigurement during the course of preparation for the experiment, thus priming them to the reactions of others to it. The main value of the Kleck & Strenta study is to demonstrate that, even under carefully controlled conditions, drawing conclusions about reactions to disfigurement in social situations is problematic and drawing such conclusions from small, uncontrolled reports is even more difficult.

Nevertheless, a body of research appears to offer objective support for the subjective experience of stigma described by disfigured or visibly disabled people. We know, for example, that disfigured people are likely to be helped less than non-disfigured and that the disfigurement, rather than fear or negative attributions to the person, is the source of this effect (Piliavin et al 1975). Whilst some later studies have suggested that, under certain circumstances, disfigured individuals are more likely to be helped, these are generally unreliable owing to methodological shortcomings (Newell 1998). Studies which require any major level of personal contact suggest that the disfigured person is afforded no advantage (Bull & Stevens 1981, Doob & Ecker 1970, Rumsey 1983) or is discriminated against (Levitt & Kornhaber 1977, Piliavin et al 1975 Soble & Strickland 1974, Ungar 1979).

It has been suggested that people avoid contact with disabled people because such individuals give rise to autonomic arousal and uncomfortable feelings of uncertainty (Kleck et al 1966). Building on Bernstein's (1976) observation that people tend to choose no closer than 'neutral' distance from disfigured people, Rumsey (1983) observed the distance consecutive arrivals at a pedestrian crossing chose when standing next to a confederate waiting there, apparently with no visible facial defect, a birthmark, or scarring and bruising. Early arrivals stood significantly further from the confederate in both the birthmark and the scarring condition than the non-disfigurement condition and further in the birthmark than the scarring condition. Furthermore, first arrival subjects chose significantly more often to stand next to the non-disfigured side of the disfigured confederates. This experiment suggests that subjects prefer greater distance from disfigured individuals than non-disfigured. In a later study, Houston & Bull (1994) also investigated proximity preferences of members of the public, by examining train seat occupancy in seats surrounding a confederate apparently with no visible defect, a birthmark, scarring or bruising. They found an overall effect of facial appearance on occupancy of seats accounted for by the difference between the birthmark and no defect conditions.

The above studies together support the notion that disfigured individuals are indeed stigmatised in public social situations, at least if we regard avoidance of contact as an indicator of stigmatisation. It should be noted, however, that these studies involved relatively superficial contact. There are no field studies which directly demonstrate avoidance of disfigured people in more intimate social situations although anecdotal accounts are frequent.

There is, however, some indication that judgements of attractiveness interact with judgements of social competence. Rumsey et al (1986b) explored the effect of the *behaviour* of facially disfigured people on the reactions of others in a videotaped study of a confederate with or without a port wine stain who demonstrated either good or bad social skills with 12 female subjects. The socially competent confederate was rated as more warm and friendly by subjects and as more warm, friendly, likeable, interesting and competent by independent observers regardless of whether or not the confederate was disfigured. Moreover, subjects smiled more and showed lower response latencies towards the socially competent confederate. Rumsey et al concluded that social skill might exert sufficient influence to override the negative influence of stigmatisation as a result of facial disfigurement. This suggestion is supported to some degree by findings from Bull & Brooking's (1986) study, in which male disfigured participants were judged to be significantly more intelligent and attractive when represented to subjects as being married. Similarly, disfigured females were judged as less attractive than non-disfigured only when represented as unmarried. If we regard being married as a testimony to a person's social competence, this experiment may offer further evidence that social skill influences ratings of attractiveness.

ADDRESSING THE PSYCHOSOCIAL DIFFICULTIES OF FACIALLY DISFIGURED PEOPLE

Despite growing recognition of the psychological distress associated with disfigurement, treatment studies are rare. Indeed, even the provision of psychosocial intervention seems unusual. Wallace (1988), in a study of 43 UK burns units, found that of the 28 replies received, only two units provided specialist counselling whilst only seven had some form of lay support. Less than 25% of the patients in Wallace's sample reported *any* useful contact with any professional with regard to their burns. Yet Newell's (1998) survey of plastic surgery ex-patients found that psychological distress was widespread, with 31% showing as cases on the General Health Questionnaire and 45% showing at least mild anxiety on the Hospital Anxiety and Depression Scale (HAD).

Nevertheless, accounts of treatment are infrequent and are almost exclusively restricted to single case studies or collections of such studies (Bernstein 1976, 1982, Cohen et al 1991, Jacobson et al 1961, Shakin Kunkel et al 1995) or to general descriptions of therapeutic approaches (Bronheim et al 1991). These studies do not always differentiate between preexisting psychological difficulties and the consequences of disfigurement, nor between the consequences of the disfiguring aspects of impairments and functional aspects, such as difficulty with speech and eating following oral surgery.

Lefebvre & Arndt (1988) suggested tactics which might be employed to increase life skills in adolescents with facial disfigurements, based on 15 years of liaison psychiatry in this area. These included: helping strangers handle shock and fear, handling teasing and name-calling, making new friends, talking to members of the opposite sex, handling job interviews. Unfortunately, this study is inadequate to allow any conclusion to be drawn about the effectiveness or otherwise of the treatment suggestions the authors make, which are further weakened by lack of description of the interventions undertaken. Griffiths (1990) suggested a similar range of tactics but did not supply either a rationale for their use or citations as to their effectiveness.

Feigenbaum (1981) specifically tackled the social skills difficulties of disfigured people, using a 'social training' programme which also included elements of Meichenbaum's (1977) stress inoculation approach to CBT. There were significant differences both between pre- and posttraining scores for the experimental group and between the experimental and control groups posttreatment across a variety of measures of anxiety. The analysis would have been strengthened by the inclusion of data from the initial time point for the control group and by the examination of any possible effects of differences between experimental and control groups pretreatment.

James Partridge is a burns survivor who has developed an approach to treatment based on a group approach which involves social skills training of the kind advocated by Rumsey (1983) but also such diverse elements as role modelling, imitation, instruction, brainstorming, role plays, creative problem solving and feedback. Workshops based on his methods are now being evaluated (Partridge et al 1994) and and some 88% of attenders found them useful, whilst 77% reported using the skills and information they had gained on the course in real-life situations. In a more formal evaluation, Robinson et al (1996) found that, in a group of 64 treatment completers, 6 weeks after the workshops, HAD anxiety had fallen significantly and was no longer different from normative samples. Moreover, high levels of social avoidance and distress had significantly reduced after treatment and attenders felt significantly more confident in the presence of strangers and when meeting new people. Improvements were maintained or increased at 6-month follow-up. Unfortunately, this study lacks a control group but is a promising initial examination of the potential for social skills training in this area.

A COGNITIVE BEHAVIOURAL APPROACH TO BODY IMAGE DISTURBANCE

Earlier in this chapter, we noted that there are a number of difficulties with existing major models of body image. However, Slade's model has the potential to be revised to provide a model for body image disturbance in general, rather than simply within the context of eating disorders. Whilst Slade's model is largely untested, it has major points of similarity to Lethem et al's (1983) 'fear avoidance' model of exaggerated pain perception, which has shown some predictive value in the treatment of pain states (Rose et al 1992).

The development of a comprehensive cognitive behavioural formulation of disturbed body image is of potential importance because cognitive behavioural approaches are associated with considerable therapeutic success in many areas (see, for example, Fonagy & Roth 1996, Parry 1996, Rachman & Wilson 1980). If the factors which initiate and maintain the difficulties experienced with body image (particularly in social situations) are, for example, similar to those involved in the initiation and maintenance of phobic behaviour, then a successful approach to treatment and, arguably, prophylaxis exists for people experiencing an actual or potential threat to the integrity of their body image. Indeed, in the psychiatric context, cognitive behavioural interventions already have a considerable track record in addressing difficulties with body image, for example, in eating disorders (e.g. Fairburn & Cooper 1989) and in BDD (e.g. Gournay et al 1997). Moreover, it has been argued that the cognitive behavioural approach to BDD might be extended to help those whose disturbance of body image is the consequence of some actual change to body appearance or function (Gournay et al 1997, Newell 1991, 1997).

Newell (1991) proposed such a model, strongly based on Lethem et al's (1983) approach to chronic pain. In essence, Lethem et al propose that increased incapacity, distress and pain perception result from the fear of pain, rather than the experience of pain itself. Those who make adequate recovery from illness are those who tend to exhibit confrontation rather than avoidance and that tendency to confront rather than avoid is determined by interacting factors from the individual's background and environment. The key contributing elements (life events, personality, pain history and coping strategies) produce a psychosocial context for the pain event, which determines the individual's response to it along a continuum from avoidance to confrontation of potentially pain-producing situations. The patient predicts that pain is likely to occur if a particular behaviour is performed and consequently avoids that behaviour. Similarly, if an activity is being performed and the patient predicts that pain is likely to ensue, then that activity will be ceased. Cognitive behavioural accounts of the genesis and maintenance of anxiety through passive and active avoidance predict that, in consequence, the range of permissible activities will become more and more restricted and increasingly innocuous stimuli will be interpreted as threatening.

Newell's (1991) approach assumes that many of the psychological difficulties experienced by people who have suffered a threat to body image are similar to those suffered by phobics. In other words, they are mediated primarily by fear and avoidance, which are themselves primarily maintained by conditioning and the dysfunctional thoughts which often accompany avoidance learning in phobias (Butler 1989). Newell's (1991) cognitive behavioural formulation asserts, for disfigured people, that activities associated with the lost or damaged part of the body are avoided, because they give rise to autonomic features of anxiety and to anxiety-provoking thoughts. Further activities which remind the person of the lost or damaged area, even though not directly associated with it, are likewise avoided. For example, following mastectomy, a woman might avoid reading women's magazines in which articles about cancer, breast augmentation, swimsuits or lingerie might be present. Similarly thoughts associated with the damaged area are resisted, since they also come to be associated with autonomic arousal and anxiety.

This formulation was limited in that it described only the development of disturbance in detail, although the accompanying treatment example described the use of exposure therapy and the action of the process of habituation in leading to a diminution of fear (Marks 1987). Lethem et al (1983) describe a psychosocial context leading to either disturbance or recovery. Newell (1998) suggested that this psychosocial context is equally applicable to body image, with the following amendments. 'Pain history' is replaced with 'history of changes to body image', following Slade's (1994) model of body image in eating disorders. 'Fear of pain' is changed to 'fear of changed body and reactions of others', whilst 'pain coping strategies' is changed to 'body image coping strategies'. The rationale for these amendments is further reported in Newell (1998, 1999).

The fear avoidance model of response to disfigurement was originated to account for difficulties following insults to body image as a result of surgery, trauma or disease. In a slightly altered form, the model accounts equally well for such occurrences and for body image disturbance as a result of disfigurement from birth. In this latter case, since the disfigurement is present from birth, the potential for confrontation or avoidance likewise exists from this time, rather than from the time of occurrence of disfigurement at some later date. Thus, in the case of the person disfigured from birth, elements of the psychosocial context of disfigurement do not predate the occurrence of disfigurement. Instead, the disfigurement itself may be a major contributing factor in the psychosocial development of the individual. Also, specific elements such as enforced avoidance, which may be present following injury, are unlikely to be a major factor. Newell's (1998) fear avoidance model of disturbed body image is shown in Figure 10.3.

Figure 10.3 uses social avoidance as the key example of avoidance or confrontation. This has been chosen because of its potentially damaging consequences across a range of activities such as work, leisure and dating but

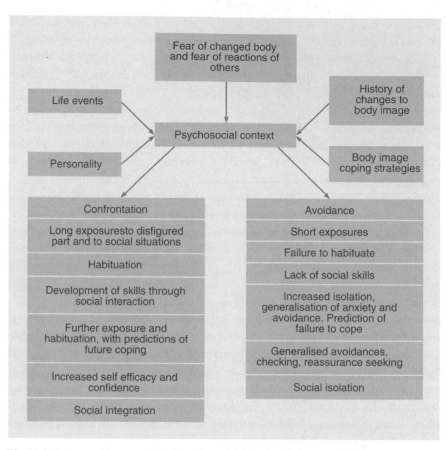

Fig 10.3 A fear-avoidance model of psychosocial difficulties following disfigurement

it is by no means the sole example of avoidance in disturbed body image. Certainly an examination of the behaviour of BDD sufferers reveals a great deal of anxiety and specific avoidances, albeit in the context of the overvalued idea, and these avoidances are a source of significant handicap to the sufferer. Similarly, avoidance and anxiety may be widespread amongst sufferers from facial disfigurement. Thus, Gamba et al (1992) report avoidance of examining operation sites and looking in mirrors by head and neck cancer patients, whilst social difficulties are the most frequently reported complaints amongst disfigured people (Kalick et al 1981, Macgregor 1951, Malt 1980, Partridge et al 1994, Robinson et al 1996, Rubinow et al 1987, Rumsey 1983). Newell (1998) found a wide range of avoidances reported by facial disfigurement sufferers, including: walking in the street, wearing certain clothes, having sexual intercourse, averting the affected side, eye contact, wearing glasses/sunglasses/heavy make-up as camouflage, being photographed.

Just as the notion of fear of pain and consequent avoidance is the key aspect of Lethem et al's (1983) fear avoidance model of exaggerated pain perception, Newell's (1998) has as its central feature fear of the changed body and the responses of others. It is apparent from many of the above studies that the *actual* responses of people to the disfigured individual are mainly negative and it is likely that these reactions will have a profound effect in terms of increasing the disfigured person's fear of such reactions. The fear avoidance model attempts to account for why such reactions contribute to greater psychosocial disturbance in some individuals than others.

SUPPORT FOR THE FEAR AVOIDANCE MODEL

Whilst Newell's (1991) model was, like those of Price (1990a,b) and Slade (1994), almost entirely speculative there are a number of reasons to suggest that particularly in the 1998 formulation presented here, it may be regarded as a useful approach to problems of body image disturbance.

First, as we noted earlier, there is considerable anecdotal evidence of anxiety amongst disfigured people. This is supported by some of the studies of their social difficulties (Robinson et al 1996, Williams & Griffiths 1991). Moreover, the Newell (1998) study found not only high levels of anxiety as measured by the HAD but the avoidances noted above. Furthermore, correlations were found between a measure of body image disturbance (adapted from Probst et al 1995) and a broad range of measures of avoidance and anxiety, suggesting that disturbance of body image, anxiety and avoidance are linked in this group.

The promise offered by social skills-based approaches (which contain elements of confrontation of the feared situations) offers a further source of support for the fear avoidance model, since we would expect exposure to give rise to habituation and, therefore, to decreased anxiety and distress (e.g. Marks 1987), as it does in phobic patients. In Newell (1998) a minimal intervention treatment strategy was employed, involving the use of self-help leaflets along cognitive behavioural lines, emphasising confrontation of the feared situations. Participants who received the leaflet did significantly better than controls in three of nine measures. More importantly, two of these significantly different measures specifically examined phobic and general anxiety.

In a final test of the model, Newell & Marks (2000) compared facially disfigured people with agoraphobic and socially phobic patients using the fear questionnaire (Marks & Mathews 1979). It was noted that the facially disfigured group (who were matched for global problem severity with the phobics) scored lower than agoraphobics on a measure of agoraphobic avoidance but significantly higher on a measure of social phobic avoidance. The disfigured group did not differ from the social phobics on either score. Thus it appears that facially disfigured people resemble social phobics in terms of their pattern of avoidance and are more severely socially handicapped than agoraphobics.

In summary, the fear avoidance model is potentially useful in addressing the psychosocial difficulties of facially disfigured people because it is related to an approach to human difficulties (the cognitive behavioural approach) which has demonstrable efficacy in addressing these difficulties. This is particularly so of social anxiety, a major source of distress to disfigured people. Moreover, the cognitive behavioural approach is effective in addressing disorders of body image in the context of psychiatric disorder (eating disorders and BDD). Finally, there is some empirical evidence which directly supports the model. Anxiety and avoidance occur in disfigured people. It seems that disfigured people are helped by treatment approaches which contain an element of confrontation of the feared situation (exposure therapy) and skills acquisition (social skills training). Disfigured people apparently resemble phobic patients, in particular social phobics, whose difficulties are maintained, to a considerable extent, by anxiety and avoidance of the feared situations.

IMPLICATIONS FOR TREATMENT

The problem of body image disturbance is potentially vast. For example, Robinson et al (1996) estimate the number of people in the UK suffering disfigurement at a level likely to be regarded as disabling as 400 000. Clearly, this does not include those suffering from 'invisible' threats to body image, such as the removal of internal organs. Given the findings of Wallace (1988), it is unlikely that many disfigured people will be in contact with psychological services, although numerous researchers note that the level of handicap can be severe in a small but significant subgroup of sufferers. There is thus a need for intervention at a range of levels: prevention, preparation, general advice and specific interventions. The fear avoidance model, used in conjunction with an awareness of the areas of functioning likely to be affected (see, for example, Macgregor 1951, Newell 1998, Partridge 1990, Price 1990a,b, Rumsey 1983), leads to an approach which is potentially valuable across all these levels.

Prevention

There is a pressing need for a greater understanding of the difficulties encountered by people facing threats to body image. In this connection, the role played by Changing Faces (a group founded by James Partridge) is of considerable importance since, in addition to its therapeutic work, the group works with clinicians, researchers and through the media to increase awareness of the challenges faced by disfigured people. The group also publishes newsletters and maintains a website and helpline. A further group, Let's Face It, founded by Christine Piff, a cancer surgery survivor, takes a similar support and educational role. Nurses and other health-care professionals are frequently in contact with these groups, seeking advice and information, but are also in a position to make an important educational and preventive contribution as part of their public health role.

More generally, education of the public regarding the role of cognitive behavioural factors in the genesis and maintenance of psychological problems such as phobias is at a rudimentary level, although a number of self-help publications (e.g. Marks 1980) have brought cognitive behavioural interventions to a wide audience. The dissemination of this kind of information could prove important both to the general public and to those who go on to experience a challenge to their body image, simply by increasing awareness that their difficulties are normal, widespread and, to an extent, understood and amenable to treatment.

Preparation for surgery and general advice

The issue of education also arises in the context of preparation for surgery or medical intervention which is likely to result in a marked challenge to body image. Clearly this would include any visibly mutilating surgery or any treatment which alters bodily appearance or function, such as radiotherapy However, interventions which result in the loss of an internal organ or bodily function may also result in profound threats to body image and will thus likewise require considerable preparatory intervention by health professionals. However, although a considerable amount has been written about preparation for surgical and other procedures in general, there is little which addresses the issue of preparation for changes in body image specifically. This may be because there are other issues to be covered, because clinicians believe (mistakenly) that patients will cope (Holmes 1986) or because psychological difficulties resulting from life-threatening illness other than those related to body image are felt to be of greater importance.

Careful explanation of the nature and results of the intervention is important before any procedure. In cases where a challenge to body image is likely, such preparation should emphasise this element. Although a precise description of what will happen to the patient is necessary, it is important, from a cognitive behavioural perspective, to combine this with an account of the likely psychological consequences of an unwanted alteration in appearance. Thus, the patient needs to know that the change may lead to fear, a desire to escape from, avoid or deny the change which has occurred, specific examples of situations or activities which may be avoided, the likely reactions of the patient and others in social situations. Much of this information can be gained from patients themselves, with the two additional advantages of allowing them to ventilate their own fears and giving an early example of the way in which exposure works; describing fears is itself a form of confrontation and confrontation (exposure) in imagination is associated with improvement by exactly the same process as exposure in real life. Meeting with patients who have undergone similar procedures can be another source of this exposure.

Following a discussion of such possible psychological and behavioural changes, an account of steps patients can take to help themselves may be given and will aim to be specific to the difficulties foreseen or reported by the patient. From a cognitive behavioural perspective, this will mean explaining how exposure to feared consequences leads to a decrease in distress. Complicated explanations are not needed here, since most people have experienced anxiety in unfamiliar situations and the enormous but transitory relief which comes from escaping from such situations. Similarly, most people recognise that such escape tactics usually lead to further distress if the situation has to be entered again. By contrast, we all have experience of remaining in an uncomfortable situation, noticing that anxiety decreases relatively quickly and that following such confrontation, subsequent situations tend to be less discomforting. Common examples such as speaking in a meeting, being interviewed for a job, meeting people for the first time all convey the message of anxiety reduction as a consequence of confrontation and repetition far better than appeals to conditioning or cognitive theories. Price (1990a) identifies three styles of coping following threats to body image integrity: frank coping, modified coping and avoidance. Newell (1991) recommends that the first of these styles be encouraged with patients whenever possible, since avoidance is maladaptive and fast exposure is associated with greater improvement than slow.

Some level of avoidance may be inevitable following surgery or other intervention since the affected area may be covered in bandages or the person may be unable to use the affected area. However, the fear avoidance model suggests that this avoidance should be limited as far as possible and that patients should be encouraged to examine the affected area as soon as possible. Usually this involves a process of negotiation with the patient, in which the health-care professional seeks to involve the patients with the maximum level of exposure they can tolerate at any particular time. A series of tasks to be performed can be agreed, often in ascending order of difficulty, so that the patient experiences early successes in confronting anxiety. The patient may also be offered some coping tactics, such as relaxation exercises or positive self-statements, whose main purpose is to enable the patient to remain in contact with the feared situations. Typically, the nurse will want to emphasise with the patient four crucial components of this general cognitive behavioural approach: anxiety decreases as a result of confrontation (exposure); anxiety decreases more reliably the longer the exposure; anxiety decreases the more frequent the exposure; reduction in anxiety generalises from the specific situations in which exposure is practised to other, similar situations.

It is worth remembering that the majority of patients will do well with this level of general preparation and advice. Indeed, many participants in the treatment part of the Newell (1998) study had been considerably handicapped for a number of years, but still made gains as a result of a simple self-help leaflet. This type of intervention should be well within the expertise of most experienced general nurses, occupational therapists or physiotherapists and the provision of further self-help information would be valuable. Changing Faces produces a number of information leaflets which are a useful supplement to the advice of the nurse. General self-help information such as Marks (1980) may also be suggested. Clinicians who are interested in pursuing the cognitive behavioural approach further will find readable accounts in Marks et al (1977), Richards & McDonald (1990) and Newell (1994).

SPECIFIC TREATMENT

For individuals experiencing severe difficulties with body image disturbance and its associated behavioural avoidances and social difficulties, the fear avoidance model and the cognitive behavioural approach in general possess considerable advantages, as we have noted earlier. Dealing with complex cases of this kind is generally regarded as the role of specialist therapists, usually psychologists, nurses and psychiatrists who have undertaken specialist training in this discipline. Newell & Dryden (1991) provide a readable general introduction to the cognitive behavioural approach, whilst Marks (1987) presents an extensive review of the effectiveness of the approach in general and of exposure therapy in particular and Richards & McDonald (1990) provide a good practical introduction. A detailed discussion of treatment is beyond the scope of this chapter but specialist intervention will usually involve the following elements.

◆ Detailed functional analysis of the person's difficulties, often using an ABC (antecedents, behaviour, consequences; autonomic/physical system, behavioural system, cognitive system) approach.
◆ Detailed description of the cognitive behavioural approach.
◆ Definition and measurement of treatment targets to which both therapist and patient can subscribe.
◆ Involvement of family and friends in treatment tasks with the client.

◆ Planning and executing a series of exposure tasks, often with an emphasis on social situations.
◆ Specific training and practice in social skills if these are lacking.
◆ Generation of coping tactics and of rewards for successful completion of exposure tasks.
◆ Identification and challenging of dysfunctional beliefs surrounding body image.
◆ Planning to prevent relapse.

Unfortunately, CBT is a scarce commodity and is unlikely to be widely available outside major clinical centres. Even for those suffering quite severe consequences of body image disturbance, this is a considerable problem, particularly since, as we noted earlier, many people who have suffered a challenge to their body image are not in touch with any psychological services. This is particularly unfortunate given that many of the difficulties they experience, most notably social avoidance, have been well addressed by CBT.

Guidelines for assessment and intervention

Key issues at assessment

◆ Avoidance of situations (e.g. social situations, particular clothes, speaking/eating in public, sexual intercourse, meeting new people)
◆ Taking precautions (e.g. wearing sunglasses, standing with the light behind you, averting the face)
◆ Particular thoughts asociated with the appearance (e.g. attitudes of others, fear of inability to cope)
◆ Physical symptoms of anxiety (e.g. racing heart, nausea, shaking)
◆ Experience of relief on leaving fear-evoking situations
◆ Skill deficits (e.g. conversing with others, answering questions about one's disfigurement)
◆ Increasing life handicap as a result of negative thoughts, social avoidance, other avoidance
◆ Desired goals

Key issues at intervention

◆ Clear treatment explanation and goal definition
◆ Agreed, graded exposure assignments
◆ Involvement of family/friends
◆ Experimentation to prove that anxiety reduces
◆ Generation and rehearsal of appropriate coping tactics and social skills
◆ Regular expert supervision

CONCLUSION

Numerous commentators (Bull & Stevens 1981, Houston & Bull 1994, Macgregor 1990) have noted the lack of research into facial disfigurement, its psychosocial sequelae and their treatment. Despite the work of a number of theorists and the considerable rise in popular writings in nursing concerning body image, there is also little systematic research with regard to this more general topic. This is interesting given the importance placed on the psychosocial experiences of patients by nurses and other non-medical health professionals in particular. Perhaps most importantly, studies of treatment for disturbed body image are rare outside the psychiatric literature although, in the field of facial disfigurement, the work of the Rumsey/Partridge group shows considerable promise, as does the cognitive behavioural approach described in this chapter. Both these treatment approaches now require further investigation.

In the area of facial disfigurement, further systematic investigation of the characteristics of those who experience psychosocial difficulties would be welcome. In other areas of body image disturbance, specific tests of the fear avoidance model would be a useful further step in examining this model. More generally, all patients' difficulties in which body image disturbance is an issue require continuing systematic examination. In terms of service delivery, we know the size of the task and suspect that there is a massive shortfall in provision: a great increase in public awareness and concern will be required to produce the will amongst service providers to address this imbalance.

ANNOTATED BIBLIOGRAPHY

Bull R, Rumsey N 1988 The social psychology of facial appearance. Springer-Verlag, London

Now slightly old, but consists of an excellent review of a broad range of issues surrounding facial appearance, disfigurement and stigma. Contains accounts of the major empirical studies in this field.

Hawton K, Salkovskis P M, Kirk J, Clark D M (eds) 1989 Cognitive-behaviour therapy for psychiatric problems. A practical guide. Oxford University Press, Oxford

This is a general text outlining cognitive behavioural interventions for a variety of common mental disorders. The chapters related to assessment and to phobias are particularly relevant.

Newell R 2000 Body image and disfigurement care. Routledge, London

Explores the issues raised in this chapter in considerable detail, with detailed chapters on models of body image, the fear avoidance model, psychological aspects of disfigurement and treatment.

Price R 1990 Body image: nursing concepts and care. Prentice Hall, New York

Whilst Price's model of body image has a number of flaws, this text remains an extremely comprehensive introduction to body image issues across a broad range of clinical settings.

REFERENCES

Bernstein N R 1976 Emotional care of the facially burned and disfigured. Little, Brown, Boston

Bernstein N R 1982 Psychological results of burns. The damaged self-image. Clin Plast Surg 9(3):337–346

Bronheim H, Strain J J, Biller H F 1991 Psychiatric aspects of head and neck surgery. Part II: Body image and psychiatric intervention. Gen Hosp Psychiatry 13:225–232

Brown T A, Cash T F, Mikulka P J 1990 Attitudinal body-image assessment: factor analysis of the Body-Self Relations Questionnaire. J Pers Assess 55(1&2):135–144

Bruch H 1962 Perceptual and conceptual disturbances in anorexia nervosa. Psychosom Med 24:187–194

Bruchon-Schweitzer M 1987 Dimensionality of the body image: the body image questionnaire. Percept Mot Skills 65:887–892

Bull R, Brooking J 1986 Does marriage influence whether a facially disfigured person is considered physically unattractive? J Psychol 119(2):163–167

Bull R, Stevens J 1981 The effects of facial disfigurement on helping behaviour. Ital J Psychol 8:25–33

Butler G 1989 Phobias. In: Hawton K, Salkovskis P M, Kirk J, Clark D M (eds) Cognitive-behaviour therapy for psychiatric problems. A practical guide. Oxford University Press, Oxford

Carlisle D 1991 Face value. Nurs Times 87(42):26–28

Cash T F 1989 Body-image affect: gestalt versus summing the parts. Percept Mot Skills 69:17–18

Cash T F, Winstead B A, Janda L H 1986 The great American shape-up. Psychol Today 20(4):30–37

Cohen C G, Krahn L, Wise T N, Epstein S, Ross R 1991 Delusions of disfigurement in a woman with acne rosacea. Gen Hosp Psychiatry 13:273–277

Cumming W J K 1988 The neurobiology of the body schema. Br J Psychiatry 153(suppl 2):7–11

Dewing J 1989 Altered body image. Surg Nurse 2(4):17–20

Doob A N, Ecker B P 1970 Stigma and compliance. J Pers Soc Psychol 14(4):302–304

Dropkin M J 1989 Coping with disfigurement and dysfunction after head and neck surgery: a conceptual framework. Semin Oncol Nurs 5(3):213–219

Dropkin M J, Scott D W 1983 Body image reintegration and coping effectiveness after head and neck surgery. J Soc Otorhinolaryngol Head Neck Nurs 2:7–16

Fairburn C G, Cooper P 1989 Eating disorders. In: Hawton K, Salkovskis P M, Kirk J, Clark D M (eds) Cognitive-behaviour therapy for psychiatric problems. A practical guide. Oxford University Press, Oxford

Feigenbaum W 1981 A social training program for clients with facial disfigurations: a contribution to the rehabilitation of cancer patients. Int J Rehabil Res 4(4):501–509

Fonagy A, Roth P 1996 What works for whom? Guilford, New York

Gamba A, Romano M, Grosso I M, Tamburini M, Cantu G, Molinari R, Ventafridda V 1992 Psychosocial adjustment of patients surgically treated for head and neck cancer. Head Neck 14:218–223

Gournay K, Veale D, Walburn J 1997 Body dismorphic disorder: pilot randomized controlled trial of treatment; implications for nurse therapy, research and practice. Clin Effectiveness Nurs 1(1):38–43

Griffiths E 1990 More than skin deep. Nurs Times 85(40):34–36

Holmes P 1986 Facing up to disfigurement. Nurs Times 82(34):16–17

Houston V, Bull R 1994 Do people avoid sitting next to someone who is facially disfigured? Eur J Soc Psychol 24:279–284

Jacobson W E, Meyer E, Edgerton M T 1961 Psychiatric contributions to the clinical management of plastic surgery patients. Postgrad Med 29:513–521

Kalick S M, Goldwyn R M, Noe J M 1981 Social issues and body image concerns of port wine stain patients undergoing laser therapy. Lasers Surg Med 1:205–213

Kleck R, Strenta A 1980 Perceptions and impact of negatively valued physical characteristics on social interaction. J Pers Soc Psychol 39(5):861–875

Kleck R, Ono H, Hastorf A H 1966 The effects of physical deviance upon face-to-face interaction. Hum Relat 19:425–436

Lacey J H, Birchnell S A 1986 Body image and its disturbances. J Psychosom Res 30(6):623–631

Lang P 1971 The application of psychophysiological methods to the study of psychotherapy. In: Bergin A E, Garfield S L (eds) Handbook of psychotherapy and behavior change. John Wiley, New York

Lazarus R S 1966 Psychological stress and the coping process. McGraw-Hill, New York

Lefebvre A M, Arndt E M 1988 Working with facially disfigured children: a challenge in prevention. Can J Psychiatry 33(6):453–458

Lethem J, Slade P D, Troup J D G, Bentley G 1983 Outline of a fear-avoidance model of exaggerated pain perception – I. Behav Res Ther 21(4):401–408

Levitt L, Kornhaber R C 1977 Stigma and compliance: a re-examination. J Soc Psychol 103:13–18

Macgregor F C 1951 Some psychosocial problems associated with facial deformities. Am Sociol Rev 16:629–638

Macgregor F C 1990 Facial disfigurement: problems and management of social interaction and implications for mental health. Aesthetic Plast Surg 14:249–257

Malt U 1980 Long term psychosocial follow-up studies of burned adults: review of the literature. Burns 6.190–197

Malt U, Ugland O M 1989 A long-term psychosocial follow-up study of burned adults. Acta Psychiat Scand 355 (8)(suppl):94–102

Marks I M 1980 Living with fear. McGraw-Hill, New York

Marks I M 1987 Fears, phobias and rituals. Oxford University Press, New York

Marks I M, Mathews A M 1979 Brief standard self-rating for phobics. Behav Res Ther 17:263–267

Marks I M, Hallam R S, Connolly J, Philpott R 1977 Nursing in behavioural psychotherapy. Royal College of Nursing, London

McCrea C W, Summerfield A B, Rosen B 1982 Body image: a selective review of existing measurement techniques. Br J Med Psychol 55.225–233

Meichenbaum D 1977 Cognitive behavior modification. General Learning Press, Morristown, NJ

Newell R 1991 Body image disturbance: cognitive-behavioural formulation and intervention. J Adv Nurs 16:1400–1405

Newell R 1994 Interviewing skills for nurses and other health professionals. Routledge, London

Newell R 1997 Commentary. Body dismorphic disorder: pilot randomized controlled trial of treatment; implications for nurse therapy research and practice (Gournay K, Veale D, Walburn J). Clin Effectiveness Nurs 1(1):44

Newell R 1998 Facial disfigurement and avoidance: a cognitive-behavioural approach. Unpublished PhD thesis, University of Hull

Newell R 1999 Altered body image: a fear-avoidance model of psychosocial difficulties following disfigurement. J Adv Nurs 30(5):1230–1238

Newell R, Dryden W 1991 Clinical problems: an introduction to the cognitive-behavioural approach. In: Dryden W, Rentoul R (eds) Adult clinical problems: a cognitive-behavioural approach. Routledge, London

Newell R, Marks I M 2000 Phobic nature of social difficulty in facially disfigured people. Br J Psychiatry 176:177–181

Parry G 1996 NHS psychotherapy services in England. Review of strategic policy. NHS Executive, London

Partridge J 1990 Changing faces: the challenge of facial disfigurement. Penguin, London

Partridge J, Coutinho W, Robinson E, Rumsey N 1994 Changing Faces: two years on. Nurs Standard 8(34).54–58

Piliavin I M, Piliavin J A, Rodin J 1975 Costs, diffusion and the stigmatized person. J Pers Soc Psychol 32:429–438

Price R 1990a A model for body image care. J Adv Nurs 15:585–593

Price R 1990b Body image: nursing concepts and care. Prentice Hall, New York

Probst M, Vandereycken W, Van Coppenolle H, Vanderlinden J 1995 The Body Attitude Test for patients with an eating disorder: psychometric characteristics of a new questionnaire. Eat Disord 3(2):133–144

Rachman S J, Wilson G T 1980 The effects of psychological therapy. Pergamon, Oxford

Richards D, McDonald R 1990 Behavioural psychotherapy: a handbook for nurses. Heinemann, London

Robinson E, Rumsey N, Partridge J 1996 An evaluation of the impact of social interaction skills training for facially disfigured people. Br J Plast Surg 49:281–289

Rose M J, Klenerman L, Atchison L, Slade P D 1992 An application of the fear avoidance model to three chronic pain problems. Behav Res Ther 30(4):359–365

Rubinow D R, Peck G L, Squillace K M, Gantt G G 1987 Reduced anxiety and depression in cystic acne patients after successful treatment with oral isotretinoin. J Am Acad Dermatol 17(1):25–32

Rumsey N 1983 Psychological problems associated with facial disfigurement. Unpublished PhD thesis, North East London Polytechnic

Rumsey N, Bull R, Gahagan D 1986a A developmental study of children's stereotyping of facially deformed adults. Br J Psychol 77:269–274

Rumsey N, Bull R, Gahagan D 1986b A preliminary study of the potential of social skills for improving the quality of social interaction for the facially disfigured. Soc Behav 1:143–145

Schilder P 1935 Image and appearance of the human body. Kegan Paul, London

Scott D W, Oberst M, Dropkin M J 1980 A stress-coping model. Adv Nurs Sci 3:9–23

Secord P F 1953 Objectification of word association procedures by the use of homonyms: a measure of body cathexis. J Pers 21:479–495

Secord P F, Jourard S M 1953 The appraisal of body-cathexis: body-cathexis and the self. J Consult Psychol 17(5):343–347

Shakin Kunkel E J, Rodgers C, Field H L et al 1995 Treating the patient who is disfigured by head and neck cancer. Gen Hosp Psychiatry 17:444–450

Sigelman C K, Singleton L C 1986 Stigmatization in childhood: a survey of developmental needs and issues. In: Ainley S C, Becker G, Coleman L M (eds) The dilemma of difference: a multidisciplinary view of stigma. Plenum, New York

Slade P D 1988 Body image in anorexia nervosa. Br J Psychiatry 153(suppl 2):20–22

Slade P D 1994 What is body image? Behav Res Ther 32(5):497–502

Slade P D, Troup J D G, Lethem J, Bentley G 1983 The fear-avoidance model of exaggerated pain perception – II. Preliminary studies of coping strategies for pain. Behav Res Ther 21(4):409–416

Soble S L, Strickland L H 1974 Physical stigma, interaction and compliance. Bull Psychon Soc 4(2B):130–132

Ungar S 1979 The effects of effort and stigma on helping. J Soc Psychol 107:23–28

Veale D, Bookock A, Gournay K et al 1996 Body dysmorphic disorder: a prospective survey of 50 cases. Br J Psychiatry 169(2):196–201

Wallace L A 1988 Abandoned to a social death. Nurs Times 84(10):34–37

Williams E E, Griffiths T A 1991 Psychological consequences of burn injury. Burns 17(6):478–480

RESOURCES

Changing Faces

1–2 Junction Mews

London W2 1PN

Tel: 020 7706 4232

email: info@faces.demon.co.uk

A national organisation founded by burns survivor James Partridge which offers resources for people who have experienced changes to their facial appearance.

11

Posttraumatic stress disorder: assessment and intervention strategies in trauma, critical care and general medical settings

David Hannigan   Stephen Regel

KEY ISSUES

◆ Posttraumatic symptoms and posttraumatic stress disorder (PTSD) often present in general medical settings

◆ Severe physical illness or its treatment may cause posttraumatic symptoms

◆ Although 75% of individuals exposed to a traumatic event do not go on to develop PTSD, in those that do, the condition can be chronic and extremely debilitating

◆ Structured early interventions following serious injury with regular follow-up are often beneficial in helping individuals understand and normalise their reactions

◆ Thorough and comprehensive assessment with appropriate measures is essential

◆ There is strong empirical support for cognitive behavioural therapy (CBT) as a therapy of choice for PTSD

INTRODUCTION

Posttraumatic stress disorder (PTSD) is a common source of morbidity after traumatic events, e.g. road traffic accidents, burn trauma, major disasters and violent crime. This chapter aims to address assessment, primary management and specific therapeutic strategies for individuals who have been exposed to a variety of traumatic stressors. These will be discussed in the context of trauma and critical care settings, with an emphasis on the role of practitioners who have mental health liaison responsibilities in the above settings.

An overview of the literature on trauma and PTSD will be presented, with particular attention paid to the prevalence of posttraumatic responses in medical and critical care settings. Consideration will also be given to some of the main theoretical perspectives that contribute to our understanding of the development and maintenance of PTSD, together with vulnerability factors and co-morbid psychiatric conditions. The chapter will also focus on cognitive behavioural therapy (CBT) for trauma and PTSD as the outcome research is impressive. For example, Blake & Sonnenberg (1998) reviewed 29 studies on CBT for PTSD and found compelling evidence that PTSD symptoms can be ameliorated using CBT. The chapter will also draw upon case material to illustrate assessment and intervention strategies.

POSTTRAUMATIC STRESS DISORDER AS A CONCEPT

There have been descriptions of symptoms and syndromes with PTSD-like features reported in a variety of literature throughout the centuries (Trimble 1985). Perhaps the earliest account of war neurosis was by the Greek historian Herodotus, who described the psychogenic blindness suffered by the Athenian warrior Epizelus at the battle of Marathon in 490 BC.

One of the most detailed early accounts of the effects of a traumatic incident can be found in the 17th-century diarist Samuel Pepys's accounts of the psychological sequelae he experienced after witnessing the Great Fire of London. In a detailed analysis, Daly (1991) identified a variety of symptoms of PTSD from Pepys's account of the disaster which befell London in 1666.

The concept of PTSD was not officially recognised as a serious mental health problem until 1980 when it was included in the psychiatric diagnostic handbooks, most notably the American Psychiatric Association's *Diagnostic and Statistical Manual of Mental Disorders* (DSM, APA 1980). The diagnostic criteria were revised in 1987 and underwent a further revision in 1994 (DSM-IV, APA 1994). The current edition (DSM-IV) states that the diagnostic criteria of PTSD are:

> *The development of characteristic symptoms following exposure to an extreme traumatic stressor involving direct personal experience of an event that involves actual or threatened death or physical injury, or other threat to*

*one's physical integrity; or witnessing an event that involves death, injury or
a threat to the physical integrity of another person; or learning about
unexpected or violent death, serious harm, or threat of death or injury
experienced by a family member or other close associate. (APA 1994, p 424)*

In addition, the person has been exposed to a traumatic event in which both
the following were present. Criterion A: (1) the person experienced, witnessed
or was confronted with an event or events that involved actual or threatened
death or serious injury or a threat to the physical integrity of others and (2)
the person's response involved intense fear, helplessness or horror.

Furthermore, three distinct groups of symptoms are known to arise following a traumatic event: Criterion B, reexperiencing intrusive imagery; Criterion
C, avoidant symptoms and Criterion D, arousal symptoms. In order to fulfil
the diagnostic criteria of PTSD, the individual must experience at least one (or
more) symptoms from B, at least three (or more) from C and at least two (or
more) from D (Box 11.1).

Box 11.1 Criteria for posttraumatic stress disorder (adapted from DSM-IV
1994 Diagnostic classification of posttraumatic stress disorder)

Both the following criteria need to be met in order for this diagnosis to be
made.
1. The person has experienced, witnessed or been confronted with an
   event/events that involved actual or threatened death or serious injury
   or a threat to the physical integrity of themselves or others.
2. The person's response involved intense fear, helplessness or horror

The following symptom clusters must also be present for more than 1
month, with disturbance causing significant distress/impairment in social,
occupational or other important areas of functioning.

REEXPERIENCING SYMPTOMS (1 or more needed)	AVOIDANCE AND DISSOCIATIVE SYMPTOMS (3 or more needed)	INCREASED AROUSAL SYMPTOMS (2 or more needed)
◆ Recurring, upsetting intrusive memories of the event (e.g. images, thoughts)	◆ Avoidance of thoughts & feelings or conversations reminiscent of the trauma	◆ Difficulty falling/ staying asleep
◆ Recurrent distressing dreams of the event	◆ Avoidance of activities, people or situations reminiscent of the trauma	◆ Increase in irritability/anger, generally short-tempered

Box 11.1 Cont'd		
REEXPERIENCING SYMPTOMS (1 or more needed)	AVOIDANCE AND DISSOCIATIVE SYMPTOMS (3 or more needed)	INCREASED AROUSAL SYMPTOMS (2 or more needed)
◆ Behaving/feeling as if the traumatic event were recurring (e.g. flashbacks)	◆ Inability to recall an important aspect of the trauma	◆ Difficulties in concentration
◆ Intense/psychological distress on exposure to internal or external reminders of the trauma	◆ Diminished interest in usual activities	◆ Hypervigilance
◆ Intense physiological arousal to internal or external reminders of the trauma	◆ Feeling detached or estranged from others	◆ Exaggerated startle response
	◆ Restricted range of affect	
	◆ Sense of foreshortened future	

PTSD has also often been described as a 'normal reaction to an abnormal response', the implication being that symptoms of PTSD are indicative of normal processes. This can be a major issue, as if this were the case, then the prevalence would undoubtedly be much higher. Joseph et al (1997) argue that whilst PTSD provides a useful framework for conceptualising psychological reactions to trauma, the symptoms of PTSD should be viewed as indicative of unresolved processing of the traumatic event (an issue that will be considered later).

There have been studies which attempted to identify pretrauma risk factors, including familial history of psychiatric illness on childhood trauma, for example sexual assault or separated or divorced parents before the age of 10 (Davidson et al 1991). McFarlane (1989) also identified neuroticism: introversion, prior psychiatric disorder and adverse life events before and after the trauma (often referred to as secondary trauma). Although McFarlane (1989) reported that previous stressors were particularly influential in the development of chronic rather than acute PTSD, studies suggest that immediate posttraumatic stress is also influenced by recent stress. It appears that one's vulnerability to developing posttraumatic stress may be greater when the trauma occurs in the context of accumulating stressful events that represent a threat to the individual (Bryant & Harvey 1996, Hannigan & Regel 1996). Whilst these studies have attempted to identify pretrauma risk factors, there is as yet no consensus regarding these factors. Therefore, they should be at best regarded as 'potentially' increasing the odds of developing PTSD and not as a guarantee of it.

Another important issue is that of co-morbidity. The DSM encourages multiple diagnoses and recognises that there are often other conditions which either overlap or occur as a result of PTSD. High levels of depression are common among survivors of traumatic events (Loughrey et al, 1988, North et al 1994). In addition, substance abuse (Joseph et al 1993) and enduring personality changes (Horowitz 1986) are also common co-morbid features.

ACUTE STRESS DISORDER

Acute stress disorder (ASD) was recently included as a new diagnosis in DSM-IV to describe posttraumatic stress in the first month after a trauma. ASD consists of reexperiencing, avoidance, arousal and dissociative symptoms. The disturbance must last for a minimum of 2 days and a maximum of 4 weeks, after which time a diagnosis of PTSD should be considered. The main difference between ASD and PTSD is that for a diagnosis of the former, three dissociative symptoms must be present. The premise underpinning ASD is that dissociation is a central coping mechanism that minimises awareness of the adverse emotional consequences of trauma (Van der Kolk & Van der Hart 1989).

The reason for including ASD is that the condition may present in the client population under discussion in this chapter and, more importantly, may serve as a predictor of PTSD. Recent studies, particularly with road traffic accident (RTA) survivors, have shown that between 18% and 24% display severe stress reactions (Bryant & Harvey 1996, Mayou et al 1993). Whilst much of the research into ASD as a predictor of PTSD has been carried out with RTA victims, the findings may be generalised to other areas, e.g. burn trauma (where there is also an overlap with serious assault). As yet, the research into ASD as a predictor for PTSD in other traumatic events is lacking but the evidence thus far indicates that it is worthy of assessment in the stages following exposure to a traumatic stressor.

THE EPIDEMIOLOGY OF TRAUMA AND POSTTRAUMATIC STRESS DISORDER

Norris (1992) studied a community sample from four cities in the south eastern United States and estimated current rates of PTSD in individuals exposed to traumatic events to range from 5% to 11%. One of the most recent epidemiological surveys (The National Co-morbidity Survey), designed to study the distribution, correlates and consequences of psychiatric disorders in the United States, estimated lifetime prevalence of PTSD at 7.8%. Survival analysis showed that more than one third of people with an index episode of PTSD fail to recover even after many years (Kessler et al 1995).

A recent community study in Germany of 3021 young adults, between the ages of 14 and 24, yielded a low incidence of PTSD: 1% for males and 2.2% for females. This is much lower than the previous US studies but the conditional probability for PTSD after experiencing traumas and risk factors and co-morbidity patterns was quite similar (Perkonigg et al 2000). There are, of course, cultural factors which need to be taken into consideration. At the time of writing, there have been no similar studies in the UK.

THE PREVALENCE OF TRAUMA AND POSTTRAUMATIC STRESS DISORDER IN CRITICAL CARE AND GENERAL MEDICAL SETTINGS

Having considered the epidemiology and prevalence surrounding trauma and PTSD in a wider context, we will now focus on the specific prevalence of trauma and PTSD in the above areas. Liaison mental health nurses and other healthcare professionals will often be called upon to address the psychological impact of physical injury and illness on the individual and their carers in the above settings. In addition, PTSD symptoms have also been described after medical illness and treatment (Mayou & Smith 1997, Shalev et al 1993). This section will present an overview of some of the most likely (and less obvious) areas where issues of ASD and PTSD may present as part of a broader picture of psychological distress (see Box 11.2).

Modern medicine often uses invasive procedures, for which the individual has little real preparation or understanding. Health professionals are not infallible and mistakes and accidents unfortunately can and do occur during medical procedures. A complication occurring during a procedure or a medical accident can have profound effects upon the individual. In addition to the trauma and shock that a complication or error has caused, the individual also has to contend with the fact that the very people who they felt were there to help them have played a part in this (see Case Study 11.2). This can give rise to feelings of helplessness and lack of control, as well as a future loss of trust in health professionals, distrust of future diagnosis and advice and fear of future treatments. Shalev et al (1993) concluded that posttraumatic stress is prolonged after medical events, presumably due in part to the individual's lack of control of the situation.

Road traffic accidents

The most common presentations in trauma and orthopaedic units are those arising from a variety of accidental injuries, ranging from road traffic accidents (RTAs) to industrial accidents. The range of RTA survivors will include drivers, pedestrians, motorcyclists and cyclists. However, the literature on RTAs has tended to focus on motor vehicle accidents per se (the literature in this area is extensive and for a comprehensive recent review, see Hickling & Blanchard, 1999). The rates for PTSD following RTAs vary from 11% to 46%.

Probably the best designed prospective study was that conducted by Mayou et al (1993). In a study of a consecutive series of 188 RTA victims, they found that a quarter described long-term psychiatric consequences of three overlapping types: mood disorder, PTSD and phobic anxiety about travel. In addition, a fifth of subjects complained of persistent and disabling anxiety. One fifth of the sample with major or minor injuries experienced severe initial distress characterised by altered mood and horrific memories. Nineteen of the sample (11%) met the criteria for PTSD at 1 year. Regel et al (1997) found significantly lower rates of psychological distress and PTSD in a sample of severely injured RTA victims at 6-months follow-up.

Burn trauma

Within the last decade there has been an emerging interest in the multifaceted nature of posttraumatic psychopathology (Roca et al 1992, Sturgeon et al 1991, Taal & Faber 1997) and PTSD following burn injury (Bryant 1996, Perry et al 1990). Whilst the above studies have indicated that posttraumatic psychopathology is not uncommon in burn survivors, long-term prospective outcome studies to assess the prevalence of PTSD, using standardised measures and clinical interviews, based on the current DSM-IV diagnostic criteria for PTSD are lacking. In addition, many of the studies are retrospective with an absence of standardised assessment of psychopathology and PTSD posttrauma.

Box 11.2 Prevalence rates of PTSD in relation to different medically related traumatic incidents

Burn injury	7–45%
Child's life-threatening illness	10%
Child's unexpected death	45%
Myocardial infarction	9%
Obstetric/gynaecological procedures	1.7–6%
Road traffic accidents	10–46%
Stroke (TIA/CV)	9.8%
Sudden death of a 'loved one' (adult)	14%

Nevertheless, this area of critical care has a high degree of psychological and psychiatric morbidity and there is often a need for consistent psychological input from the liaison services (Regel et al 1997). We have found that psychological care in this area is not consistent across the speciality in the UK. However, in other parts of Europe it is an important aspect of care and viewed as an essential part of an integrative care package.

Trauma and PTSD in general medical settings

Traumatic reactions have also been found to occur in other general medical contexts and settings as indicated by the literature, e.g. cardiac arrest survivors (Kutz et al 1994, Ladwig et al 1999, Van Driel & Op Van den Velde 1995), general surgical units (Shalev et al 1993), stroke patients (Sembi et al 1998) and breast cancer (Cordova et al 1995). There is clearly a need for more research in these areas as many of the above studies do have methodological shortcomings, e.g. small sample sizes, inconsistent use of psychometric measures.

PTSD resulting from obstetric trauma

The effect that obstetric experiences can have on individuals has been mostly overlooked in the area of PTSD research, with only a few studies taking place to date. Menage (1993) reviewed 500 women's experiences of obstetric and gynaecological procedures; over 100 described their experiences as being 'very distressing' or 'terrifying'. Of these women, at follow-up, 30 met the criteria for PTSD. These women identified that they experienced feelings of powerlessness during the procedure, a lack of information about the procedures taking place, the experience of physical pain and a perceived 'unsympathetic' attitude on the part of the staff.

A small case series described PTSD resulting from obstetric trauma, where the labour was medically complicated, painful, prolonged and threatening to the life of the mother and the baby (Ballard et al 1995). A more recent study of childbirth experiences in Sweden found that 28 women (of 1640) met the criteria for PTSD, related to their recent delivery experiences; amongst other things, they cited the contact with delivery staff in negative terms. The authors also reviewed posttraumatic stress reactions after emergency caesarean sections. Twenty-five women were interviewed a few days and a few months after emergency section. Nineteen had experienced their delivery as a traumatic event but at 1 and 2 months postpartum none of the women met the criteria of PTSD. However, 13 women had various forms of posttraumatic stress reaction and some of these had high levels of intrusive thoughts (Wijma et al 1997).

ASSESSMENT OF POSTTRAUMATIC STRESS

Assessment is essential before any therapeutic intervention can begin. Alexander (1996) suggested that a major focus for ongoing trauma research should be the evaluation of prevention and treatment methods. In addition, he also suggested (personal correspondence) that inadequate assessment prior to intervention often leads to poor outcomes. He stresses the need to identify:

◆ trauma-specific normal and pathological reactions in the absence of preexistent psychopathology
◆ preexistent psychopathology which has been triggered by a recent trauma
◆ co morbidity (the presence of another major psychiatric disorder, e.g. depression) in response to trauma.

Therefore a multimodal approach to assessment is advocated and needs to include these four main areas:

◆ structured interview
◆ formal mental state examination
◆ three systems cognitive behavioural assessment (cognition, behavioural and physiological responses)
◆ the use of appropriate measures (see Appendix).

The interview should begin with a pretrauma history which has a number of functions: to establish the individual's premorbid functioning; to determine the individual's baseline of functioning; to examine the common themes of the individual's life struggles or conflicts as although the PTSD may be largely due to a current stressor, the manifestation of the symptoms and their

Box 11.3 Assessment issues – general

◆ Pretrauma history

◆ Immediate pretrauma psychosocial context

◆ The event and immediate coping response

◆ Objective factors

◆ The frequency, duration, intensity and nature of the trauma

◆ Was it single or multiple trauma?

◆ Were traumas clearly delineated incidents?

◆ Was the trauma a culmination of a number of experiences?

◆ Was trauma human induced or an act of nature?

◆ Did it occur to only one individual or a group?

◆ Active/passive role – the degree of passivity or activity can have a powerful influence on the meaning of the trauma and the development of PTSD, for example:

◆ Was the individual a helpless victim?

◆ Was he/she active in any way to alter the situation?

◆ Were there any options for acting differently?

◆ How do they perceive the meaning and outcome of their actions?

influence on the individual will be significantly influenced by their characteristic modes of coping and attribution. Therefore, in addition to standard questions related to general mental health issues, there needs to be a series of questions covering trauma-specific variables (Box 11.3).

The posttrauma psychosocial context, the environment in which the individual recovers and the responses from community, social agencies and the family are also influential and significant in terms of recovery. For example, it is often asked of individuals in A&E departments, 'Have you someone to go home to?'. What is rarely asked is 'What are you going home to?'. Therefore, areas of consideration should be the presence of ongoing stressors, e.g. the person is acting as the main carer for an elderly relative or the recent occurrence of stressful life events such as a break-up of a long-term relationship, etc. Many victims of trauma also come into contact with a variety of social agencies, e.g. criminal justice system, insurance companies, etc. and can often become traumatised a second time, through the insensitive handling of the initial and subsequent distress. Family responses can and do have a major impact on the individual. Figley (1988) described four healing functions that a family can undertake in the readjustment process of PTSD. These also have pathological variables which need to be considered. See Box 11.4.

Box 11.4 Assessment issues – recovery environment

Family responses following traumatic events

Healing
◆ Detecting symptoms of trauma

◆ Confronting trauma

◆ Encouraging revisiting of the trauma

◆ Facilitating resolution of conflict

Pathological
◆ Denying existence or significance of symptoms

◆ Denying need to deal with trauma

◆ Reinforcing avoidance

◆ Active avoidance of conflict resolution

Responses from social agencies and the community
◆ Were they treated with respect?

◆ Were they satisfied with treatment?

◆ Were there elements of secondary victimisation?

Janoff Bulman (1985) proposed that PTSD following victimisation, e.g. rape and criminal assault, results in the shattering of basic assumptions that the victims hold about themselves, others and the world. She identified three basic assumptions that are commonly shared by most people affected:

◆ the belief in personal invulnerability
◆ the perception of the world as meaningful and comprehensible
◆ the view of self and others in a positive light.

Therefore the assessment of attribution and meaning is vital in understanding an individual's reactions following traumatic events (see Box 11.5). The cognitive appraisal model of PTSD emphasises the importance of individuals' basic assumptions and beliefs about the self and the world that usually are not challenged at a deep level. Traumatic events have the potential to shatter these basic assumptions. There is growing empirical support for the importance of cognitive appraisal in trauma (Epstein et al 1998, Kilpatrick et al 1989). The relevance of shattered assumptions and fragmented personal theories of the self and the world corresponds to the experiential realities of PTSD sufferers. This model has the added benefit of being compatible or complementary with other views of PTSD.

> **Box 11.5** Assessment issues – attribution and meaning
>
> ◆ To what extent has their trauma altered their basic beliefs and assumptions?
> ◆ What are their new views of self and the world?
> ◆ Are there new personal outlooks in place?
> ◆ What does the trauma mean in terms of the victim's plans for the rest of their life?
> ◆ Is the person focused on the unfairness of the past or on the possibilities of the future?

> **Box 11.6** Assessment issues – strengths and resources
>
> ◆ When does the person feel better, even when it is only the exception and not the rule?
> ◆ What thoughts, feelings and behaviours do they have at those times?
> ◆ What coping strategies have been tried that were even partially successful?
> ◆ What other difficult situations have they overcome in the past?

Another area for consideration is the significance of anger. Anger is a common emotional reaction in victims of trauma. It can also be an extremely debilitating emotion. It often focuses on the lack of concern or apology from those believed to be responsible and the lack of recognition of the suffering and disability caused. When anger is a prominent issue it can often influence attitudes to the pursuit of compensation. The individual often becomes preoccupied with the lack of concern or apology, rather than gaining financial reward. Careful clinical assessment is indicated, as whilst these individuals may score highly on clinical tests and measures, indicating high levels of distress or PTSD, they may not necessarily meet the diagnostic criteria for PTSD; in fact, a diagnosis of depression is more likely in such cases. Therefore, if the above issues are not highlighted, clinical assessments and reports may need to be treated with some degree of caution.

EARLY INTERVENTIONS FOLLOWING EXPOSURE TO TRAUMATIC EVENTS

There is considerable controversy surrounding early interventions following exposure to traumatic events and recent studies with injured individuals following burn trauma (Bisson et al 1997) and RTAs (Hobbs et al 1996) have shown negative effects. These studies, however, do have limitations and methodological shortcomings. Essentially, these studies utilised a psychological debriefing (PD) model. This process comprises a series of consecutive phases through which various aspects of the traumatic incident are explored and worked through. The aim of the debriefing process is to enable individuals to ventilate and explore their thoughts, feelings and reactions, ultimately facilitating emotional reprocessing and thereby helping them to come to terms with their experience and prevent psychological problems occurring in the future (Dyregrov 1989).

It has been argued (Dyregrov 1998, Richards 1997) that PD was originally designed for groups and not individuals and therefore these studies were an unfair test of the efficacy of PD. In essence, this only serves to confuse the issue. However, we are prepared to admit to subscribing to the principles and practice of PD and, whilst acknowledging doubts as to whether it prevents the development of PTSD, are inclined to the belief that it leads primarily to earlier help seeking, because of the educative component. If this is found to be true, then the psychoeducational benefits alone of the PD process should be actively utilised, within a supportive framework, though further carefully designed studies with groups and individuals are needed.

An explanation, information giving and education are crucial components, especially in the early stages of an individual's traumatic experience, as people are often confused and frightened by their experience and symptomatology. There may also be physically related aspects compounding their distress, which may need assessing.

Some of this distress can be diffused by a simple, straightforward explanation of their difficulties, that they are responding in a normal way to a distressing experience and what course their symptoms may take, i.e. that the

---

Box 11.7 Assessment issues – physically related aspects

◆ Did the person experience/witness any procedures in hospital that they felt traumatised by?

◆ Are there any ongoing stressors resulting from their medical condition?

◆ Is there the threat that the medical condition may recur, be exacerbated in the future or be life threatening?

◆ Are any symptoms better explained by physical causes rather than psychological trauma (e.g. pain related causing disturbed sleep, irritability; radiotherapy causing depressed mood and lethargy)?

majority of individuals return to normal emotional functioning within a few days or weeks.

We have utilised early interventions which draw on elements of a PD model but are carefully structured and focus on:

◆ normalisation of reactions, symptoms and emotional responses
◆ education surrounding normal and abnormal responses to trauma, together with advice and guidance on coping strategies
◆ follow-up and support.

For a more detailed discussion of early intervention and the arguments around efficacy see Chapter 12.

Case Study 11.1 Early intervention

Jane was a 28-year-old professional woman who was admitted following a serious RTA and had suffered severe multiple injuries. She had stopped on the motorway to help at an accident. She saw another driver running towards her waving at her to stop and help. As she stopped on the hard shoulder and was preparing to get out of the car, her car and the other driver were hit by a lorry travelling at speed which could not stop in time. The other man was killed instantly and she was trapped in the car and had to be cut out by the emergency services. After 3 weeks in hospital, she was having tearful episodes, experiencing problems sleeping (unrelated to pain), was low in mood and expressing feelings of guilt at having survived when someone else had died. When originally offered help by the ward staff, she had declined but then later requested to be seen.

She was seen for 1 hour, in which time she was given the opportunity to discuss the circumstances of the accident (which she had previously not done in any depth for fear of upsetting her relatives), her thoughts and emotional reactions at the time, her current difficulties and reactions, e.g. her guilt feelings. She also expressed her anxieties about what she had been told by friends and relatives about the accident as she had a poor memory of events. As a consequence she had formed her own narrative based on what she'd been told; thus she had reconstructed memories, some of which were inaccurate, as confirmed by the police and eyewitnesses. The issue of 'reconstructed memory' (Joseph & Masterson 1999) was discussed in some depth and she was able to develop a more accurate narrative which helped her deal with the guilt she had been feeling over the death of the other driver. She was provided with education, advice and guidance as described above and encouraged to ask questions about her reactions and responses. Her reactions were normalised in the context of her experience She was later seen once on the ward for follow-up and then in the outpatients department. Six months later, she was making a good recovery with no psychological ill effects. She reported that the early session and the follow-up had helped make sense of her feelings and reactions at the time and in the subsequent days and weeks.

A COGNITIVE BEHAVIOURAL MODEL OF POSTTRAUMATIC STRESS DISORDER

A cognitive behavioural approach can be viewed as a flexible, integrative model which provides a wider contextual understanding of the development and maintenance of PTSD and the implications this has in pragmatic terms for the client for any subsequent psychotherapeutic interventions. The CBT model takes the view that the meaning and interpretation of a traumatic event play a significant role in the development and maintenance of PTSD. This utilises an information-processing and cognitive model of dealing with controllability and predictability of perceived threat in trauma situations (Foa et al 1989). Exposure to the feared or avoided situations, either in real life or in imagination, is often a key therapeutic intervention, playing an important if not crucial role in the reduction of intrusive thoughts and hyperarousal. Cognitive restructuring strategies are used to help the individual deal with their shattered beliefs and assumptions brought about by the traumatic stressor (Foa et al 1991).

Current treatment strategies for PTSD

As discussed previously, whilst the efficacy of early interventions for the prevention of posttraumatic reactions has yet to be convincingly demonstrated, there is evidence to suggest that there are effective treatment strategies for established PTSD (for a comprehensive recent review, see Sherman 1998). However, there is considerably less orthodoxy in the field of psychotherapy and psychiatry than in general medicine and so psychological/psychotherapeutic interventions can and do vary considerably.

There has always been a competitive element between various psychotherapeutic approaches and this has been highlighted when comparisons have been made between the effectiveness of cognitive behavioural psychotherapy and psychodynamic psychotherapy. Research into the treatment of PTSD is no exception to this. Andrews (1991) put the scientific cat amongst the psychotherapy pigeons with a metaanalysis of the psychotherapy literature. He concluded that psychoanalytically orientated therapies, when contrasted with CBT, 'are no better than placebo or clinical care and unlikely to be ever demonstrated to be so' (p. 381).

This then begs the question of which psychotherapeutic option is likely to be the most effective for PTSD. Whilst the contribution of psychoanalytic thinking to our understanding of the development PTSD should be acknowledged (Horowitz 1986), there are no outcome studies to indicate the effectiveness of psychoanalytic or psychodynamic therapy for PTSD. The efficacy of psychodynamic therapy for PTSD has typically been demonstrated through qualitative case reports and single case studies (Kellett & Beail 1997). Non-directive or supportive counselling has also been shown to be of general rather than specific use in the treatment of PTSD (Duckworth & Charlesworth 1988). In addition, despite the rapid increase in counsellors, especially within primary care, there is little evidence that generic counselling, provided by itself, is particularly effective and there was '... merit in increasing access to specialist services which provide cognitive behavioural therapy for the purposes of prevention' (NHS Centre for Reviews and Dissemination 1997, p 9).

There is, however, a growing body of evidence highlighting the effectiveness of cognitive behavioural strategies (Foa et al 1991, Hannigan & Regel 1996, Marks et al 1998, Richards & Rose 1991, Richards et al 1994) and eye movement desensitisation and reprocessing (EMDR) (a technique which sits comfortably in the cognitive behavioural repertoire) in the treatment of PTSD (Shapiro 1995, Wilson et al 1995). Despite the ongoing debate surrounding the use of EMDR, there is now a growing body of scientific literature on the technique and a number of studies are confirming its effectiveness in the treatment of PTSD (Spector & Read 1999).

Specific cognitive behavioural treatment strategies

It is important to give individuals a credible rationale and explanation for the complexity of their response to the traumatic event. We use the analogy of 'inadequately packed emotional luggage' with individuals to describe the process of therapy (Box 11.8). Many individuals have reported finding this useful during the evaluation phase of therapy. Therapy will often consist of the following.

Education

This involves three important components.

◆ An explanation, rational and discussion around the range and nature of posttraumatic stress symptoms.
◆ The processes involved in the development and maintenance of PTSD, including the importance of the role of beliefs, assumptions, attributions and life events.
◆ An explicit description and rationale for any proposed therapeutic interventions.

> **Box 11.8** The 'inadequately packed emotional luggage' analogy
>
> *'When someone is exposed to or experiences a traumatic event, they experience a range of thoughts and emotions which they are unable to deal with or make sense of at the time of the trauma, for various reasons. As a result, this is often hurriedly packed in an imaginary bag and taken away with them from the scene of the trauma. However, this 'emotional luggage', because it has been badly packed, frequently bursts open from time to time. This is often experienced as distressing thoughts, images and feelings, which you have tried to push out of your mind because you find them so upsetting. Common examples would be when you may be exposed to situations or events which resemble aspects of the trauma or the trauma itself.'*
>
> Here examples of the individual's specific cognitive and behavioural avoidances could be cited, together with other relevant examples.
>
> *'The various aspects of therapy and the processes involved are aimed at helping you unpack and then repack this emotional luggage, thereby helping you to come to terms with and make sense of your traumatic experience. Inevitably there are things you have to keep, for example the traumatic experience. You will be able to dispense with some items and rearrange others. The aim is to eventually be able to carry the bag without it bursting open unexpectedly and that you can open it and view the contents at any time without undue distress. However, the unpacking and repacking is a painful process, though this becomes easier over time.'*
>
> At this point an explanation of the nature of cognitive therapy would also be given, as well as a rationale, if appropriate, for the use of exposure therapy or EMDR.

Anxiety management training

Often the most straightforward aspect of any treatment package for PTSD, this may include relaxation, breathing exercises, problem solving and elements of stress inoculation training (SIT) (Meichenbaum 1985).

Exposure in imagination

This involves the patient being asked to relive their traumatic memories, in first person and present tense, giving as much detail as possible about the traumatic event and their thoughts, emotions and responses; attention would be paid to specific aspects, e.g. smell, sounds, etc. Often it is possible to construct a hierarchy, using less distressing material first. At specific points a rewind and hold technique is used, whereby the person is asked to concentrate on the worst aspect of the traumatic event, to freeze and hold the image, whilst repeatedly describing in detail all they can remember about this element of the trauma. This is repeated till habituation occurs. The session is audiotaped and they are asked to practise this between sessions, till habituation occurs. A 50–70% reduction in anxiety is desirable for effective reduction in symptomatology and as with any exposure therapy, consistency and regular practice are essential (Richards & Lovell 1999).

Exposure in vivo

This would involve exposure in real life to feared/avoided situations, either directly related to the traumatic event or which resembled it in some way. This could be either graded or prolonged and either therapist aided or unaccompanied. Partners or significant other family members are usually encouraged to act as co-therapist if possible. Patients are given specific instructions and guidelines for exposure therapy, with emphasis being placed on the research evidence to support its effectiveness. Foa et al (1989) argue that while exposure to the trauma memories may allow reevaluation of threat and habituation, there may be no change in the emotional reactions other than fear without direct confrontation of conflicts, misattributions or expectations.

Cognitive psychotherapy

The focus here is on the identification of the shattered beliefs and assumptions and the rebuilding of these through cognitive restructuring. Generally, a cognitive approach based on a straightforward Beckian model (Beck & Emery 1985) is effective. However, more PTSD-specific cognitive approaches, such as Janoff-Bulman's (1985) cognitive appraisal model and cognitive processing therapy (CPT) (Resick & Schnicke 1993), based on the information processing theory, are also extremely effective. This model was originally developed to help victims of rape but can be adapted to a variety of other traumatic stressors. It aims to facilitate the integration of a traumatic event with previously constructed schemata. Cognitive restructuring was also recently evaluated by Thrasher et al (1996) in two case studies. Both clients improved significantly within ten 90-minute sessions of cognitive restructuring, using Beckian-style cognitive techniques.

EMDR

In essence, EMDR involves pairing memories/disturbing thoughts and the resultant emotions with repeated saccadic (rapid and rhythmic) eye movements, resulting in the desensitisation of the memories. A similar pairing of memory and a chosen positive cognition, with further eye movements, constitutes the reprocessing component. The precise mechanism for clinically reported change is as yet unclear and is still the subject of considerable ongoing research. The available evidence is that the treatment effects of EMDR are maintained at follow-up. There is also clear evidence that exposure to both avoidance situations and traumatic memories are clinically significant areas for treatment interventions in PTSD. A cognitive behavioural approach which also utilises EMDR (if appropriate) therefore offers a cost-effective, integrative, pragmatic and flexible framework for the treatment of PTSD.

Case Study 11.2 Exposure in imagination

Linda developed PTSD following a traumatic obstetric experience, during the birth of her second child. There had been complications during her first pregnancy, resulting in Linda requiring a caesarean section. She was terrified that this would occur again but had been reassured that this would not be needed. However, during her labour, complications arose and eventually the decision was made to carry out an emergency caesarean section. After her son was delivered Linda was informed that there had been a complication during the operation and that her uterus had accidentally been ruptured and she had lost a considerable amount of blood.

Eight months later Linda was referred for treatment. A full CBT assessment took place over two sessions and included the use of standardised rating scales and questionnaires. Linda presented with a full range of PTSD symptomatology and co-morbid depression. Treatment followed of nine sessions in total and included: education, imaginal exposure, cognitive restructuring and activity scheduling.

The main component of treatment was imaginal exposure. Linda was asked to write about her experience and completed 11 pages of A4 to describe her experiences! This was then audiotaped and Linda was instructed to listen to the tape 2–3 times per day through headphones. Linda's hospital records were obtained and reviewed with her, enabling her to gain a greater understanding of the decision-making process involved in her care. This element was useful in assisting Linda to cognitively restructure her experiences.

Linda showed an 85% improvement on subjective and objective measures, which were all maintained, and further improved upon when she was last seen at a 1-year follow-up.

Case Study 11.3 Exposure in vivo

Fay, 47, underwent a planned admission to a surgical ward for a hysterectomy. She had been an inpatient previously, during which she found all the staff she encountered to be helpful and supportive and was left with a positive view of 'hospitals'. Consequently she had a positive outlook prior to her admission.

Case Study 11.3 Cont'd

Unfortunately during the operation problems occurred, resulting in her being admitted to an intensive care unit (ICU) for 6 days, following which she developed an infection requiring a total hospital stay in excess of 3 weeks. Fay felt that staff on the ward that she went to from ICU treated her unsympathetically, as she believed that the staff thought she was 'overreacting' about the amount of pain and discomfort she was experiencing.

Four months later Fay was referred for treatment of PTSD. Symptoms included flashbacks, nightmares, avoidance of hospitals (and of all media triggers concerning medical matters), a sense of foreshortened future and a high level of irritability/anger.

Treatment followed a detailed CBT assessment, which showed that Fay's prior beliefs concerning hospitals and medical procedures had been 'shattered' by her recent experiences. Treatment focused on rebuilding her shattered assumptions, imaginal exposure to her intrusive memories of the event and in vivo (real life) reminders of her experience. Elements of anger management and problem solving were also included in her treatment package.

To help Fay carry out in vivo exposure, a graded hierarchy was devised so that she could commence by facing less distressing stimuli before moving onto more distressing reminders of her trauma. This culminated in her visiting the ward on which she stayed and discussing her experiences with the staff there. Overall, Fay received 12 sessions of therapy; subjective and objective measures showed an improvement in functioning and a decrease in symptomatology of 90%, which was maintained at 6-months follow-up.

CONCLUSION

PTSD is a debilitating and disabling psychiatric condition which often presents with high levels of co-morbidity, e.g. depression. It is a mental health problem which can often present in individuals in general health-care settings, as a preexisting condition or as an additional condition resulting from traumatic injuries which have necessitated admission. It can also result from invasive and potentially life-threatening medical procedures and interventions.

Liaison mental health nurses and other health-care professionals will encounter both the acute and chronic forms of the condition in a variety of critical care and general medical settings. Early intervention must be carefully structured, focusing on normalisation, education and follow-up support. For established PTSD, careful assessment followed by appropriate cognitive behavioural interventions will often effect significant and lasting change.

QUESTIONS FOR DISCUSSION

◆ You are asked to give advice to staff on the burns unit about a man suffering from a serious electrical burn which occurred 8 days previously. He is highly agitated and is experiencing nightmares and flashbacks. What advice do you give?

◆ A staff nurse on the trauma/orthopaedics ward asks you to visit immediately to assess a man who was involved in a RTA 4 days previously, in which his partner was killed. They are concerned that despite his partner's death he appears calm and not unduly distressed. What action do you take or what advice do you give?

◆ Four months after a traumatic incident, if a person is suffering with PTSD, should they be persuaded to seek brief non-directive counselling in the hope that the symptoms will resolve or should more formal treatment be suggested?

ANNOTATED BIBLIOGRAPHY

Follette V M, Ruzek J I, Abueg F R (eds) 1998 Cognitive behavioural therapies for trauma. Guilford, New York

Useful chapters on CBT for trauma-related anger and guilt and substance abuse and concurrent PTSD.

Joseph S, Williams R, Yule W 1997 Understanding post traumatic stress – a psychosocial perspective on PTSD and treatment. John Wiley, Chichester

A very good (and affordable) introductory text on trauma. Useful chapters on assessment and theoretical underpinnings.

Van der Kolk BA, McFarlane A C, Weisaeth L (eds) 1996 Traumatic stress – the effects of overwhelming experience on mind, body and society. Guilford, New York

*Considered by some to be **the** textbook on trauma at the time of writing, it is weighty and comprehensive in scope. There are six sections which include chapters on developmental and cultural issues, the psychobiology of PTSD, memory and PTSD, and current treatments. The best sections by far are the chapters on memory and dissociation.*

Yule W (ed) 1999 Post traumatic stress disorders – concepts and therapies. John Wiley, Chichester

Very good all-round text for health professionals working with trauma survivors, whatever the setting or context. The book includes chapters on theory, treatment, cultural aspects, PTSD in children, EMDR and psychological debriefing. It is accessible and comprehensive. The chapter on CBT for trauma is particularly useful.

REFERENCES

Alexander D A 1996 Trauma research: a new era. J Psychosom Res 41(1):1–5

Andrews G 1991 Evaluation of psychotherapy. Curr Opin Psychiatry 4:379–383

American Psychiatric Association 1980 Diagnostic and statistical manual of mental disorders, 3rd edn. American Psychiatric Press, Washington DC

American Psychiatric Association 1994 Diagnostic and statistical manual of mental disorders, 4th edn. American Psychiatric Press, Washington DC

Ballard C G, Stanley A K, Brockington I F 1995 Post traumatic stress disorder (PTSD) after childbirth. Br J Psychiatry 166:525–528

Beck A T, Emery G 1985 Anxiety disorders and phobias: a cognitive perspective. Basic Books, New York

Bisson J I, Jenkins P L, Alexander J 1997 Randomised controlled trial of psychological debriefing for victims of acute burn trauma. Br J Psychiatry 171:78–81

Blake D, Weathers F, Nagy L M et al 1992 Clinician Administered PTSD Scale. National Centre for Post Traumatic Stress Disorder, Boston

Blake D D, Sonnenberg R T, 1998 Outcome research on behavioural and cognitive treatments for trauma survivors. In: Follette V M, Ruzek J I, Abueg F R (eds) Cognitive behavioural therapies for trauma. Guilford, New York

Bryant R A 1996 Predictors of post-traumatic stress disorder following burns injury. Burns 22(2):89–92

Bryant R A, Harvey A G 1996 Initial posttraumatic stress responses following motor vehicle accidents. J Trauma Stress 9(2):223–234

Cordova M, Andrykowski M, Redd W et al 1995 Frequency and correlates of posttraumatic stress disorder like symptoms after treatment for breast cancer. J Consult Clin Psychol 63:981–986

Daly R J 1991 Samuel Pepys and post traumatic stress disorder. Br J Psychiatry 143:64–68

Davidson J R T, Hughes D, Blazer D 1991 Post traumatic stress disorder in the community: an epidemiological study. Psychol Med 21:1–9

Duckworth D H, Charlesworth A 1988 The human side of disaster. Policing 4:194–210

Dyregrov A 1989 Caring for helpers in disaster situations: psychological debriefing. Disaster Manage 2(1):25–30

Dyregrov A 1998 Psychological debriefing – an effective method? Traumatology: www.fsu.edu/trauma

Epstein R S, Fullerton C S, Ursano R J 1998 Posttraumatic stress disorder following an air disaster: a prospective study. Am J Psychiatry 155(7):934–938

Figley C R 1988 Post traumatic family therapy. In: Ochberg F (ed) Post traumatic therapy and victims of violence. Brunner/Mazel, New York

Foa E B, Steketee G, Rothbaum B O 1989 Behavioural/cognitive conceptualisation of post-traumatic stress disorder. Behav Ther 20:155–176

Foa E B, Rothbaum B O, Riggs D, Murdock T B 1991 Treatment of PTSD in rape victims: a comparison between cognitive-behavioural procedures and counselling. J Consult Clin Psychol 59:748–756

Goldberg D 1981 The General Health Questionnaire 28. NFER–Nelson, Windsor

Hannigan D J, Regel S 1996 An audit of PTSD referrals to an acute mental health service in the UK. Paper presented at the British Association for Behavioural and Cognitive Psychotherapies Annual Conference, Stockport, England.

Hickling E J, Blanchard E B 1999 The international handbook of road traffic accidents and psychological trauma: current understanding, treatment and law. Elsevier Science, Oxford

Hobbs M, Mayou R, Harrison B 1996 A randomised controlled trial of psychological debriefing for victims of road traffic accidents. BMJ 313:1438–1439

Horowitz M J 1986 Stress-response syndromes: a review of posttraumatic and adjustment disorders. Hosp Community Psychiatry 37(3):241–249

Horowitz M, Wilner N, Alvarez W 1979 Impact of Events Scale: a measure of subjective stress. Psychosom Med 41:209–218

Janoff-Bulman R 1985 The aftermath of victimisation: rebuilding shattered assumptions. In: Figley C R (ed) Trauma and its wake: the study and treatment of post traumatic stress disorder. Brunner/Mazel, New York

Joseph S, Masterson J 1999 Posttraumatic stress disorder and traumatic brain injury: are they mutually exclusive? J Trauma Stress 12(3):437–453

Joseph S, Yule W, Williams R, Hodgkinson P 1993 Increased substance use in survivors of the Herald of Free Enterprise disaster. Br J Med Psychol 66:185–191

Joseph S, Williams R, Yule W 1997 Understanding post traumatic stress – a psychosocial perspective on PTSD and treatment. John Wiley, Chichester

Kellett S, Beail N 1997 The treatment of chronic post traumatic nightmares using psychodynamic – interpersonal psychotherapy: a single case study. Br J Med Psychol 70:35–49

Kessler R C, Sonnega A, Bromet E 1995 Posttraumatic stress disorder in the national comorbidity survey. Arch Gen Psychiatry 42:1048–1060

Kilpatrick D G, Saunders B E, Amick-McMullan A et al 1989 Victims and crime factors associated with the development of crime related posttraumatic stress disorder. Behav Ther 20:199–214

Kutz I, Shabtai H, Solomon Z, Neumann M, David D 1994 Posttraumatic stress disorder in myocardial infarction patients: prevalence study. Isr J Psychiatry Relat Sci 31(1):48–56

Ladwig K-H, Schoefinius A, Dammann G, Danner R, Gürtler R, Herrmann R 1999 Long-acting psychotraumatic properties of a cardiac arrest experience. Am J Psychiatry 156(6):912–919

Loughrey G C, Bell P, Kee M 1988 Post-traumatic stress disorder and civil violence in Northern Ireland. Br J Psychiatry 153:554–560

Marks I, Lovell K, Noshirvani II 1998 Treatment of posttraumatic stress disorder by exposure and/or cognitive restructuring. Arch Gen Psychiatry 55:317–325

Mayou R, Smith K A 1997 Post traumatic symptoms following medical illness and treatment. J Psychosom Res 43(2):121–123

Mayou R, Bryant B, Duthie R 1993 Psychiatric consequences of road traffic accidents. BMJ 307(6905):647–651

McFarlane A C 1989 The prevention and management of the psychiatric morbidity of natural disasters: an Australian experience. Stress Med 5:29–36

Meichenbaum D 1985 Stress inoculation training. Pergamon, New York

Menage J 1993 Post-traumatic stress disorder in women who have undergone obstetric and/or gynaecological procedures: a consecutive series of 30 cases of PTSD. J Reprod Infant Psychol 11(4):221–228

NHS Centre for Reviews and Dissemination 1997 Effective health care: mental health promotion in high risk groups, 3:3. University of York

Norris F 1992 The epidemiology of trauma: frequency and impact of different potentially traumatic events on different demographic groups. J Consult Clin Psychol 60(3):409–418

North C S, Smith E M, Spitznagel E L 1994 Posttraumatic stress disorder in survivors of a mass shooting. Am J Psychiatry 151(1):82–88

Perkonigg A, Kessler R C, Storz S 2000 Traumatic events and post-traumatic stress disorder in the community: prevalence, risk factors and comorbidity. Acta Psychiat Scand 101:46–59

Perry S, Difede J, Musngi G 1990 Predictors of posttraumatic stress disorder after burn injury. Am J Psychiatry 149(7):931–935

Regel S, Duggan C, Hannigan D, Dewey M, Dunn K 1997 A six month follow-up of victims of serious road traffic accidents (RTA's). Paper presented at the Fifth European Conference on Traumatic Stress, Maastricht, Netherlands

Resick P A, Schnicke M K 1993 Cognitive processing therapy for rape victims – a treatment manual. Sage Publications, London

Richards D 1997 The current status of psychological debriefing and PTSD. Keynote address to the South Yorkshire Trauma and Debriefing Network, Doncaster Royal Infirmary

Richards D, Lovell K 1999 Behavioural and cognitive behavioural interventions in the treatment of PTSD. In: Yule W (ed) Post traumatic stress disorders – concepts and therapy. John Wiley, Chichester

Richards D, Rose J S 1991 Exposure therapy for post traumatic stress disorder: four case studies. B J of Psychiatry 158:836–840

Richards D, Lovell K, Marks I M 1994 Post-traumatic stress disorder: evaluation of a behavioural treatment program. J Trauma Stress 7(4):669–680

Roca R P, Spence R J, Munster A M 1992 Post traumatic adaptation and distress among adult burn survivors. Am J Psychiatry 149(9):1234–1238

Sembi S, Tarrier N, O'Neill P 1998 Does post-traumatic stress disorder occur after stroke? A preliminary study. Int J Geriatr Psychiatry 13:315–322

Shalev A Y, Schreiber S, Galai T 1993 Post-traumatic stress disorder following medical events. Br J Clin Psychol 32:247–253

Shapiro F 1995 Eye movement desensitisation and reprocessing: basic principles, protocols and procedures. Guilford Press, New York

Sherman J J 1998 Effects of psychotherapeutic treatments for PTSD: a meta-analysis of controlled clinical trials. J Trauma Stress 11(3):413–435

Spector J, Read J 1999 The current status of eye movement desensitization and reprocessing (EMDR). Clin Psychol Psychother 6:165–174

Sturgeon D, Rosser R, Shoenberg P 1991 The King's Cross fire. Part 2: the psychological injuries. Burns 17(1):10–13

Taal L A, Faber A W 1997 Dissociation as a predictor of psychopathology following burns injury. Burns 23(5):400–403

Thrasher S M, Lovell K, Noshirvani M, Livanou M 1996 Cognitive restructuring in the treatment of post-traumatic stress disorder – two single cases. Clin Psychol Psychother 3(2):137–148

Trimble M R 1985 Post-traumatic stress disorder: history of a concept. In: Figley C R (ed) Trauma and its wake: the study and treatment of post-traumatic stress disorder. Brunner/Mazel, New York

Van der Kolk B A, Van der Hart O 1989 Pierre Janet and the breakdown of adaptation in psychological trauma. Am J Psychiatry 146(12):1530–1540

Van Driel R C, Op Van den Velde W 1995 Myocardial infarction and post-traumatic stress disorder. J Trauma Stress 8(1):151–159

Wijma K, Soderquist J, Wijma B 1997 Posttraumatic stress disorder after childbirth: a cross sectional study. J Anxiety Disord 11(6):587–597

Wilson S A, Becker L A, Tinker R H 1995 Eye movement desensitisation and reprocessing (EMDR). Treatment for psychologically traumatised individuals. J Consult Clin Psychol 63(6):928–937

Zigmond A, Snaith R 1983 The Hospital Anxiety and Depression Scale. Acta Psychiatry Scand 67:361–370

RESOURCES

Victim Support
Cranmer House
39 Brixton Rd
London SW9 6DZ
Provides support to victims of crime.

Brake
PO Box 548
Huddersfield HD1 2XZ
Tel: 01484 559909
Promotes the awareness of safer driving, by reducing speed, eliminating drink/driving and trying to offer support and advice to victims of road traffic accidents.

Action for Victims of Medical Accidents (AVMA)
44 High Street
Croydon
Surrey CR0 1YB

Offers independent advice, information and support to individuals who feel they have suffered a medical accident. AVMA runs a regional support network with meetings, newsletters and an annual conference.

APPENDIX: MEASURES FOR TRAUMA AND PTSD

The Hospital Anxiety and Depression Scale (HADS): Zigmond & Snaith (1983)

This is a brief 14 item self-report questionnaire used for detecting states of depression and anxiety. A cut-off score of 11 in each subscale indicates a 'definite' case of anxiety or depression. In an inpatient setting, this would be more sensitive than the GHQ-28

General Health Questionnaire (GHQ-28): Goldberg (1981)

This is a self-rating scale for screening for psychiatric morbidity in the general population. The threshold/cut-off point for identifying 'psychiatric caseness', i.e. the likelihood that the individual could be classified as a psychiatric case, is 7. However, if used with a physically injured population it would be more appropriate to raise the threshold/cut-off point to 13 or above. A note of caution is advised with the GHQ-28. If given in the early stages post-injury, it is often inevitable that the patient will score a false positive as the questionnaire asks about the individual's general health and well-being 'over the past few weeks'.

Impact of Events Scale (IES): Horowitz et al (1979)

This self-rating scale is also widely used in research and clinical practice and measures the degree of psychological distress caused by exposure to traumatic events. The time frame for the frequency of symptoms is over the 'past 7 days'. It has two subscales: **Intrusion** corresponds to the first axis of PTSD, Reexperiencing Phenomena, and **Avoidance** corresponds to the second axis, the Avoidance/Numbing criteria. Whilst there are various published cut-off points, a useful guide is 30.

The Clinician Administered PTSD Scale (CAPS): Blake et al (1992)

The CAPS is a diagnostic tool and is more appropriate as a research instrument but it is nevertheless well validated and was developed to measure cardinal and hypothesised signs and symptoms of PTSD. It also provides a method to evaluate the frequency and intensity of individual symptoms as well as the impact of the symptoms on social and occupational functioning, the overall intensity of the symptoms and the validity of the ratings obtained. It uses a time frame of 1 month in keeping with the diagnostic criteria for the presence of PTSD symptoms.

PTSD symptom checklists (even if adhering to the DSM-IV criteria) are not a satisfactory method of assessing the absence or presence of PTSD as there is a danger of over- or underdiagnosis without careful attention to the patient's self-report of frequency and intensity of symptoms.

Staff support in trauma and critical care settings

Stephen Regel

KEY ISSUES

- ◆ Trauma and critical care settings are inherently stressful environments
- ◆ The impact of stressors on staff in these areas can have profound and lasting effects
- ◆ Stressors can also be cumulative over time
- ◆ Stressors in trauma and critical care environments are often multifactorial and multifaceted
- ◆ Assessment and consultation of staff support needs are essential when considering the provision of support groups
- ◆ The support framework for professional carers should be tailored to the culture and needs of the group
- ◆ Critical Incident Stress Debriefing (CISD) is a useful tool within the context of a comprehensive critical incident stress management programme

INTRODUCTION

Stress experienced by health professionals in the NHS is an area attracting increasing attention, not only out of concern for the individuals involved but because of the inevitable impact on the quality of care. While no health-care professional is immune to the pressures and stressors in a health-care environment, there is evidence to suggest that many areas of nursing, particularly critical care environments, e.g. A&E, intensive care and burns units, are vulnerable to stress and may benefit from support (Foxall et al 1990, Regel 1997, Walsh et al 1998).

This chapter will therefore focus on critical care areas and examine the impact of stressors on staff. Comparisons and parallels will be drawn with other workers in similar situations, e.g. the emergency services. Issues related to secondary traumatisation and 'compassion fatigue' (Figley 1995) resulting from work in the above areas and its implications on the carer will also be discussed. Given the nature of the work in critical care areas, there will also be a focus on issues surrounding exposure to 'critical incidents'. The chapter will also examine early interventions such as Critical Incident Stress Debriefing (CISD) following critical incidents (or traumatic events) and provide an overview of such interventions in the light of recent developments and controversies. It will also examine the case for staff support and issues related to the delivery of effective support strategies.

PREVALENCE OF STRESS IN NURSES IN CRITICAL CARE AREAS

Workplace stress among nurses has been consistently identified in the literature as significant (Wheeler 1997a,b). In addition, it is likely to have negative impact on health, job satisfaction, absenteeism, workplace injuries, attrition rates and clinical outcomes (Buchan 1995, Huber 1995). Descriptive studies of stressful workplace situations have also been conducted. Results indicate that workload, conflict, role preparation and death and bereavement are key areas where nurse stress occurs. In addition, the cost of stress-related illness to health systems has been assessed at an annual £7 billion (Farrington 1995).

In the first of a series of review papers on nurse occupational stress research, it was argued that there were weaknesses and gaps in current nurse stress research (Wheeler 1997a). The author also suggested that a substantial number of studies had focused on high-dependency and intensive care areas within general nursing at the expense of other areas, e.g. mental health, learning disability and midwifery.

It was also suggested that as studies of stress within nursing appeared to concentrate on intensive care units (ICUs) and other similarly highly specialised areas, this may have led to the unfounded view that individuals working in these areas face greater frequency and degree of stress than those working in other areas (Wheeler 1997b). A few studies in the UK have attempted to determine the prevalence of stressors in critical care areas (Walsh et al 1998). Some authors have written about the impact of burnout on critical care nurses (Hudak & Gallo 1994, Millar & Burnard 1994). Adomat & Killingworth (1994) identified organisational rather than clinical issues as primary drivers of stress in intensive care nurses.

The studies on stress and nursing, whether aimed at critical care or more general areas, are fraught with methodological difficulties (Wheeler 1997b). Whilst the above is true to some extent, the situation is by no means clear in relation to the prevalence, nature and intensity of stressors within critical care environments; absence of evidence is not evidence of absence. Despite the observations of Wheeler (1997b), there is clearly a need for further research in this area with a specific focus on nurses working in high dependency and areas of critical care.

Critical care units accommodate patients who are very ill and highly dependent on acute care. In addition there are other variables to consider. In a burns unit, for example, nursing staff have to contend with a variety of stressors. These range from problems faced when administering difficult medical and surgical procedures to the stress of dealing with the psychosocial factors which often accompany burn trauma. For example, a significant proportion of burn trauma occurs in the context of stressful life events, which include the following:

◆ adults with burn injury who also have psychiatric conditions
◆ many victims are single, unemployed and from disadvantaged backgrounds
◆ a number come from dysfunctional family backgrounds in which employment, poor housing and relationship problems complicate the situation (Kolman 1983, Regel 1997).

In an intensive care environment there are different contextual stressors. In the main these are related to ethical dilemmas, e.g. being involved in discussions and decisions surrounding the termination of ventilation or dealing with bereaved and distressed relatives. The author's recent clinical experience has also identified a number of other events which have acted as traumatic stressors. Occasionally individuals working in critical care or high-dependency environments may experience events that could be defined as 'critical incidents' – situations that cause them to experience unusually strong emotional reactions which may affect or interfere with their ability to function, either immediately after the event or in the days that follow (Mitchell 1983).

Mitchell (1983) sought to classify critical incidents among emergency service personnel and suggested the following.

◆ Any case which is particularly poignant or emotionally charged, e.g. the sudden death of a child in tragic circumstances.
◆ Any incident in which the circumstances are so unusual or the sights or sounds so distressing as to produce a high level of immediate or delayed emotional reactions that overwhelm normal coping mechanisms.

◆ Any incident which attracts unusual and intensive media attention.
◆ Injury or death of a staff member whilst on duty.

Many of the above may equally be applied to those working in critical care environments. The case studies below illustrate the nature of critical incidents.

Case Study 12.1

A young woman suffering from severe burn trauma was admitted to the adult intensive care unit as a result of a serious assault by her husband. Following a row in the family home, he poured gasoline over her and set light to her in front of their three young children. Whilst seriously injured she nevertheless managed to summon help from the emergency services, but sustained almost 95% burns. She was brought to the unit by air ambulance, though was by this time in a critical condition and not expected to live more than a few hours. However, she survived almost 24 hours following admission and was cared for by staff on the night shift. Two members of staff in particular spent time with her and her extended family. During that time, through talking with the family, they learnt much about her life, family and personality. Despite her terrible injuries (she was almost unrecognisable), the staff reported that she had begun to take on a persona – they felt as though they knew her well. This inevitably resulted in a greater degree of emotional involvement and identification. The staff also reported seeing poignant images of her with her children on the TV news and special reports, which emphasised the tragedy of the situation and the contrast with her physical condition resulting from her injuries. The case had also attracted intense media coverage and the unit was besieged with phone calls for information and news. The police were also present as there had been attempts by reporters to enter the unit. All those involved in her care felt that it had been one of the most draining and stressful incidents experienced on the unit and they had requested a CISD session.

Case Study 12.2

Night staff on the high-dependency unit, during routine tasks in the early hours of the morning, discovered a patient had hung himself in the ward bathroom. He was ambulant and had informed staff of his whereabouts. This had been the first incident of its kind to occur and all the staff concerned found that they were unprepared for dealing with such an event. They felt that it challenged every belief and assumption they held about their work and the nature of the environment – 'people don't come in to hospital to commit suicide!' (see Chapter 11 on Posttraumatic stress disorder). Again, there was police involvement because of the circumstances of death, statements were taken and no one was allowed to leave till almost midday, nearly 4 hours later than usual. Stunned and shocked relatives had to be informed and comforted. One of his relatives became extremely angry and blamed staff for not being more vigilant. The event was especially difficult to handle because the patient concerned was known to everyone and well liked. Again, the unit manager and staff requested a CISD, which was attended by all present at the incident.

STRESS IN EMERGENCY SERVICES PERSONNEL

At this point it is worth considering the impact and prevalence of traumatic stressors on emergency services personnel. There are many parallels to be drawn between the impact of traumatic stressors on emergency workers and those experienced by nurses (and other disciplines) in a critical care environment. Indeed, there are often likely to be situations when they may be called upon to work together, for example following a major incident or disaster. An extensive review of the literature on workplace trauma and its management was carried out by the Institute of Employment Studies for the Health and Safety Executive (IES 1998a). The report described research that examined psychological outcomes relating to emergency work. A number of studies examined the impact of exposure to traumatic events in ambulance men (Ravenscroft 1993), firefighters (Fitzpatrick 1994) and police officers (Brown & Campbell 1990).

Early indications of psychological distress in emergency workers began in the early 1980s following a series of disasters in the UK and abroad (Duckworth 1986, Shepherd & Hodgkinson 1990, Taylor & Frazer 1982). Inevitably, this prompted the view that emergency workers should be considered secondary victims and ultimately provided with support. In addition, there was evidence that many of those studied developed a variety of other psychiatric conditions such as depression and anxiety (Raphael 1983, 1986)

The impact of secondary traumatic stress

It was clear that research was beginning to demonstrate that a variety of professionals involved in disaster and rescue work could potentially become secondary victims. However, there has been scant systematic study of the impact of exposure to traumatic stressors in nurses (and other disciplines) working in critical care environments. However, the notion of 'helper stress' has been arousing greater research interest of late. Figley (1995) has written extensively about the effect of traumatic stressors and the cost of caring on the carers. He proposed the concept of secondary traumatic stress (STS) and coined the term 'compassion fatigue', defining STS as 'the natural consequent behaviours and emotions resulting from knowing about a traumatising event experienced by a significant other and the stress resulting from helping or wanting to help a traumatised or suffering person' (p 7). Another term for STS is vicarious traumatisation; essentially this is taken to mean becoming traumatised or experiencing high levels of stress *through the experience of others*. The most comprehensive concept of vicarious traumatisation appears to be that presented by Pearlman & Saakvitne (1995), who describe the phenomenon as '… the cumulative transformation in the inner experience of the therapist that comes about as a result of empathic engagement with the client's traumatic material' (p 31).

Whilst the above authors were drawing upon their work with trauma therapists, the similarities with emergency workers and nurses working in critical care areas are clear. However, there is little evidence from the studies on vicarious traumatisation that individuals develop conditions such as Post-Traumatic Stress Disorder (PTSD). However, they may experience some of the following:

◆ emotional numbing
◆ feelings of despair, hopelessness, shame and guilt
◆ a loss of belief in justice or in a sense of balance, resulting in cynicism and bitterness
◆ sleep problems, irritability and impatience
◆ loss of trust in others.

The implications from the work on vicarious traumatisation are important in any consideration of the impact on carers in the contexts described above. The most obvious is the potential negative impact and effect on the quality of care delivery.

STAFF SUPPORT: ISSUES TO CONSIDER

There are a number of general issues for consideration prior to the implementation and facilitation of support groups and these will be considered below. Antebi (1993) described the work of the psychiatrist on a burns unit and the setting up of a consultation-liaison service. The model for staff meetings and support was multidisciplinary (excluding medical staff; no reasons are given other than to say that they approached the psychiatrist separately for discussions). The meetings were held weekly; the content was decided by staff and was usually based around teaching on a specific psychological or psychiatric problem, followed by discussion of 'problem' patients. No pressure was exerted for staff to attend, although there appeared to be a core group of regular attenders. However, psychiatrists at registrar and senior registrar levels rotate, so consistency and continuity may be a problem, as may their availability in any given circumstances.

The literature on providing support for staff in critical care settings is sparse and often tends to be of a psychodynamic orientation (Parish et al 1997). The authors describe a reflective practice group in an ICU. There was no planned agenda and the nature of the sessions were very non-directive, with the facilitators often acting as a 'mirror'. A typical question might be 'What is the atmosphere like in here at the moment?'. It is clear that the authors adapted a fairly psychodynamic perspective, indicating influences from Yalom (1985). Interestingly, they also describe that the hospital chaplain had facilitated previous support work and whilst there had never been any criticism of the chaplain's abilities and qualities, some individuals experienced difficulties with the religious connotations of his role. There was little objective measure of the group's success other than the fact that the group continued to meet for over 2 years (Parish et al 1997). A number of other authors (Burnard 1991, Nichols & Jenkinson 1991, Wright 1991) have described supportive interventions and these are worthy of scrutiny for those readers considering either setting up or leading a support group. However, Llewelyn (1989) quite rightly advises caution in applying some of the techniques advocated, as they can be beneficial if chosen as individual coping strategies but counterproductive if imposed on people without consideration for individual circumstances.

Before setting up or facilitating a support group, it is essential to make an assessment of need within the context of the environment. Liaison mental health nurses may be called upon to facilitate support groups in areas with which they have regular contact. However, as yet there has been little in the consultation-liaison literature that describes such involvement (Regel & Davies 1995). There is the potential for a significant demand for mental health skills in critical care areas. Our clinical experience of staff support in critical environments such as intensive care and burn trauma over the past decade has indicated that knowledge and skills in the assessment and management of problems that manifest in these areas have been invaluable. These include:

◆ knowledge of normal and pathological responses to trauma and bereavement
◆ knowledge and skills in management of acute anxiety responses
◆ crisis intervention, defusing and debriefing skills.

Assessment should involve detailed discussions of perceived need with unit staff of all grades and disciplines and the support groups should ideally be multidisciplinary in nature, though this may not always be possible for a variety of reasons (Antebi 1993). A working knowledge of the environment and the stressors experienced will provide an invaluable insight into that environment, not to mention a 'feel' for the dynamics and personalities within the unit. Parish et al (1997) also highlighted the importance of management support for such ventures, e.g. in the form of funding for the facilitators and, most importantly, 'permission' to leave the workplace. Without this type of support, such ventures are doomed to failure.

The next section describes some practical strategies for implementing staff support groups.

STAFF SUPPORT: A WORKING MODEL FOR PRACTICE

Whilst there are different models for facilitating staff support groups (as outlined above), we favour a pragmatic approach designed to be compatible with the nature and context of the environments under discussion. General medical environments are by their very nature task orientated. Staff are problem focused and there are often significant constraints on time, given the unpredictable nature of the environment. In addition, we have found that a pragmatic, practical approach which adopts a problem-solving framework is effective and acceptable to the majority of individuals who work in these environments who will often have little knowledge of psychological concepts and processes, just as mental health professionals will have little detailed knowledge of the physical care provided. We suggest that a model for staff support could adopt the principles underpinning a cognitive behavioural model:

◆ a focus on the 'here and now'
◆ the use of explicit, agreed goals
◆ problem solving
◆ adopting an active, directive but collaborative approach (adapted from Hackman 1993).

It is often helpful to use a current case that has presented problems and ethical dilemmas as a frame of reference for a support session. A notable incident involved the death of a child. An approach utilising the principles described above was used with the group. From the original discussion a number of themes emerged, which allowed for the discussion of emotions and personal reactions of those team members involved (Box 12.1).

If a request is received from a critical care area for staff support, it is worth working through a series of stages as part of the initial assessment. Some of the suggestions below may prove helpful. The list is by no means inclusive and there may be other variables to consider depending on the context. Many of these may seem like common sense but it is always best not to assume or presume anything!

◆ Arrange a time to meet key members of staff. If a mutually convenient time is not possible for the first occasion, meet them at their convenience. This is often good for relationship building, especially when there have been problems with previous facilitators. Meet more than once if necessary.

◆ Prepare a mental list of questions beforehand that can be asked in an informal discussion.

◆ If they have had previous support sessions, discuss their experiences. What was the most and least helpful and why? What were the frequency

> **Box 12.1** Support group–example of case discussion and emergent themes
>
> ### Case
> Death of a child from 85% burns
>
> ### Theme 1
> Junior staff members' first experience of a severe injury
> What ways are there of dealing with this?
>
> ↓
>
> ### Theme 2
> Ethical dilemma/issues discussed, e.g. is getting involved purely spectatoring
> or a valuable learning experience?
>
> ↓
>
> ### Theme 3
> The role of students in a case like this
> What are the issues regarding their support and preparation?
>
> ↓
>
> ### Theme 4
> Discussion of organisational stressors and areas of conflict/responsibility
>
> ↓
>
> General discussion and feedback of the emergent themes including
> thoughts, feelings, reactions, discussion of lessons learnt

and duration of sessions? How long had these been running? Why did they stop?

◆ What do the team feel their needs are? If this is the first time that they have requested support sessions, why now? What are their expectations? Do they have any preconceived ideas about support groups?

◆ Be open and honest with the team. Describe your intended model of working. Check this with their understanding and expectations of what will be involved.

◆ Invite questions from the team.

◆ Discuss any reservations or concerns they may have. Discuss a possible format and practicalities, e.g. times, venue, number of participants and ground rules (see below).

◆ The constituency of the group is important. Will it be multidisciplinary? Will all grades of staff be involved?

◆ What else might they be seeking? Is it worth considering a 'package' of which the support group may be a part? Do some preparation – read up on the area if necessary and be aware of some of the common problems, themes and issues that may come up.

◆ Finally, don't be precious! You will be dealing with a group of knowledgeable and highly skilled professionals so view this as an opportunity to share knowledge and skills. Don't be rigid – be prepared to be flexible and adaptable. The opportunity to apply mental health knowledge and practice in a general setting is immensely rewarding and a mutually beneficial experience for all concerned.

If the above has been productive and a decision is made to provide some input, it is recommended that a time be agreed for evaluation and feedback. It is also useful, as mentioned previously, to acquire a reasonable working knowledge of the area before starting the sessions and to this end it is worth spending as much time as possible trying to understand the environment, familiarising yourself with common procedures and terminology, establishing a rapport and relationship with the ward or unit team, attending team meetings as appropriate. The easiest way to achieve this is by spending a shift or two on the unit. It is also our view that facilitators should be trained and experienced in psychosocial and psychological models of care and involved in clinical practice. They should possess counselling or psychotherapy skills in both group and individual settings. Training or experience in cognitive behavioural therapy is desirable. They should also have a knowledge, in general terms, of the clinical environment in which support is to be provided; for example the client group, the types of psychosocial and psychological problems experienced and an awareness of relevant literature and research, e.g. on trauma and PTSD for critical care settings. A technical knowledge is not always essential, especially if the facilitator is only providing staff support; however, if she or he is to fulfil a number of other functions, as mentioned earlier, some knowledge is desirable.

Certain practical problems have to be acknowledged and worked around, given the intrinsic nature of the environment. Therefore the basic format or ground rules of the group setting could be as follows.

◆ Confidentiality is paramount, especially if the group at any point deals with the personal issues of those present at the time.
◆ Interruptions are, within reason, acceptable (given the demands of the unit).
◆ Staff members will not be discussed in their absence.
◆ Managerial and organisational aspects will be discussed only if all those concerned are present.
◆ The format of the group is flexible but the main focus is the presentation of a case history and the discussion of problems and any emergent themes.
◆ Specific teaching requests can be made and planned in advance.

In addition to the above, other features, for example problem solving (Meichenbaum 1985, Sobel & Worden 1981), form an essential part of staff support.

Common to many problem-solving programmes is a formula that involves the following steps and is useful for case management.

◆ Define the stress or stress reaction to be dealt with.
◆ Establish realistic goals.
◆ Generate a wide range of alternative solutions.
◆ Imagine or consider others' reactions to similar stressors.
◆ Evaluate the pros and cons of each proposed solution and rank solutions in order, from the least to the most practical and desirable.
◆ Possibly rehearse chosen strategies.
◆ Try out the most acceptable and feasible solution.
◆ Reconsider the original problem in the light of the attempt at problem solving.
◆ Expect some failures but reward effort.

CRITICAL INCIDENT STRESS DEBRIEFING AND PSYCHOLOGICAL DEBRIEFING

Another important aspect of staff support is critical incident stress debriefing (CISD). This is essentially based on a crisis intervention model, developed by Mitchell (1983). The technique was further articulated and refined by Dyregrov (1989), who coined the term 'Psychological Debriefing' (PD). These two terms are often used interchangeably to describe the same process (for the purposes of clarity, PD will be used throughout this section). PD or a variant of the model is now widely used with emergency services personnel (Mitchell & Dyregrov 1993), the armed forces (Jones & Roberts 1998) and in a variety of other situations where individuals or groups have been exposed to a traumatic event (Flannery & Penk 1996, Tehrani 1994).

Dyregrov (1989, p 25) defined PD as: '... a group meeting arranged for the purpose of integrating profound personal experiences both on the cognitive, emotional and group level, and thus preventing the development of adverse reactions'.

Thus, when used appropriately, it could be an invaluable tool in the repertoire of a support group facilitator. The aim of a debriefing is to minimise the occurrence of unnecessary psychological suffering after a traumatic incident, by allowing the ventilation of emotions, reactions and experiences. Although designed for groups, it can also be extremely helpful for individuals who have been involved in any way in a serious trauma; for example, staff involved in a major incident or dealing with seriously injured adults and children (as in the examples used earlier). However, there has been considerable controversy of late as to the efficacy of PD, prompting calls for use of the technique to be stopped (Wessely et al 1998). The debate surrounding the efficacy and utility of PD with survivors and professional groups following exposure to traumatic events has become confused, primarily because of the methodology of the recent research. This is an important issue and an attempt will be made here to disentangle some of the issues for the sake of clarity and in view of the implications for practice in the context of staff support.

Psychological Debriefing (PD) in context

Mitchell (1983) described CISD as a structured intervention utilising six phases (not seven, as is so often referenced), which were:

1. the introductory phase
2. the fact phase
3. the feeling phase
4. the symptom phase
5. the teaching phase
6. the re entry phase.

He did not describe a seven-stage model till 5 years later (Mitchell 1988a,b). It was to be used as an organized approach to the management of stress responses in the emergency services. He stated that it '... entails either an individual or group meeting between the rescue worker and facilitator who is able to help the person talk about his feelings and reactions to the critical incident' (Mitchell 1983, p 37). He went on to state that '... follow-up CISD may be performed with the entire group, a portion of it, or with an individual' (p 39). Note the use of the word 'individual' as this is important for the debate and we will return to this later.

All through the 1980s PD was widely used with the emergency services and a number of other survivor and professional groups in the USA, Australia, New Zealand, Scandinavia and throughout Europe, including the UK. In Mitchell's defence, he never claimed that it would prevent PTSD, merely help to ameliorate its long-term consequences.

The debate on the evidence

In 1994, the first questions were raised about PD's efficacy, with calls for more research into its application, using randomised controlled trials (RCTs) (Bisson & Deahl 1994, Raphael et al 1995). Finally two RCTs were published. The studies were carried out with injured burn trauma (Bisson et al 1997) and road traffic accident (RTA) survivors (Hobbs et al 1996). Both studies demonstrated negative effects among the intervention groups. The influential Cochrane Review, a systematic review of the published literature in this area, concluded 'There is no current evidence that psychological debriefing is a useful treatment for prevention of post traumatic stress disorder after traumatic incidents. Compulsory psychological debriefing for victims of trauma should cease' (Wessely et al 1998).

Advocates of PD argued that these studies were an unfair test of PD/CISD as they applied a technique meant for groups to individuals and that 'debriefing conducted individually is essentially single shot exposure and has considerable potential to harm the individual by sensitising them to their memories' (Richards 1997). Moreover, these were injured individuals and therefore there were a number of other variables to consider. For example, it was suggested that early interventions following serious illness or injury should be discouraged as physical healing needs to take place before psychological healing can begin (Dyregrov 1998). However, there is ample evidence that early interventions following serious injury or illness can be effective, especially the psychoeducative components (Bennett & Carroll 1993, Bordow & Porritt 1979, Bunn & Clarke 1979, Clare & Singh 1994, Raphael 1977). The educational aspect of PD is one of the most important elements of the process as it provides a framework for understanding normal and pathological responses to the illness or traumatic event.

Detractors of PD argued that here at last was evidence that PD as an early intervention was ineffective and therefore should cease, especially in this age of clinical governance and evidence-based practice. However, this has only served to blur the issues surrounding the nature and process of PD. The recent RCTs with burn trauma and RTA victims are not without their limitations. In the Bisson et al (1997) study on burn trauma, the authors admitted that the vagaries of randomisation meant that all the subjects with the highest levels of subjective life threat, previous psychological morbidity and previous psychological treatment ended up in the intervention group. In addition, the authors viewed PD as a treatment and described it as 'intense imaginal exposure to a traumatic incident' (Bisson et al 1997, p 80). Intense imaginal exposure is a therapeutic technique, which is often used in the treatment of trauma survivors (Richards & Lovell 1999). Anyone familiar with PD, trained and experienced in the process knows full well that it involves discussion about the event, rather than an intense imaginal reliving of the experience. Clearly, this is a significant issue, particularly as PD was never intended as a treatment or counselling strategy; nevertheless, the notion of counselling has become synonymous with PD. Again, this only serves to cloud the issue further. PD is not counselling and the differences are clear (Box 12.2) (Dyregrov 1997).

Box 12.2 Differences between debriefing and therapy (or counselling)

Debriefing is…

◆ a support procedure

◆ based on crisis intervention theories and models

◆ always a short-term approach

◆ usually a group process, but can be used with individuals

◆ an approach which assists personal defences

◆ a one-off procedure, but should include follow-up and be part of a comprehensive stress management package.

Therapy is…

◆ a treatment procedure

◆ usually based on classic therapeutic models

◆ often a long-term initiative

◆ usually an individual process

◆ an approach which may alter personal defences

◆ may continue until the problem resolves.

The Hobbs et al (1996) study was also not without limitations. Hobbs & Adshead (1997), in a later chapter describing the study in detail, acknowledged that 'After the first ten subjects, the interventions were undertaken instead by the research assistant. The intervention therefore immediately followed the screening interview, with which it became merged to some degree, and interviewer "blindness" was inevitably compromised' (p 167). This aspect of the study, however, was never published in the original paper. A study with ambulant RTA survivors also showed no differences, though the sample was small and the study has some serious flaws (Conlon et al 1998). A more recent study with crime victims has also shown neutral results though again the authors acknowledge limitations in the study and, somewhat curiously, separate education from the PD process itself, despite the fact that it is an integral part of the intervention (Rose et al 1999).

Therefore the debate will continue, but the evidence as described above cannot in itself be sufficient to warrant discontinuing PD as a crisis intervention or a tool for facilitating support in areas such as critical care environments. At the time of writing a few studies are under way with the aim of evaluating the effects and impact of PD on the development of psychological sequelae following exposure to traumatic events. More research is needed with groups and with individuals as the existing studies leave much to be desired and are at variance with practice. Whilst there are a number of other methodological issues that are worthy of consideration, the lack of standardisation in the debriefing process itself is something that needs to be addressed in any future research. Inevitably, these subtle differences in method and process introduce a variety of confounding variables, which has significant implications for the methodology of any outcome studies or evaluative research into PD. Nevertheless there is some evidence that interventions with some groups, e.g. burn trauma victims, can be effective, especially when a structured PD approach is utilised and includes follow-up (Regel 1998).

Therefore, whilst it appears the jury is still out, there is also substantial evidence that a number of organisations will continue to provide PD or a variant of the model as a measure of staff support (IES 1998b, Jones & Roberts 1998). The author will continue to subscribe to the principles and practice of PD and, whilst acknowledging some doubts as to whether it prevents the development of PTSD, is strongly inclined to the belief that it leads to *earlier help seeking*. If this is found to be true, as some evidence suggests (Regel 1998), then the psychoeducational benefits alone of the PD process should be actively utilised, within a supportive framework.

CONCLUSION

Staff support is starting to be recognised as an important area of need in many challenging critical care environments. A further acknowledgement is that the demands of today's rapidly changing NHS and the pressures created by those changes make providing a framework for staff support even more urgent. In the caring professions, we are notorious for not looking after those who provide the care. In a report published by the Health and Safety Executive, Cox (1993) argues that at least part of the effect of any stress management programme (whatever its nature) is due to the way it alters workers' perceptions of and attitudes to their organisations and hence organisational culture. He also argues that poor organisational culture might be associated with an experience of stress, while a good organisational culture might weaken the effects of stress on health. Therefore senior managers and clinicians should consider a variety of measures in order to provide a comprehensive integrative staff care approach in line with the current HSE recommendations (IES 1998b).

ANNOTATED BIBLIOGRAPHY

Dyregrov A 1997 The process in psychological debriefings. J Trauma Stress 10(4):589–605

A readable paper which addresses many of the process and practical issues related to PD, including composition of groups, problems in the process, group culture, etc.

Mitchell J T, Everly G S 1997 Critical incident stress debriefing: an operations manual for the prevention of traumatic stress among emergency services and disaster workers, 2nd edn. Chevron Publishing, Ellicott City, Maryland

A fairly comprehensive text on CISD and practice. It has useful guidelines and covers a fair amount of ground on some of the key issues. It does have a US perspective but is nevertheless informative.

Tehrani N 1994 Debriefing individuals affected by violence. Counsel Psychol Q 7(3):251–259

Useful paper describing a model aimed at individual PD, utilised by the Royal Mail in the UK. Offers a different and useful perspective.

Meichenbaum D 1985 Stress inoculation training. Pergamon Press, New York

A systematic study of stress inoculation, a treatment modality aimed at the reduction and prevention of stress. A useful resource.

REFERENCES

Adomat R, Killingworth A 1994 Care of the critically ill patient: the impact of stress on touch in intensive therapy patients. J Adv Nurs 19:912–922

Antebi D 1993 The psychiatrist on the burns unit. Burns 19(1):43–46

Bennett P, Carroll D 1993 Intervening with cardiac patients. Health Psychol Update 14:3–6

Bisson J, Deahl M 1994 Psychological debriefing and prevention of post-traumatic stress. Br J Psychiatry 165:717–720

Bisson J I, Jenkins P L, Alexander J 1997 Randomised controlled trial of psychological debriefing for victims of acute burn trauma. Br J Psychiatry 171:78–81

Bordow S, Porritt D 1979 An experimental evaluation of crisis intervention. Soc Sci Med 13A:251–256

Brown J M, Campbell E A 1990 Stress and policing: sources and strategies. John Wiley, Chichester

Buchan J 1995 Counting the cost of stress in nursing. Nurs Standard 9(10):30–32

Bunn T A, Clarke A M 1979 Crisis intervention: an experimental study of the effects of a brief period of counselling on the anxiety of relatives of seriously injured or ill hospital patients. Br J Med Psychol 52:191–195

Burnard P 1991 Coping with stress in the health professions – a practical guide. Chapman and Hall, London

Clare L, Singh K 1994 Preventing relapse in psychotic illness: a psychological approach to early intervention. J Ment Health 3:541–550

Conlon L, Fahy T J, Conroy R 1998 PTSD in ambulant RTA victims: a randomised controlled trial of debriefing. J Psychosom Res 46(1):37–44

Cox T 1993 Stress research and stress management: putting theory to work. Health and Safety Executive Contract Research Report No. 61/1993. HMSO, London

Duckworth D H 1986 Psychological problems arising from disaster work. Stress Med 2:315–323

Dyregrov A 1989 Caring for workers in disaster situations: psychological debriefing. Disaster Manage 2:25–30

Dyregrov A 1997 The process in psychological debriefings. J Trauma Stress 10(4):589–605

Dyregrov A 1998 Psychological debriefing – an effective method? Traumatology: www.fsu.edu/trauma

Farrington A 1995 Stress and nursing. Br J Nurs 4(10):574–578

Figley C 1995 Compassion fatigue – coping with secondary traumatic stress disorder in those who treat the traumatised. Brunner Mazel, New York

Fitzpatrick J 1994 Traumatic stress in the emergency services. Disaster Manage 6(1):9–11

Flannery R B, Penk W E 1996 Program evaluation of an intervention approach for staff assaulted by patients: preliminary inquiry. J Trauma Stress 9(2):317–324

Foxall M J, Zimmerman L, Standley R, Bene B 1990 A comparison of frequency of sources of nursing job stress perceived by intensive care, hospice and medical/surgical nurses. J Adv Nurs 15:577–584

Hackman A 1993 Behavioural and cognitive psychotherapies: past history, current application and future registration issues. Behav Cogn Psychother 21(suppl 1):7–12

Hobbs M, Adshead G 1997 Preventative psychological intervention for road crash survivors. In: Mitchell M (ed) The aftermath of road accidents. Routledge, London

Hobbs M, Mayou R, Harrison B 1996 A randomised controlled trial of psychological debriefing for victims of road traffic accidents. BMJ 313:1438–1439

Huber D 1995 Understanding the sources of stress for nurses. Aust J Nurs 92(12):16J–16P

Hudak C, Gallo B 1994 Critical care nursing: a holistic approach, 6th edn. J B Lippincott, Philadelphia

Institute of Employment Studies 1998a Workplace trauma and its management. A review of the literature. Health and Safety Executive. HMSO, Norwich

Institute of Employment Studies 1998b From accidents to assaults: how organisational responses to traumatic incidents can prevent post traumatic stress disorder in the workplace. Health and Safety Executive, Contract Research Report. HMSO, Norwich

Jones N, Roberts P 1998 Risk management following psychological trauma: a guide for Royal Marine Corps combat stress trauma practitioners, 4th edn. Headquarters Royal Marines, Whale Island, Portsmouth

Kolman P 1983 The incidence of psychopathology in burned adult patients – a critical review. J Burn Care Rehabil 416:430–436

Llewelyn S 1989 Caring: the cost to nurses and relatives. In: Broome A (ed) Health psychology – processes and applications. Chapman and Hall, London

Meichenbaum D 1985 Stress inoculation training. Pergamon Press, New York

Millar B, Burnard P 1994 Critical care nursing. Baillière Tindall, London

Mitchell J T 1983 When disaster strikes … The critical incident stress debriefing process. J Emerg Med Serv January: 36–39

Mitchell J T 1988a Development and functions of a critical incident stress debriefing team. J Emerg Med Serv November:43 46

Mitchell J T 1988b The history, status and future of critical incident stress debriefings. J Emerg Med Serv December:47–52

Mitchell J T, Dyregrov A 1993 Traumatic stress in disaster workers and emergency personnel. In: Wilson J P, Raphael B (eds) International handbook of traumatic stress syndromes. Plenum Press, New York

Nichols K, Jenkinson J 1991 Leading a support group. Chapman and Hall, London

Parish C, Bradley L, Franks V 1997 Managing the stress of caring in ITU: a reflective practice group. Br J Nurs 6(20):1192–1196

Pearlman L A, Saakvitne K W 1995 Treating therapists with vicarious and secondary traumatic stress. In: Figley C R (ed) Compassion fatigue: coping with secondary traumatic stress disorder in those who treat the traumatised. Brunner Mazel, New York

Raphael B 1977 Preventive intervention with the recently bereaved. Arch Gen Psychiatry 34:1450–1454

Raphael B 1983 Who helps the helpers? Effects of disaster on rescue workers. Omega 14:9–20

Raphael B 1986 When disaster strikes: a handbook for the caring professions. Hyman, London

Raphael B, Meldrum L, McFarlane A C 1995 Does debriefing after psychological trauma work? BMJ 310:1479–1480

Ravenscroft T 1993 Post traumatic stress disorder in the London Ambulance Service. Unpublished BSc thesis, London University

Regel S 1997 Staff support on the burns unit. In: Bosworth C (ed) Burn trauma – nursing management and care. Baillière Tindall, London

Regel S 1998 A case for early interventions following road traffic accidents and burn trauma. Paper presented at the European Society for Traumatic Stress Studies, Regional European Conference, St Catherine's College, Oxford

Regel S, Davies J 1995 The future of mental health nurses in liaison psychiatry. Br J Nurs 4:1052–1056

Richards D 1997 The current status of psychological debriefing and PTSD. Keynote address to the South Yorkshire Trauma and Debriefing Network, Doncaster Royal Infirmary

Richards D, Lovell K 1999 Behavioural and cognitive behavioural interventions in the treatment of PTSD. In: Yule W (ed) Posttraumatic stress disorders: concepts and therapy. John Wiley, Chichester, pp 239–266

Rose S, Brewin C, Andrews B 1999 A randomised controlled trial of individual psychological debriefing for victims of violent crime. Psychol Med 29:793–799

Shepherd M, Hodgkinson P E 1990 The hidden victims of disaster: helper stress. Stress Med 6:29–35

Sobel H, Worden J 1981 Helping cancer patients cope: a problem solving intervention for health care professionals. MBA/Guilford Press, New York

Taylor A G, Frazer A G 1982 The stress of post disaster body handling and victim work. J Hum Stress December:4–12

Tehrani N 1994 Debriefing individuals affected by violence. Couns Psychol Q 7(3):251–259

Walsh M, Dolan B, Lewis A 1998 Burn-out and stress among A&E nurses. Emerg Nurse 6(2):23–30

Wessely S, Rose S, Bisson J 1998 A systematic review of brief psychological interventions ('debriefing') for the treatment of immediate trauma related symptoms and the prevention of post traumatic stress disorder. Cochrane Library. Issue 4

Wheeler H H 1997a A review of nurse occupational stress research: 1. Br J Nurs 6(11):642–645

Wheeler H H 1997b Nurse occupational stress research: 4. The prevalence of stress. Br J Nurs 6(21):1256–1260

Wright B 1991 Sudden death – intervention skills for the caring professions. Churchill Livingstone, Edinburgh

Yalom I D 1985 The theory and practice of group psychotherapy. Basic Books, New York

Index